BIG CITY HOSPITALS DON'T LIKE COWARDS

A View of the Nursing World by an Autistic Man

Copyright by Brian Evans 2014

To contact Brian call…
870-416-1030 or
870-416-0553

PREFACE

It is my desire that by reading this book you will be enlightened as to how emotionally traumatizing it can be for someone not to have their needs met. During Brian's life, he has endured many medical procedures, most of which were not handled properly, which resulted in a genuine fear of people in the medical field.

There are more and more children being diagnosed with autism every day and these children will be adults someday. The medical field needs to be prepared for that day and right now they most certainly are not. Nurses may think, "I have my personal space and I don't want anyone in it except for my spouse." If much of what you do as a nurse is based on sympathy, empathy, and compassion as well as your desire to care for the patient I wonder how that's done.

Autism is a fascinating disorder because every person with autism will need different things to be done that brings them comfort in order to avoid a meltdown. It is definitely the responsibility of the caregiver, or spouse in my case, to inform you of exactly what that need is and then it is your responsibility to meet that need. If you are not willing to meet that need...I wonder why be a nurse when to nurse is to provide comfort with compassion. You may ask me why I don't do it. It's because my husband needs someone in the medical field to do it. No matter how scared he is, at least he will have one of "them" on his side. I would love to be the one Brian turns to for comfort, and I am. In this area of his life however it is different.

Please find it in your heart to continue reading even though parts of this book are repetitive because that is a part of autism. Chapter 38 is a very enlightening list of things involved in being a nurse that are being neglected in preparing nurses for their job. Special needs patients, like my husband, are suffering the consequences. Nursing is a very difficult job; I can only imagine the stresses you endure daily. But please for the sake of people in your care; remember that they are in desperate need of your compassion."

In Christian Love,
Bertha Marie Evans

BRIAN GENE EVANS

Dedication

This book is dedicated to anyone who is disabled and/or has a needle phobia and/or has oversensitivity to pain.

I wish to explain in this book several scenarios of ways I have been treated horrible in several of the bigger hospitals in Arkansas and Missouri. Even in Texas from when I was younger because of my fear of needles and my need to be comforted and consoled by nurses I'm comfortable with. Their lack of compassion and willingness to do this for me has caused me major emotional trauma.

I would like to show you what happens in all the bigger hospitals where the nurses refuse to meet my needs or give me people I'm comfortable with. It was traumatic for me to deal with them. Especially since, not only do they not meet the needs I desperately need met but they also yell at me, make derogatory comments to me, even do things to punish or humiliate me. They can't stand it that I have a fear of needles, and it bugs them that I cannot handle getting through an IV stick as easily as the last person does. That goes for anything else invasive too. No matter what it is, if I scream, act scared, or start breathing hard because I am afraid of what they are doing, it makes them mad. They think that I ought to just grow up and be able to take it like a man like everyone else. They don't understand that I can't, because I have oversensitivity to pain. I am not misbehaving myself when I scream and cry in pain. I'm really in pain. I need their help, and they're not giving it to me. Instead they're yelling at me, griping at me, and threatening me. My wife, Bertha Marie, and I both have been interrogated by these people, and even by a security guard before.

They obviously did not understand the importance of meeting my needs by comforting me and consoling me through the procedures I have done, like the needle sticks they do on me in the way I need them to do it. I really do need them to give me the people I need to comfort me in a way that works best for me.

I also would like to show you what, in my instance, has been done to see to it that my needs are met. The smaller hospitals, like Dreamer's Hope Regional in Arkansas, who have dealt with me, actually understood me after my wife advocated for me.

As a matter of fact, the last time I had a three day stay in their hospital, which I love, the nurses were very nice to me there. They did not give me any nurses that made me uncomfortable. We told them that I have a fear of *male* nurses because I was tortured by men in the hospital setting as a child. We also told them that the more serious, mediocre acting *female* nurses made me nervous. We also told them that even if they did not make me nervous they were still boring to me and did not bring me comfort. If they did not have the peppy, motherly like personality that brings me comfort, they would not know what to do for me, even if they were nice to me.

We told this hospital several things. I was autistic, wanted *bubbly acting*; happy go lucky *female* nurses only that would allow me to hug them. A hug to me is putting my right ear to the other person's cheek. When I have to have an IV, blood test or a shot, I need to have a *bubbly acting*, happy go lucky *female* nurse to rub my head to calm me down while a different happy go lucky *female* nurse does the stick. I also need to be able to apply Emla (Lidocaine/Prilocaine) cream on one hour before the stick as thick as possible in order to help numb the site of the stick. I would also need to be knocked out completely for any invasive procedures, such as surgeries, catheter insertions, tests that involve needles, tubes, and blades, etc. I would not be able to handle anything this sharp or painful awake at all.

For several years, over a decade now, these people have met me with full eagerness and compassion, by giving me everybody I asked for, and needed who did everything I needed them to exactly the way I asked them to do it.

These were the most wonderful people I ever met in the hospital setting.

The last time I was in there hospital they had a horrible time re-adjusting my IV in the inpatient ward. Even though I was worried sick they would be upset about it, they were not.

It took five girls several minutes to get it fixed. When I told them how worried I was one of them said, "You may have trouble getting through needle sticks and other invasive procedures, but your difficulty with getting through painful situations like this one is a far cry from what we have to put up with from other patients who do better at getting through the painful stuff, but yet gripe and complain about other things continually that are nothing but trivial. I want you to know that regardless of what happened here today that you are the most well behaved patient we have ever had and we really appreciate that."

So you see everybody did exactly what I wanted here and what I needed and we had a win-win situation in the end. If every hospital would do this we would have a far better situation for everyone.

I hope that this book will help to stop the abuse of vulnerable patients in the hospital setting of the bigger hospitals that have a fear of needles that cannot defend themselves.

I want this book to cause bigger hospitals to be more reluctant to treat me in the abusive and discriminatory manner they have and anyone else who has fallen victim to the ones in the nursing field who wish to punish, intimidate, humiliate, and interrogate those who are lesser than they are, that are afraid of needles, and have trouble getting through IV sticks, and invasive procedures.

It is not our fault we are like this. We need to be able to have the privilege of getting who we need to do what we need in order to comfort and console us through anything too scary for us to handle ourselves. You can't make a person not have a need he has, it will always be a need no matter what you think about it.

Everything was wonderful for years with this hospital that handled me so well.

Unfortunately for now, all that has changed, because many new people have come on board that did not know me before. They don't understand me nor are they willing to meet my needs.

My wife went to talk to them and they suggested she find a doctor who specialized in Special Needs.

They also said that they were not trained to handle Special Needs patients so she should also see if the Children's Hospital would take me. They do not understand my differences, idiosyncrasies or needs.

They have never seen anyone quite like me before with legitimate needs to be treated like a child by all his nurses and *chipper acting*, cheerful *female* ones at that. I feel like the new nurses feel like, "Why me?" They do not understand my situation at all.

If the cheerful, *chipper acting female* nurses, that aren't currently familiar with me, only knew what my situation really entailed and what I have already been through they might see things differently. They would still have to be willing to comfort me not just feel sorry for me for what other *male* nurses and *serious trended female* nurses have done to me to hurt me.

It is not good enough that the *chipper acting female* nurses I like so much just be nice and smile. They need to be willing to give me hugs, rub my head to calm me down through needle sticks, and be as gentle with their needles as possible, and try to cheer me up when I am anxious and hyperventilating. They need to also allow me to put Lidocaine/Prilocaine 2.5% Cream on 1 hour before the stick.

This Lidocaine cream usually knocks out most of the pain, sometimes even all of it, but not always. Sometimes the Lidocaine doesn't always work as well on certain days and I may feel the pain almost as loudly, so they have to be ready for that. And they always need to be willing to knock me completely out for all invasive procedures. They also need to knock me out for any catheter insertions, urinary or heart. I cannot handle it awake.

A shot and a blood test feel like someone sticking a steak knife in me. An IV feels like someone stabbed me with a butcher knife. And a catheter feels like a sword being run through me. Keep that in mind when you get to be my nurse. You can see why I would need comforted just seeing this being the situation. Who wouldn't if it was this bad?

Most people do not feel pain this loudly, but I have sensory issues because I am autistic and I have needs that need to be met and the only thing that works is what works for me. It doesn't work for you to do what works for you; it's what works for me that will help, nothing else will do. If you are not willing to meet these needs the way I need them met, I cannot do anything for you. I need nurses that will meet all these needs with *chipper acting*, cheerful personalities and with full compassion and happiness. Please, if you are a nurse I like and I get you for a nurse, you need to be willing to do all this for me and comfort me the way I need comforted that works for me because I will not be able to handle it if you do not. Like I said I cannot handle it any other way. I need my nurses to be like mommies and buddies to me. Please have mercy on me and do things for me the way I am asking you to do them.

You need to be a cheerful acting, *chipper acting female* nurse and you need to give me hugs, rub my head to calm me down and hold my hand through needle sticks, be gentle with the needles, and do everything you can to cheer me up and keep me calm. That's the only thing that works. I hope something can work out. I'm looking forward to some day when I find a place that understands.

If they do not, I'm not going. Do not try to trick me. You either meet my needs from the start or I'm not coming, plain and simple.

Prepare to read this book and be enlightened. You are about to find out the horrible truth about why I am the way I am, not because of anything I've done, but because of what others have done me. I hope you continue reading to explore my life witnessing all the nightmares I lived through with doctors and nurses.

Dear Nurses,

There are some chapters in this book that some individuals may consider to be graphic in nature. Please do not hold this against me. I am not doing this to be inappropriate. I am trying to point out the truth about what other *male* doctors, *male* nurses, and *serious trended female* nurses have done to me in the past and how far they would go. Most of the people I've talked to do not think it is graphic because it is tame compared to what is normally considered graphic out there.

The events that did happen, that may be considered graphic in nature, were during my childhood years.

The events I mentioned I suspected *might* happen during my adult years that may be considered graphic in nature by some individuals were based on how nurses during my adult years with controlling personalities acted like those I had when I was a child with the same personality type who did the very things to me I suspected these nurses might do.
\
Chipper acting cheerful female nurses need to know, I am not talking about you. The people that did this to me were *male* doctors, *male* nurses, and *serious trended* fe*male* nurses. They were all mean. They were all controllers. And they were all grumps. We're talking stern men, cunning men that like to make fun and serious trended women who don't like it when their patients are scared of needles and scream in pain.

I hope this clears up any misunderstandings that may occur when I mention these subjects.

Please understand there are nice nurses out there but not all nurses that are out there are nice, so if you are a nice nurse, please don't take any of this to heart, because it is not about you.

Thank you.

Brian Gene Evans

Disclaimer

The stories in this book are actual events.

Some names in this book have been changed to protect the guilty and the innocent.

The hospitals and doctors' offices and dentists' offices and the institution mentioned in this book have also all been given fictional names, but the doctor offices and hospitals and dentists offices them selves and the institution itself are quite real and the people in them are also real. I just gave the real people fictional names like I gave the real hospitals fictional names. Everyone mentioned in this book is a real person with a different name and everything I claimed they did really happened.

I wrote this book in hopes to help the nurses, doctors, and techs understand what has been done to me by various other doctors, nurses, or techs who were mean to me and had a lack of understanding about my Autism and my oversensitivity to pain and how other nurses, doctors, and techs that understood my situation handled everything differently to help me through all my invasive procedures. This book contains both good and bad scenarios of what has happened to me in the hospital setting throughout my lifetime as well as some doctor's offices, dentist's offices, and other clinics, and in one instance, a mental institution I told about my experience at in Chapter 3. My hope is to help these nurses, doctors, and techs that take care of me in the future to understand what works for me and what doesn't and how they can create a more positive environment for me while under their care and meet my special needs by giving me the cheery, chipper acting female nurses I am asking for only and meeting my list of needs by having these cheery female nurses comfort me in a way that comforts me through needle sticks and procedures by rubbing my head to calm me down and holding my hand during needle sticks and giving me hugs and letting me hug them when I go for procedures and appointments. Please enjoy your read.

Chapter One
Male Nurses at Tragedy AFB Hospital in Texas

I went to this hospital from March 3, 1969 all the way to June of 1990. This place felt more like a slave yard than a hospital. My experiences there were horrible.

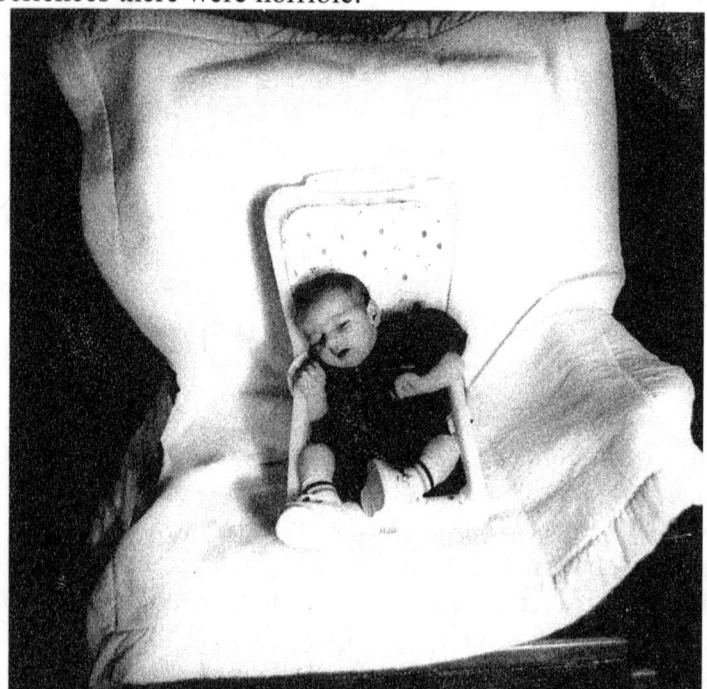

I was placed in an incubator after birth. A few minutes later a nurse told my mother I was a little blue. They never tested for brain damage or heart defects.

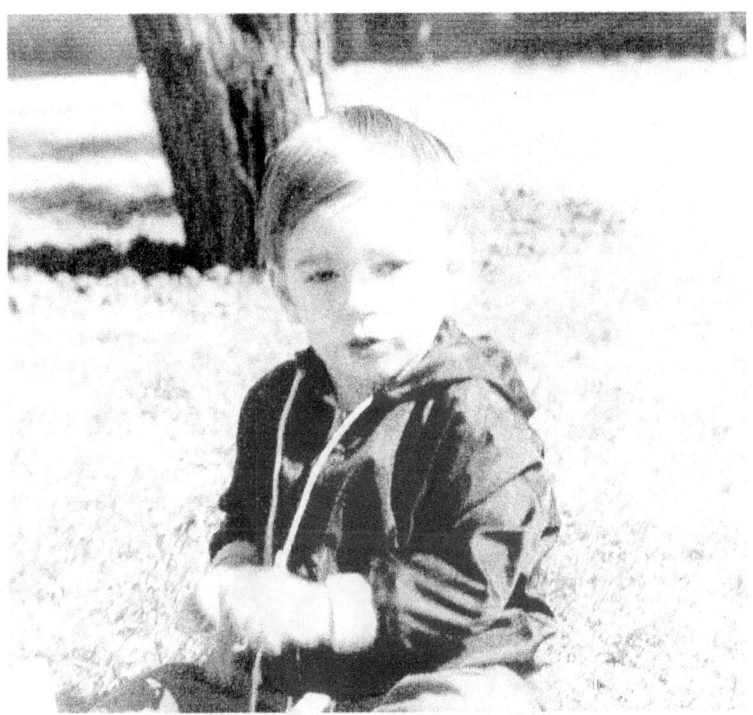

My mother found the shot record recently and said, "No wonder you were traumatized. They already started poking you left and right from two weeks old to two years old just to do the immunization shots, much less any other shots you may have had for other reasons."

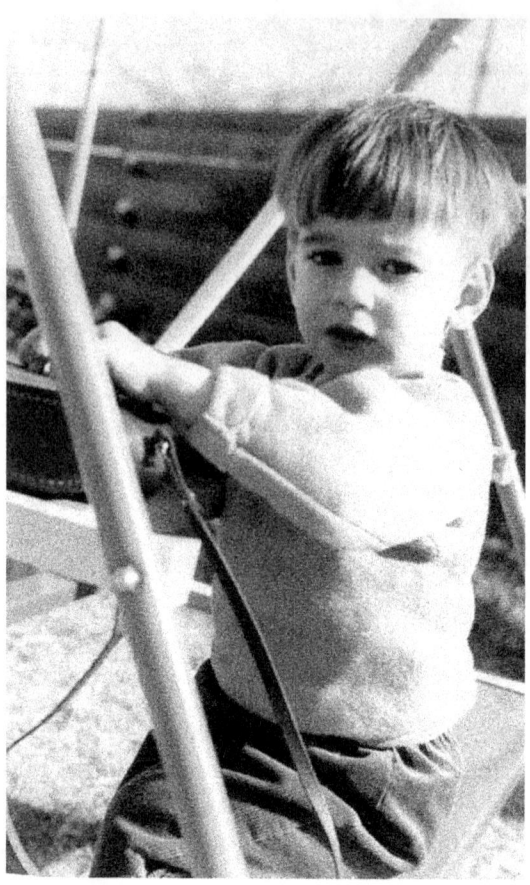

At age 3 they decided I had brain damage, and heart defects at 6 years and 9 months old. This is not even the tragic part.

Several times I went to their Emergency Room when I was a child. I remember going in there and lying on a table with those big circular operating room lights on each side of me over my head on the sides of my bed where they came at me with scalpels and needles awake. They got rough with me and were aggravated that I was scared of needles. Nearly every time they would come at me with needles possibly even stitches, or other things. I can't remember everything right off, but everything they did that involved needles of any kind scared the living tar out of me.

The stern, *male* doctors griped every time I acted squeamish over blood or scared of needles or screamed in pain over a needle stick of any kind. The nurses were *male* nurses almost every time. Some were stern. Others joked around in a very condescending way. I know for sure I had to have stitches put in my head at age 3 after running down the hall at home and hitting my head into the vent.

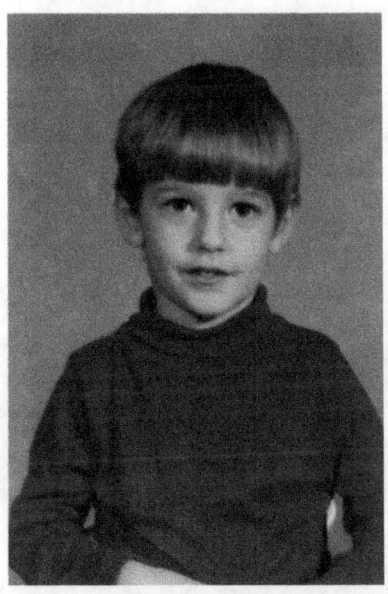

I even read in my records recently they said I fell off a tricycle when I was four. I think I remember something about falling off the hood of a car or something too. I was constantly having some kind of accident, and when I did, here it came, the nightmare of my life in the Emergency Room.

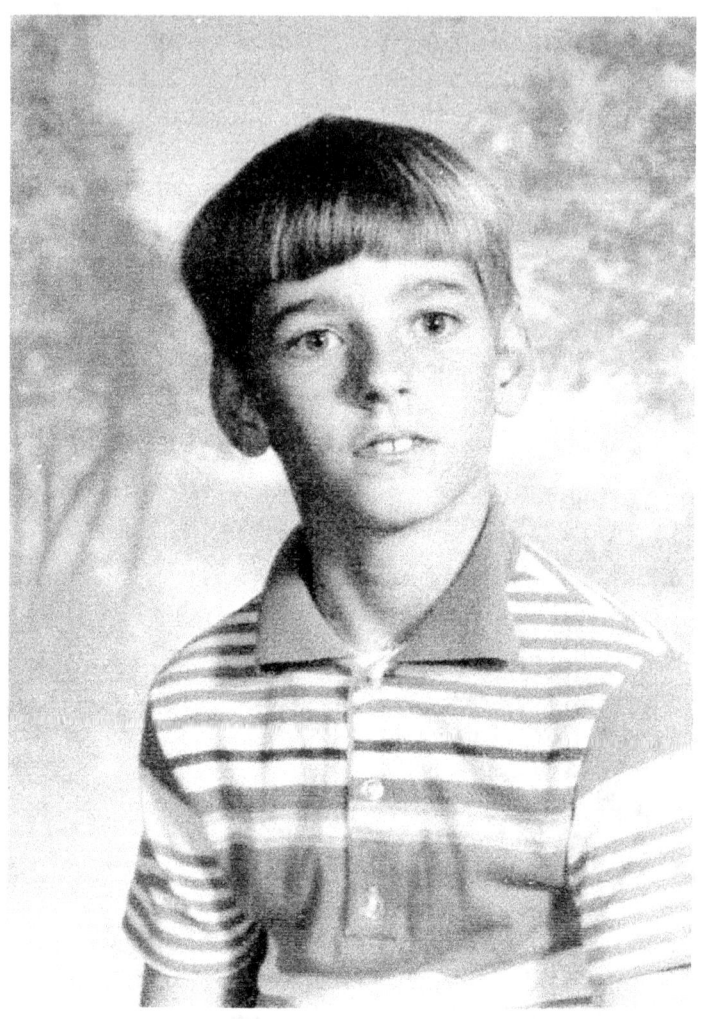

Even if I didn't have an accident I would get sick and have to have shots. Of course they were rough with the shots. I think I even remember them saying I had some respiratory problems in addition to my sinus problems and I used to get bronchitis a lot and they even came close to putting me on a respirator once. I almost forgot that experience. I think most of the cold situations were taken care of by the regular doctor in the hospital. But there were times I did go to the ER for that too. I guarantee you; they were not very nice about it. There were many other things they treated me for.

I know I had the measles and mumps once, but I don't think I went to the ER for that, just the regular doctor in the hospital. I also noticed they said I had a lot of ear infections when I was really young. Once I even had swelled tonsils. I guarantee you no matter what it was they did, they were mean about everything and came after me with needles every chance they got. They were very stern about it every time too. I wish I could remember everything. Even with what little I told you, there was far more done to me than what I'm remembering here that I'm telling you. I was constantly sent to the lab. They constantly complained I was anemic and even thought at times I had cancer of some kind and put me through all kinds of havoc with needles over that. When they finally took me seriously about the heart issue, I think they were nicer with most of that. But there may have even been things with that they did I'm not remembering that were just as bad.

If I ever got a lady nurse they would be a very serious trended nurse in a white hat that came at me in slow motion with a shot like a zombie with a straight look on her face and say, "I am going to give you a shot!" They were really creepy.

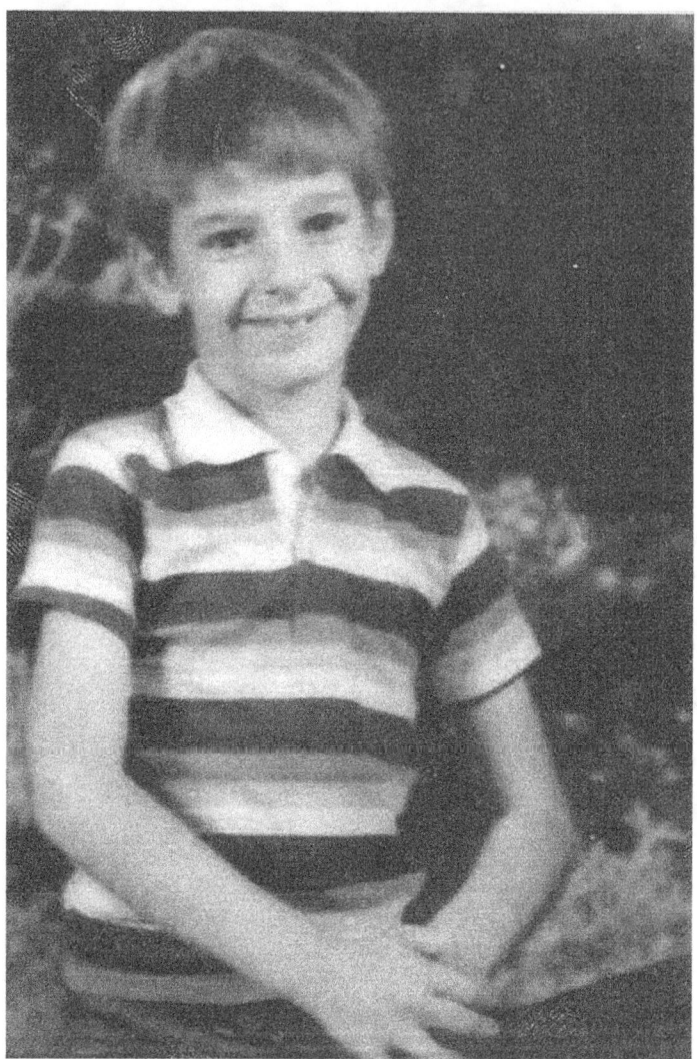

I just now accidentally remembered when I was a kid, one time I think our radiator overheated and I think I may have leaned on it with my arm or just got popped with the radiator fluid. I remember seeing fumes going up in smoke and I believe it hit my arm and left some kind of place on it.

I remember my mother saying, "I hate to say this. I think I'm going to have to take you to the Emergency Room again. I hope you don't have gangrene."

I said, "I hope I don't have gangrene. I don't want to lose my arm. I'm not about to let them cut my arm off."

My mother said, "Well, maybe it's not that bad. I hope not."

We went to the Emergency Room and they scraped at it, I think, and made me cringe.

I know I cringed at whatever they did and when they looked at it they said, "Well, there isn't any gangrene. We know that for sure."

I remember thinking, *"Good, I'm glad of that. I'm not about to let anybody cut my arm off."*

But I think I remember them possibly giving me a shot as usual and sticking me hard with some kind of injection solution into the wound and I remember them scraping at my arm making me scream. Then I think they put some kind of ointment on it and bandaged it up and said to watch it. It's hard to remember exactly what happened but I know it wasn't a very happy experience whatever they did. My memory of those experiences, though there were several, is very vague in my mind but this is what little I do remember about all of them. And like I said, there were several times this happened, not just once or twice. They were very mean every time I went in there to see them to have something done.

They would gripe at me and say, "Quit being such a baby! You need to try harder to cooperate with us! We can't take this nonsense of yours you have with your squeamishness and screaming and squirminess! You need to be still and just let us do our job! Quit being such a problem and straighten up! You need to be a man and quit being such a baby!"

They would be extremely rough with everything and scare the living tar out of me in the process. I'm pretty sure I remember some instances where men have even tackled me and restrained me to give me a shot or a blood test and rammed it in hard too.

17

The force they used to hold me down made them feel powerful beyond end and it greatly delighted them when they were able to do this to me. They acted like they were practically congratulating themselves for being this horrible because they thought it was great. I know this happened. I just cannot remember the specifics of each situation this happened in or why it happened. This is also vague in my mind but I know they acted this way toward me.

I had to go to the ER frequently as a child. There are also only a few instances I remembered any of the specifics of what happened in these situations too. This happened far more often than you would expect because I am so accident prone.

Bertha thinks if I could remember all these experiences I remember vaguely of being tortured with needles and scalpels under circular lights, considering they used no anesthesia and were very rough and mean about all of it that I would be so traumatized, as I was back then, that it would be too overwhelming for me to handle the memory of it because it was that bad.

We recently read a book by Tory Hayden about a boy named Boo that was 7 about the time I was probably 13, and I was shocked to find out that this teacher had taken this poor kid to the Emergency Room one day, and her student, Boo had to have stitches on his tongue.

The doctor in there gave the kid no anesthetic whatsoever, and the teacher said, "Excuse me! Don't you think you ought to give the boy some anesthetic?"

This doctor told Tory in this book, "Oh, he doesn't have any feelings. He'll never notice a thing."

The kid screamed and squirmed all over the place, and the teacher about had a fit at this doctor's behavior, and he threw her out of the Emergency Room.

My mother had the exact same problem with these doctors at this hospital with me and I remember this too.

I just can't remember the exact circumstances and all the details of what was being done for what conditions. As I said, I do know I was accident prone and had many accidents, so part of these experiences where for these reasons. Other experiences of this nature that took place were for reasons that did not pertain to accidents. I wish I could remember enough to tell you the details of what happened but many of these experiences have already been darkened by a deep fog in my brain causing me to have amnesias to most of what happened back there.

Some people would say, "The problem was so horrible that you're mind just blocked it out."

I think that's exactly what happened. I'm sorry I am not able to tell you all this, but what I do remember I am telling you.

Some experiences I remember intense details about that stick out in my mind like a sore thumb. Others are vague in my mind like these experiences, but I still know they happened and really took place.

The *male* doctors and *male* nurses at this military hospital had no sympathy whatsoever. They just wanted to do what they wanted to do whether it traumatized me or not.

I almost never get a female nurse at the military hospital, yes, but that wasn't always the case. There were some instances where I got a female nurse and when I did it wasn't good, because they were the "serious trended" mean acting female nurses, not the chipper ones for sure."

I remembered one day I went to a male doctor in a different hall, possibly on the second floor, and then I thought, "Didn't he tell my mother to wait in the waiting room and two ladies were going to take me to another room down the hall to do some sort of test on me or do their own examination of some kind?"

Then, I thought, "It seems like there were a few instances where this happened and not just once. It just didn't happen really often. Probably 10 times out of every 100 I ever saw the doctor."

These two "serious trended" female nurses took me to this obscure room down the hall. I remember backing away from them toward the door as the first "serious trended female nurse" yelled at me, "You want to be a problem! You want to be a problem! If you don't change into your hospital gown we will do it for you!"

I was trying to get away from them.

The first "serious trended female nurse" grabbed me by the wrist and yelled out, "Do you have the hospital gown?"

The second "serious trended female nurse" yelled, "Yes!"

The first "serious trended female nurse" yelled out to the second "serious trended female nurse", "Take his clothes off and put the hospital gown on him!"

The second "serious trended female nurse" forcibly stripped me of all my clothes except my underwear while the first "serious trended female nurse" restrained me. This second "serious trended female nurse" pulled my shirt and my pants and my shoes and socks right off of me, but left my underwear on. Then she shoved the hospital gown over my head or my chest.

The first "serious trended female nurse" grabbed my arm and dragged me to a patient bed or a table. She practically threw me on it and body slammed me to the bed.

The second "serious trended female nurse" had either an IV or shot or blood test, it may have been a booster shot or something that she was getting ready to use on me.

The first "serious trended female nurse" yelled out, "Do you have the IV?!"

The second "serious trended female nurse" yelled, "Yes!"

The first lady nurse yelled out, "Stick him!"

I screamed horrendously, "Ahhhh! Ahhhh! Ahhhh!"

The first "serious trended female nurse yelled out, "You think you're scared of us now! You'll really be scared of us here in a minute! Stick him again! Again! Again!"

I also remember a situation where I went to a room I never went to before down the smaller hall from the Hospital Pharmacy to a smaller section of the military hospital with double doors in it and two ladies did something horrible to me in there too, but it's hard to remember what. I'm pretty sure it had to do with needles.

I know they were very mean and rough and not understanding and not nice at all. I remember saying, "I don't want to go in there anymore!"

Then, in another instance when I went behind those same double doors a different day I went to two other ladies in a different room I really did like that were chipper.

The time after that they sent me to a guy right before you get to the double doors and I said, "I wish I would have got those nice ladies behind the double doors instead. I wanted them! I liked them better! I just didn't like the first two ladies I saw back there, but I liked the other two ladies."

I was sad I got stuck with a man again.

When I was ten years old some old lady doctor decided she wanted me to do a blood test three months in a row during the summer after she felt these knots on the back of my head she believed were caused by cancer. I normally got a *male* doctor who wanted to torture me.

The doctor either just had to make some serious acting *male* or *female* nurse, usually a *male* nurse, practically jab me with a shot as hard as they could just to scare me. Or send me over to the laboratory in the hospital to make me have to get a blood test so they could have their hay day. But this time it was this crazy woman who did this to me. She sent me to the lions in the laboratory to have my blood tested in June, July, and August in 1979.

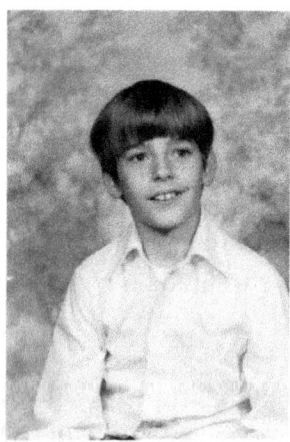

In the Laboratory these two hefty men acted like they thought they were really something. They acted like they really got a kick out of scaring vulnerable people.

I reluctantly walked in the Lab. They had me sit in the chair, and I was scared because the needles were very big and long back in those days. For those who live in my area in Arkansas have you ever seen those big fat meat marinade injectors in Country Mart with their big fat, very long needles? They were that big and that long. As a matter of fact the needles were even a little longer than those needles and just as thick as them. There wasn't any such thing as vacutaner tubes or baby IV needles yet, it was those things.

They saw I was scared, and got a big kick out of it.

They laughed at me and asked, "Do we have a baby in here? I think we have a baby in here. Do we have a baby? Do we have a baby?"

I would beg, "Please, don't hurt me!"

They would come at me with the needle acting powerful, and I'd plead with them, "Are you going to stick me with that thing?"

They'd be like, "Yeah! Yeah! We're going to stick you with it. What's the matter are you scared? Are you a baby? Are you a baby? We're putting it in right now!"

They laughed at me, and practically jabbed me with it as hard as they could, and laughed some more and I would scream loudly, "AHHHH!"

They'd just laugh and laugh and laugh.

I begged, "How much longer is it going to be? Is it going to be very long?"

In a powerful, make fun tone of voice, they jokingly said, "It's going to be a long time!" I would be like, "AHHHH!"

"Oh wow! I think he's having a hard time! We need to make a man out of this guy! Maybe you'll do better the next time!"

They were laughing and laughing and laughing and having a ball and jabbing me as hard as they could while they were at it.

"Boy, this guy is really scared! What's the matter, are you afraid? We've got a baby in here. I think we have a baby in here! What a baby! HA! HA! HA! HA! HA!"

I'd beg, "Are you done yet?"

They said, "NO, not yet! We still got a long way to go!"

After torturing me a long time they finally said," Well, looks like we're done now! I guess you made it through it anyway! Maybe you'll do better the next time?!'"

I got to where every time I had to go in there I started running out in the hallway to find places to hide. One day I went to the hallway first. Then I stopped to see if someone was looking, when the coast was clear I dashed out the door and ran as fast as I could to the car. I hid in the floor board thinking, *"Finally, no one will find me in here!"*

My mother looked all over for me and finally found me.

She said, "I've been looking all over for you. Well it looks like we're going home, if you're not going to do anything for anybody."

I would think, *"Good! I got away from those people."*

I got by without getting caught that time but one of the times a male nurse saw me running down the hall from the distance trying to catch me he yelled out, "Come back here you little twerp!" I got to where I ran away from these people a lot because of the way they acted toward me.

Another time when I went to that same Lady Doctor at the military hospital that was in a hallway behind the pharmacy and behind the immunization clinic in yet another cubby hole I did okay for that lady doctor except that I feared the blood pressure cuff might have a needle in it. But, I went to her at least 3 to 4 times, and maybe even 5 or 10.

One of the times I went to this lady, regardless of how nice she was to me, she sent me to two ladies down her hall that were also horrible to me that were "serious trended" and I had some sort of fiasco with them too.

One day, in a part of the hospital where the doctors and nurses were almost all men, there was another lady doctor in the corner of their hall and the main hall on either the first or second floor. I think it was the second floor.

I can't find where my visit with her was in my record, but Bertha saw something in my record about a fiasco I had with this lady and it started to come back to me and I remembered my experience with her was not good either.

I think she also did something horrible to me.

A "serious trended" female nurse again, of course.

If they had given me nice, chipper acting female nurses to begin with this would not have happened.

But all this was going through my mind through a dim fog, except for the one instance that stuck out more than the others.

I wonder if that's why I thought x-rays had IVs when all the ones I ever had done did not. Maybe they did a test on me that did. I don't know. I don't remember an x-ray machine though. And only the men did those, so I think they were probably just doing a shot or a blood test on me, maybe even something like a booster shot. I remember for sure I did not handle that well at all back then.

There were times when I had to go get an x-ray that I had to wait forever in the Radiology waiting room at this hospital. They had me go to a dressing room in the back to make me change into my hospital gown before they would come for me.

My mother asked these men that came for me, "Can he leave his socks on? Brian is embarrassed about his feet."

The *male* x-ray tech yelled, "NO!"

So I wound up in a hospital gown every time. I had to go barefoot in my underwear in front of everybody, embarrassed to death.

I remember one time I had fell down the concrete slab at Rose Park when I tried to climb up and down the slab from one section of the park to the other. I busted both my knees that time and had to go to Radiology to get my knees x-rayed.

One other time, I fell somewhere and I had to have my foot x-rayed to make sure I didn't break a bone and found out I had a sprained ankle. I went for chest x-rays a lot. I think I remember having to have my shoulder x-rayed because I hurt my shoulder once. I just found out by reading my records they also x-rayed those knots I had on my head around the same time I had to do that blood test three months in a row to see if I had cancer. The lady doctor that looked at it said she thought it was cancer. I also found out I had my sinuses x-rayed later. I may have even had some kind of special x-rays to take pictures of my heart considering I had that problem.

One time a kid at school punched me in the nose and I definitely went to the doctor for that, but he may have had that x-rayed as well. I know one time they took me to a room with a very fancy machine in the back. I usually went to one of the two front x-ray rooms by the waiting room which was connected to the lobby those things were in. People could see people walk back and forth into those rooms in their hospital gown even if they didn't have to sit in the waiting room wearing them. I was scared when I went to the back room for that x-ray.

It was some kind of fancy sonogram for something. I can't remember what. I think that may be the time I'm thinking of where they made me sit in the waiting area to wait on them even after I changed into my hospital gown before they took me back to the x-ray room. They said, "We're not ready yet."

Because of this I had to sit there in my hospital gown with only my underwear on, of course. And they didn't let me wear my socks either. So I was also barefooted in front of everybody too. They would take me back to do an x-ray with their machines, and my being small and not that familiar with x-rays yet, I didn't know what was going on, but they made it even scarier on purpose.

I thought sure it would involve needles when they took me back there but it didn't. These aren't the only times of course, these were only a few instances I'm remembering out of several I had to have x-rays of some kind done.   When I got to be in my 20's it no longer scared me to do an x-ray because there never seemed to be any needles involved. But then when I found out there were some x-rays that involved IVs then I really did get scared all over again.

 I also know that at age 10 I got my arm caught in a chain link fence at a school my mother visited where my sister was at.

Someone at the school found me because I was screaming like crazy in horrific pain!

They said, "Boy did you ever get lucky! That chain link that got stuck in your arm came this close to hitting that vein. If that thing would have hit your vein you would have been in serious trouble. You may have even bled to death."

I know I got stitches that time too, but I can't remember all the details of what happened. I'm pretty sure they came at me with a shot to clean or anesthetize the wound, but believe you me, when they put those stitches in I could feel it like no one's business.

I can also tell you I screamed like mad in excruciating pain when they did it too. Not only that, but I know they were rough with the needle of the shot they stuck me with in the wound and were not very nice about the way they handled me. I'm sure I screamed like crazy then too. They were always very stern when it came to doing things like this to me.

They would gripe at me and say, "Quit being such a baby! You need to try harder to cooperate with us! We can't take this nonsense of yours you have with your squeamishness and screaming and squirminess! You need to be still and just let us do our job! Quit being such a problem and straighten up! You need to be a man and quit being such a baby!"

They would be extremely rough with everything and scare the living tar out of me in the process. I'm pretty sure I remember some instances where men have even tackled me and restrained me to give me a shot or a blood test and rammed it in hard too. The force they used to hold me down made them feel powerful beyond end and it greatly delighted them when they were able to do this to me.

They acted like they were practically congratulating themselves for being this horrible because they thought it was great. I know this happened. I just cannot remember the specifics of each situation this happened in or why it happened. This is also vague in my mind but I know they acted this way toward me.

I had to go to the ER frequently as a child. There are also only a few instances I remembered any of the specifics of what happened in these situations too.

This happened far more often than you would expect because I am so accident prone. This is also true of lab, x-rays and doctor visits.

Several repeated instances of all the above situations during the first 21 years of my life at this place. Most of these experiences occurred between Birth and Junior High and only a few instances after Junior High.

These men were mean in every instance. Many men were very stern and insisted I bite the bullet. Others just made fun of me. The ones that made fun of me for sure congratulated themselves for getting by with being able to torture me and have fun with it. This happened over and over and over again.

They had no compassion for my oversensitivity to pain or fear of needles.

They rammed their shots and blood tests in me as hard as they could, some men sternly, others made fun of me. The stern ones often made me undress in front of them to examine me. So I had to change into a hospital gown when they did.

28

They would say sternly, "You need to get undressed! I need you to put on this gown!" and glared at me as they watched me undress myself.

When I was down to my underwear they looked down at me like I was an ant to them and I would reluctantly put my hospital gown on shivering to death.

I stood there in front of them naked trembling in fear, scared to death and severely embarrassed because I was self-conscious of my body. They looked at me like they loved it that they embarrassed me.

I felt ashamed of myself, standing in front of these men unclothed and felt inferior to them as they looked at me gruffly.

They would give me their stern look and proceed to come at me with the needles. And they would stick them in me as hard as they could. I was actually scared to death of them.

Then they would say, "Come here you! I can't take any of your squeamishness or squirminess! Quit giving me problems! Quit being such a baby! You're going to have to bite the bullet and take it like a man! I've got to stick you with this thing! I'm giving you a shot! Don't be giving me any problems! Be still! Don't you give me any problems! I don't need to have a baby in here! You need to take it like a man!"

I would scream horrendously every time, "Ahhhh!!! Ahhhh!!! Ahhhh!!!"

They would continue griping at me and say things like, "You want to give me problems?! Don't be giving me any problems! Come here you! Be still! I need to get this done! I can't be having a baby in here?! I need to do this! Don't be giving me any problems! Stop screaming! You need to bite the bullet! I'm not putting up with your squeamishness and screaming! Quit squirming on me! Take it like a man! Come on! You keep giving me problems and I'll really jab you hard! Be still!"

They might even do more than just a shot. It could be a whole series of things they would torture me with and they would get a big kick out of the entire thing.

I understand you have to put your patients in hospital gowns for examinations but these men went too far. It made them feel powerful to do this to me. To them it was an accomplishment to feel like they were able to force me to undress myself in front of them and make me have to stand next to them feeling petrified and humiliated and inferior to them. They acted like that make them feel big, like they were in control and they had power and they were incredibly superior to me and they loved it that I felt hopeless and helpless against them.

This made them very happy to be able to do this to me because it made them feel powerful beyond end to be able to treat me like I was their own little peon slave and I had to do everything they said and couldn't do anything about it and they could hurt me all they wanted to and make me feel like there wasn't anything I could do to stop them. They were very gruff and very mean.

These male doctors and nurses would still do these kinds of things to me even when they didn't make me undress in front of them. However, when they did get me to undress in front of them it made me feel like I was fair game to them and they could do anything they wanted to do to me and I couldn't stop them.

There were some instances where I tried to run from these men.

When these *male* doctors and *male* nurses did have me undressed to examine me I felt trapped. They usually threatened me with needles while they were at it and used them. They rammed them in me as hard as they could when they did use them.

They tried to make it hurt on purpose and yelled at me when I screamed and acted gruff. They loved to see the fear and embarrassment in my eyes when I stood naked in front of them.

They acted like they had me right where they wanted me.

30

Big City Hospitals Don't Like Cowards   Brian Evans

It was like my fear of whatever they were going to do to me was their entertainment. They acted like they felt like they were proud of themselves for getting me in that position. Now not only was I scared of them and humiliated beyond end but they figured that I wouldn't go anywhere in my gown. They knew I was too embarrassed to run from them if I was undressed and got a *power kick* out of it.

In most instances I just had to go down to my underwear and put the hospital gown on, but I noticed in some places in my records these men actually made me go completely nude in front of them and made comments in my records like *nice nude tone*. If you don't believe me I can look in the records and show it to you myself if I knew you. They really did this. I don't know what they were thinking. I figured they just thought this gave them an even bigger *power kick*. This just gave themselves an excuse in the records to do this to me as they looked gruffly at me as usual when they did this to me. They did this on purpose because they loved to embarrass me. It made them feel powerful to make me feel low.

They did this to degrade me and let me know they were in control over me. They treated me like I was their slave and looked at me as if I were their slave when they got me naked in front of them.

These men were horrible. When they did this they claimed they were making a man out of me.

They were angry that I was scared of the needles but got a kick out of it at the same time because they knew I couldn't stop them. They worked roughly with me as I stood there feeling powerless against them.

These men were control freaks and I was like a victim to them and my mother witnessed the whole thing and didn't know what to do about it or how to stop them.

As I said I am reluctant to change into a hospital gown for a *male* nurse or a *serious trended female* nurses either one.

31

Both *male* doctors and nurses and *serious trended* fe*male* nurses use making me undress for them to do their job as a tool of humiliation and control.

The people that did this to me never smiled a day in their life that I ever saw. It was these people that did this to me.

When these individuals get my clothes off of me they would say to each other, "It looks like he won't be going anywhere now! We've got him right where we want him! I don't think he'll be going anywhere! He's too embarrassed and he's scared to death of us! He won't dare run from us now!"

And then they usually said, "Now we've got him! We can do whatever we want to him now and he won't be able to stop us."

Throwing me over to these people is like throwing me over to the Romans.

The Romans usually forcibly stripped all their prisoners in front of multitudes of people in order to humiliate them and then proceeded to torture them.

These men at Tragedy AFB Hospital I am telling you about and the staff at an institution I went to for a year and a half in a later chapter were the same way. If they don't like you because you are scared of needles you are just a problem to them.

In their eyes you're just a trouble maker and they will either grab you and yell at you and ram needles in you and be stern about it and act gruff or sternly ask you to undress yourself and change into a hospital gown and then proceed to torture you with needles. If you refuse to cooperate with them, you're probably going to get stripped.

Not only would the *male* nurses do something like this, but the *serious trended female* nurses would too.

These nurses had a "You do what I say or else" kind of personality and if you refused to cooperate with them they would force you to cooperate with them whether you wanted to or not. I felt like an ant to all these nurses, but especially the stern men. I felt helpless and hopeless and powerless against all of them and continually wished I could find a way of escape from them.

These nurses wished to stomp me out and do everything they could to both hurt me and humiliate me on purpose.

They thought they were making me a man, but they are only making matters worse and they traumatized the daylights out of me in the process.

I think I vaguely remember one or two instances where I may have actually got a chipper acting female nurse because for some reason I sort of remember one being nice to me in a room full of nurses and then a "serious trended female nurse" caught them being nice to me, of course, and said, "Don't spoon feed him! He needs to bite the bullet!"

Like I said, *chipper acting female* nurses would never do this to me. Any time they ask me to change into a hospital gown I will be more than happy to do so for them, just not these people. I'm not afraid of a chipper acting female nurse manhandling me if I change into a hospital gown for them, but I am afraid of a serious trended female nurse manhandling me if I change into a hospital gown for them.

That is why I was going to refuse to change into a hospital gown for three "serious trended female nurses" you will see a story about in a later chapter in this book. When I saw how mean they looked and how straight faced they were, I thought, "I'm not falling for it this time! I'm not changing into a gown for them! They'll try to grab me and drag me and tackle me down and ram needles in me as hard as they can and gripe about it when I scream! I know how this works! I've ran into their kind before!"

Their theory is, "Get this guy undressed and then try to force him to do everything we ask and he won't be able to run because every person in the hospital will get to see him undressed with only a hospital gown on and he won't run then. We do this, and we've got him trapped!"

That's what these nurses did when I was a kid.

I think I was between ages 6 and 12 when these "serious trended female nurses did this to me" and since it seems like it occurred slightly before and slightly after meeting the female doctor that sent me to the lab to be tortured with blood tests three months in a row at age 10, I think I was around age 9 or 10 when this happened.

During the time I dealt with these "serious trended female nurses" if I refused to cooperate with them I would get stripped of all my clothes and have a hospital gown shoved on me and that was that. These "serious trended female nurses" were going to get the job done if it was the last thing they did even if they thought it meant they had to rip your clothes right off of you to get it done. That was their philosophy. They did this to put me at their mercy so they could force me to cooperate with them and torture me with needles all they wanted and make me feel like I couldn't do anything about it and couldn't do a thing to stop them.

To them I was this little peon that couldn't stop them if I wanted to and now that they had me undressed after forcibly stripping me of all my clothes and shoving a gown on me they figured I wasn't about to go anywhere if I decided I wanted to run because I was too embarrassed to let a hospital full of people see me undressed.

If I put these nurses in a position where they had to do something for me involving changing into a hospital gown and I refused to cooperate with them, they would make me change into a hospital gown whether I liked it or not. To them I was a piece of property. They felt like they owned me and could demand I do anything they ask or face the consequences, which usually meant getting stripped.

My being a piece of property to them makes them feel like they had the right to rip my clothes off at any moment that I refuse to change into a hospital gown for them because I was afraid of them. I already knew they were going to manhandle me. They would have manhandled me anyway. The only difference is now, not only would I get manhandled but I will get my clothes ripped right off my body because I refused to cooperate with them and they are going to be very ugly about it and gripe at me when they do it and force my every move and get even meaner.

These "serious trended" female nurses would literally hold me down and jerk my clothes right off of me whether I liked it or not, or grab me by the wrists while their "serious trended female nurse" partner stripped all my clothes off of me against my will. Then these "serious trended female nurses" would shove the gown on me and handle me as roughly as they could after they did it, griping and yelling at me the whole time and ramming their needles in me as hard as they could and not being nice about it at all, and not caring how it made me feel either. They just want to get the job done, and if that's what it took to get it done is to strip me off all my clothes, then so be it, they're doing it. That's the attitude they tend to have, and they will do this, because they did it to me when I was a kid when I was uncooperative with them because I was scared of them.

It was the "serious trended female nurses" that forcibly stripped me of my clothes, not the chipper ones. I almost never got the chipper ones but when I did they did not approve of the way the other ones acted.

The problem is I only got a chipper one in about two instances during my elementary school years and in one instance during my high school years. All other times I got a "male doctor or nurse" or a "serious trended female nurse".

These people never smiled a day in their life that I saw and they were the ones that did this to me, not the chipper ones.

I am not making up inappropriate stories about naked people to try to make you think about naked people. I am telling the truth.
The men that did the shots and other stuff never smiled and were always gruff, stern, and mean and demanding.

The men that did the blood tests on me, however, did smile, but they were continually cocky about hurting me with their needles acting like they found pleasure in causing pain to other patients that were more gullible and more vulnerable than they were. They were nothing but a bunch of brat tyrants wanting to have fun torturing me.

This is what they did to me at this military hospital when I did get them, and I figured years later, when I ran into "serious trended female nurses" that acted the same way that they did, that if a procedure did involve changing into a hospital gown, and I got them instead of the nurses I really wanted, and they were the ones that told me to change for them and I refused that this would begin to happen again the day I dared to refuse a "serious trended female nurse again."

So before I go on in this book, so that I don't get you confused about which nurses I will and will not cooperate with let me get it straight in your mind now.

Question: Will I change into a hospital gown for a male nurse?

Answer: No.

Question: Will I change into a hospital gown for a "serious trended female nurse"?

Answer: No.

Question: Will I change into a hospital gown for a "Chipper acting, cheery, happy go lucky female nurse"?

Answer: Yes.

36

Question: Will I go with a male nurse to my patient room?

Answer: NO.

Question: Will I go with a "serious trended female nurse" to my
           patient room?

Answer: No.

Question: Will I go with a "chipper acting, cheery, happy go lucky
           female nurse" to my patient room?

Answer: Yes.

Question: Will I let a male nurse or doctor stick me with a needle:
           A shot, blood test, IV, blade, scalpel or other sharp
           instrument?

Answer: No.

Question: Will I let a "serious trended female nurse" stick me with
           A needle: A shot, blood test, IV, blade, scalpel, or
           other sharp instrument?
Answer: No.

Question: Will I let a "Chipper Acting, Cheery, happy go lucky
           Female nurse" stick me with a needle: a shot, blood
           test, IV, blade, scalpel, or any other sharp instrument?

Answer: Yes. "Only if another chipper acting, cheery female
           nurse rubs my head to calm me down and holds my
           hand through the stick, and only if both of them give
           me hugs and let me hug them."

Question: Will I let a male nurse comfort me through a
           needle stick?

Answer: No.

Question: Will I let a "serious trended female nurse" comfort me
           through a needle stick?

Answer: No.

Question: Will I let a "chipper acting, cheery female nurse
           Comfort me through a needle stick?

Answer: Yes. Only if they comfort me the way I ask them to.
           "Rub my head to calm me down and hold my hand
           through an IV stick or other needle stick and give me
           hugs and let me hug them." They do this and we're set.

           They don't and do it a way that pleases only them and
           there's no deal. My way or not at all. That's the deal.

Question: Am I afraid of a male nurse torturing me or deliberately
           trying to hurt me if I change into a hospital gown for
           them?

Answer: Yes.

Question: Am I afraid of a "serious trended female nurse"
           torturing me or deliberately trying to hurt me if I
           Change into a hospital gown for them?
Answer: Yes.

Question: Am I afraid of a "Chipper Acting, Cheery, and happy go
           lucky female nurse" torturing me or deliberately
           trying to hurt me if I change into a hospital gown for
           them?

Answer: No.

So, all of you chipper acting, cheery happy-go-lucky female nurses that are worried about whether I will change into a gown for you because I am so reluctant to change into a gown for a male nurse or serious trended female nurse, don't be afraid to ask me to change into a hospital gown for you if you need me to.

I am willing to change into a hospital gown for you to let you examine me or prep me for a procedure anytime you ask me to, so please don't be afraid to ask. You are not the ones I am reluctant to do this for.

The "serious trended female nurses" and the "male nurses" are the ones I don't want to change for because I don't trust them not to torture me after they get me undressed thinking they have me trapped.

Also, I know the next thing you are probably going to say is, "Brian, I know you are more willing to cooperate with us because you are not afraid of us like you are these other people but we still have to stick you with needles and do biopsies on you and do other invasive stuff that might hurt you. I don't know if you know that or not. It's still going to hurt, whether we do it or not."

I know. I realize you still have to do scary stuff. I figure you're going to need to get your instruments and needles out to do what you need to do to me and it's still going to hurt, but at least you will be gentle about it and not yell and scream at me when you do it and ram your needles in me as hard as you can, but these other people will. I'm more comfortable when you do it, and I only feel comforted by chipper acting female nurses with motherly sweet personalities, not these serious types that really don't care and just act like blah all the time with a straight face that have no sweetness about them and never get excited or cheerful about anything.

These other people just make me uncomfortable even when they are someone who will not torture me like most others with their personality would.

Big City Hospitals Don't Like Cowards   Brian Evans

I need you, "the chipper acting, and cheery female nurses" and I
need you to give me hugs, and rub my head to calm me down and
hold my hand through a needle stick. You do that and we've got it
made.

For all you doctors and nurses I already go to that I already like
and get along with fine and I'm already comfortable with, please
don't let this reluctance I have to change into a hospital gown for a
"serious trended female nurse" or "male nurse" cause you to never
ask me to do this for you. You do not have to be afraid of
offending me or be afraid I'll resist you if you do this.

I understand you have to do your job and there are examinations
and procedures that have to be done where you have to ask the
patient to take off their clothes and change into a hospital gown.
I didn't want you to feel like, "Well I would ask him to do this
because I really feel like I need to but I don't think I will because I
am afraid I will offend him someway."

Here's the thing. Are you a "chipper acting female nurse"? Are
you someone I get along with great that I'm not afraid of and don't
have any riffs with? If so, you don't have anything to worry about.
The only reason I'm acting this way is because I don't want to be
bullied by a "serious trended female nurse" or a "male nurse or
doctor".

When I was a child, some of these more serious acting types
tended to use making me change into a hospital gown to make me
fair game to them in order to be able to torture me with needles in
any way they wanted to without having to worry about me running
away from them. These were mean people that did this.

If a nurse comes to me that I think is going to be mean to me, like a "straight faced female nurse" or a "male nurse or doctor" with a stern personality, I am going to back away from them and try to run from them because of how mean they are or how mean I think they might be to me, but if I like you and I'm not afraid of you and I trust you, it's okay to ask me to do this for you when you feel you need to because I will not do this to you and I will not be offended if you ask me to do this for you, so please don't refrain from doing so when you feel like you need to do so.

You will see throughout this book all the many situations where male doctors, nurses, and techs tortured me with needles and other instruments and so did all the serious trended female nurses that acted the same way they did.

But, you will also see stories here and there where I actually got the chipper acting cheery female nurses I wanted and they comforted me the way I wanted them to comfort me and needed them to comfort me and got hugs from them all as well, and all went well when they did.

All the other experiences with all the other nurses went bad, but these chipper acting cheery female nurses always saved the day when I got them.

As I said, the things listed in this chapter are not the only things that happened at this military hospital; they are just the things that pop out at me that I remember the specifics of. This happened many times over, not just two or three times.

Many more instances occurred just as horrible with all of these men and there were probably around a hundred different experiences I can't even remember all the details of that occurred at this hospital.

All the rest of what happened here is very vague in my mind but also very horrible. It was the most traumatic experience of my entire life and it lasted for twenty one years.

And there is more to come about what these male doctors, nurses, and techs and serious trended female nurses did to me at this same hospital in the coming chapters.

Because this book is being written in chronological order, I have to write about what happened in between times in other chapters, such as the dentist I went to in chapter two in the same time frame as chapter one occurred, and the institution I was in for a year and a half, from age 13 to 14/12 before I tell you what happened at the military hospital at age 15 and beyond.

When you get to a chapter that this particular hospital story continues in, it will say Part Two or Part Three after the title, so be looking for it. There's more to come.

For those nurses that are reading this book that are seeing all this stuff in these chapters of this book they may consider graphic in nature I really apologize if this makes you uncomfortable.

I felt like I needed to tell everything In all honesty that happened with every experience I ever had that is both graphic and non graphic in nature depending on the situation being told about to educate you on how some nurses that are not very nice tend to act toward their patients so you will know not to do the same things they did.

Some individuals out there reading this already know what I mean by a "serious trended female nurse" and a "chipper acting female nurse" just by the terminology I am using, but there are others that don't get what I mean at all.

One individual told me after reading this book they thought that a "serious trended female nurse" was someone that "took their job seriously" and totally missed the point altogether.

She thought because they took their job seriously, since to her "serious trended" is a word for "taking a job seriously" that I should not be complaining about what they do because they are "being serious about their work and just trying to get the job done".

This is actually not what I mean at all.

My definition of a "serious trended female nurse" is not one that takes their job seriously but is someone with a "serious trended personality".

A "serious trended female nurse" never smiles, keeps a straight face, is boring, and never gets excited about anything.

They are usually grumpy, impatient, unsympathetic, uncaring, forceful, demanding, controlling, angry acting nurses who don't care how scared you are or how much pain you are in but just want to get the job done no matter what that means.

Unlike, chipper acting female nurses, "serious trended female nurses" usually do not take "no" for an answer to anything and if you refuse to do anything for them they will grab hold of you and force your every move.

They will gripe at you, restrain you, pin you down hard, and ram needles in you as hard as they can and may even forcibly strip you of all your clothes if a procedure involves a gown and you refuse to cooperate with them.

It's been done to me before. These are the ones I am talking about that do this to me, not the chipper ones. It's the straight faced nurses that never smile that do this to me. They're the ones that act like this.

A "chipper acting female nurse" is always smiley, huggable, fun loving, adventurous, playful, encouraging, comforting, and tries to be gentle and motherly with their patients.

"Chipper, Cheery Female Nurses" usually have a lot more patience when you are struggling to get through a needle stick than a "serious trended female nurse" does.

"A serious trended female nurse" is the direct opposite of what these people are like.

Both of these take their job seriously, but "serious trended female nurses" take their job way too seriously and are forceful and controlling and dictatorial with their patients and should really find a different job and work somewhere else and not be a nurse at all because this job is not for them.

Nurses need to be encouraging, motherly, comforting, huggable, lovable, caring people with a lot of patience who care how you feel about procedures and do everything they can to help you through anything that hurts you or scares you. They are to be like a mother to you and be as compassionate as they can.

Here is the difference between how a "serious trended female nurse" would have handled a scared patient reluctant to change into a hospital gown for a procedure or examination and how "chipper acting female nurse" would have handled a scared patient that was reluctant to change into a hospital gown for them for a procedure or an examination.

A "serious trended female nurse" would have got angry when a patient acted scared and said, "Are you going to take your clothes off or are we going to take them off for you!"

With the "serious trended female nurses" if you did not undress yourself, they were going to undress you themselves, because your clothes were going to come off one way or the other, because they were going to "get the job done if it was the last thing they did".

A "chipper acting female nurse" in the same situation would have probably said, "Its okay. Don't be afraid. I'm going to be right here. You just change into your gown and I'm going to be right here for you.

44

I know this is going to be hard, but we're going to get through this. So, just change into your gown and let me know when you're ready and I'll be as gentle as I can when I stick you with needles and things, okay. It's going to be okay."

If the patient would have still absolutely refused a "chipper acting female nurse they would have probably done one of two things:

They probably would have said, "Okay, if you're not going to do this, I'll go ahead and let you go, but I really think you should do this. You really need to."

This is how they probably would have handled an adult or a child if they reacted this way to them.

In the case of a scared child who was reluctant to change into a hospital gown for them the "chipper acting female nurses" might have got another chipper acting female nurse to assist them and said, "Help me with him. He's scared to death and I need to take his clothes off and get this gown on him." if they thought they were required to force the child to cooperate with them in some form or fashion to do what they needed to do.

This is how I believe they would handle all this.

These other people, "the serious trended female nurses" and the "male nurses" that are forceful and controlling with their patients demanding they do what they say or be forced to cooperate with them and gripe at them in the process ought to get another job and quit being a nurse because the way they act is not the right way to treat your patients.

It is actually being abusive to their patients to treat them with such forcefulness and dictatorialness where they demand they take their clothes off or their going to jerk them off of them, throw them on a bed, ram them with needles in anger, and act this way toward them when they deal with them.

This is especially true when they try to keep them in the hospital with them forever so they can continue to be able to gripe at them and torture them all the more for as long as they can. This is nothing more than another alternative form of slavery.

Nurses with this attitude need to find another job and let the "chipper acting female nurses" with motherly personalities treat their patients with the comfort and the compassion and gentleness that they need.

Chapter Two
Nightmare Experience at a Dentist's Office

When I was a kid, I went to this dentist that never gave the gas. My mother kept having a hard time finding a dentist that would even give the gas. This dentist back then wanted to drill my teeth to do a filling.

My mother asked, "Can you give him gas?"

He said, "No."

Instead, he only gave a numbing shot, which was very painful to me with no gas. He also started drilling and I went absolutely ballistic on him.

My mother pleaded with him, "Can't you just give him the gas? I think he would do better if he could have the gas."

This dentist said, "No!"

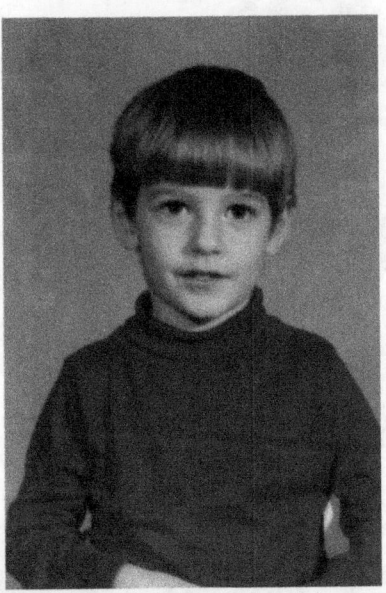

We had this problem with this man several times over and never could get anything done the way we needed it. He finally decided to admit me to the hospital to put me under the gas just to do his dental work. My mother and I both thought this was nuts, but getting the gas at the hospital was better than nothing.

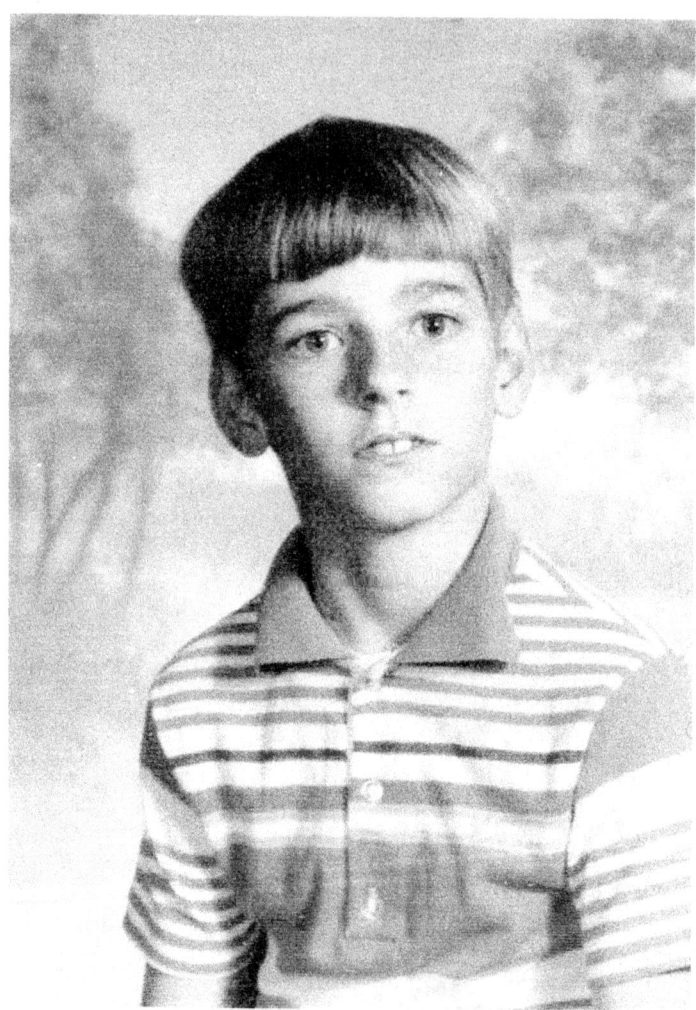

They made me change into a hospital gown and my mother said, "Brian is embarrassed about his feet. Can he wear his socks?"

The nurse said, "No. We can't do that. He'll have to take them off. I'm sorry."

Another nurse came in with a booster shot that looked like a bike pump with the biggest longest needle you ever saw.

She gave me a shot in the upper leg with it. I was shaking with fear as they approached me with the needle I was so scared. I'm sure my eyes got big as they came at me with it. I was shocked they gave me that big shot in the upper leg. I would have thought they would have done it in the arm, or the hip, but they chose the leg. I jumped, screamed and cried hysterically. Then they came in and did a few other crazy things. I can't remember what all they did. I think they even took a blood test and drove me crazy that way too. Somebody finally got a hospital bed, and told me to lay in it. Then they took me to the surgery room and gave me the gas. Finally I was out and didn't know anything else. I never felt the pain of the dental work because I was out cold when he did it. I didn't understand why in the world I had to have a booster shot and a blood test before I went and why they insisted on embarrassing me to death. This was an experience I had with a horrible dentist when I was a kid.

Big City Hospitals Don't Like Cowards   Brian Evans

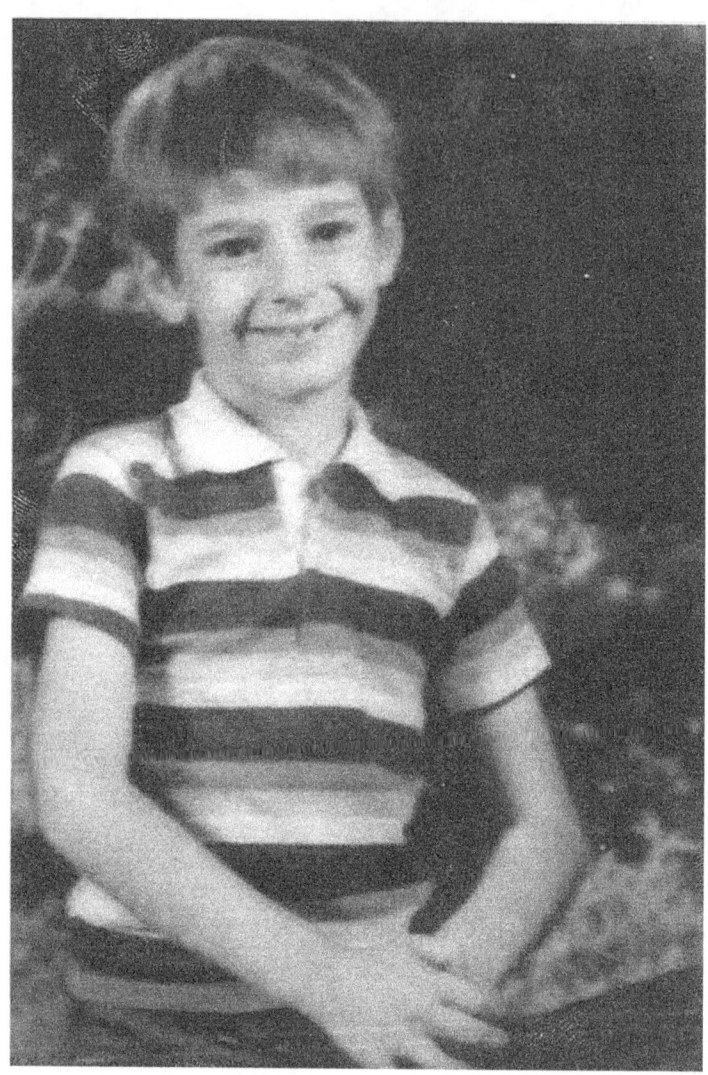

50

Big City Hospitals Don't Like Cowards   Brian Evans

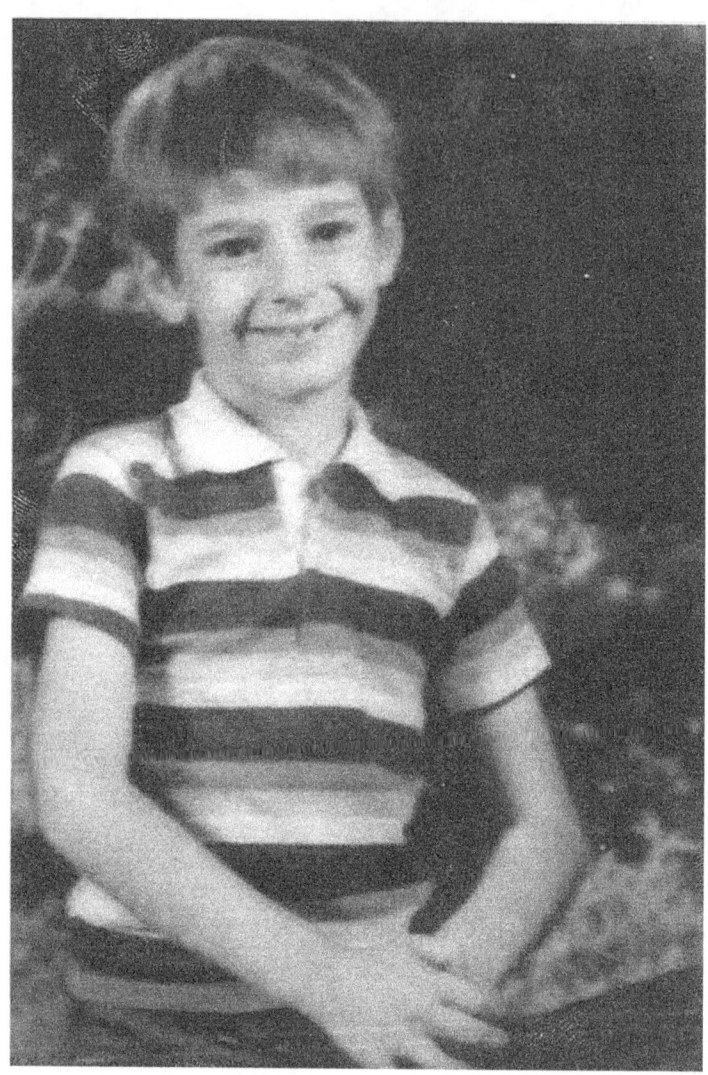

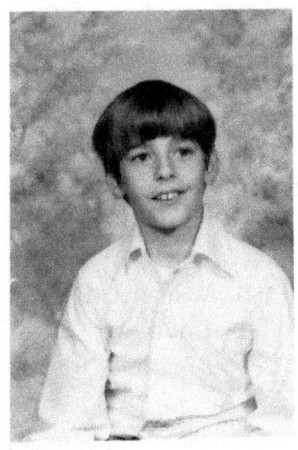

Chapter Three
Wilderness Institute
My life in a Mental Health Facility
At Age 13 to 14 1/2
June 1, 1982 to October 24, 1983

On June 1, 1982 I was put in Wilderness Institute as a kid, because I was wild and my mother could not handle me anymore. Keep in mind when you read this chapter, I was only a 90 pound, four foot seven inches tall, 13 year old boy.

This is the only chapter in this book about a mental health facility. All other chapters in this book are about medical hospitals, doctor's offices, and dentists' offices. Although this chapter is about a mental health facility and not a medical facility I wanted to further emphasize the cruelty I faced by staff in the field of health who were "males" and "serious trended" females. Even though this was not technically a medical facility, I wanted to show you the problems I had at this mental facility because it may not be considered to be in the medical field, but it is still a place you go to in the field of health. I wanted you to be able to see how like the situation at the military hospital I also had trouble with being treated with cruelty in one more place by "males" and "serious trended females" in the field of health that were over me that were responsible for my care.

When I went into the institute, at first I had a couple of my toys I had brought with me. Ryan, a staff member saw me when I started playing with them.

He told my mother, "You need to take his toys home with you because we can't have toys here and its age inappropriate for him to play with them."

My mother took the toys and said, "I'm sorry Brian, I didn't know they wouldn't let you have these here."

At first, I had a really hard time adjusting to being at the institute, because I was not used to being away from my mother. At the beginning, they started out a little more lenient with me till I got used to the place.

One day I said, "I think I'm okay now. I'm really beginning to like this place. I like being here now."

Ryan then said, "Like this place! You're not supposed to like it here! We want you to hate it here so bad you never want to come here again!"

After I admitted I was beginning to like this place my life suddenly became a living hell. They made it their number one goal to humiliate me and make me miserable.

One day, Scarlet, a lady staff person, was getting ready to have us play scheduled games for the day. I had talked to my new friend Michael, a patient, and I told him I really didn't want to play any games, but I guess I'd have to.

He said, "Oh, you don't have to play the games if you don't want to. Just tell them you don't want to play any of the games."

I went and told her I really didn't want to play the games and she said, "Did you say no? Did you say you weren't going to play any of the games?"

I said, "I really didn't want to. I thought it was optional."

Scarlet said, "Don't tell me you won't play any of the games! You have to play the games! Are you telling me no? You don't tell me no! Take your clothes off!"

I did exactly what she said. She made me take my shirt and pants and shoes and socks off in front of everyone and then handed me a white undershirt with colored sleeves that she called the *shirttail* shirt and said, "Put this on!"

I had to stand there barefooted in my underwear only, in front of everybody with the *shirttail* shirt she gave me to put on over my chest after I took my own shirt off.

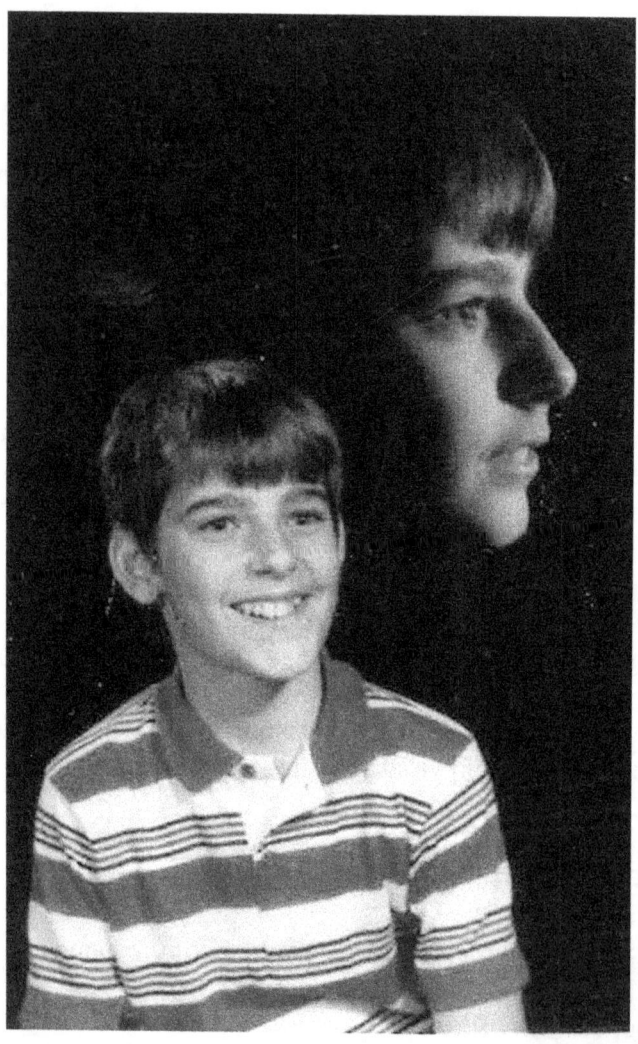

Scarlet, Ryan, and Rico got a constant power kick out of making their patients take all their clothes off except their underwear in front of a room full of people to get back at them for doing something they didn't like. Every time a patient did something they didn't like they did this to them as well.

Ryan got aggravated with my sense of humor one day when I was joking around with the other boys.

Ryan said, "Take your clothes off!"

Ryan made me take my shirt and my pants and my shoes and socks off, and told me to throw them in the floor beside me. Everyone then got to see me bare-chested, bare legged, and bare footed. All I had on was my underwear.

He then handed me a *shirttail* shirt and said, "Put this on!" He made me stand there for 30 minutes while all the other boys stared at me in my underwear because he said I was goofy. After I took all my clothes off he picked them up and locked them in the office.

Although the staff was mostly men, if there were women around, tough luck, they got to see you in your underwear too.

One day in the lobby/living room, Rico accused me of something I didn't do. As usual, he also tried to twist my words around about everything.

When I argued with Rico trying to defend myself he said, "Take your clothes off!"

Rico also made me take my shirt and my pants and my shoes and socks off in front of everybody and handed me a *shirttail* shirt to put on and said, "Put this on!"

Then Rico said, "Well! I bet you don't feel so hot about yourself now without your clothes on! What do you think of yourself now?"

Rico continually blamed me for stuff that wasn't true. He twisted my words around constantly, making me take my clothes off right in front of everybody, every time I tried to defend myself against him. I just can't remember all the instances he did this in for some reason, but they were many.

One day, Scarlet caught me wearing my socks to bed, and grabbed me by the arm, and dragged me out of my room into the lobby.

Scarlet said, "Did you wear your socks to bed! You broke the hygiene rule! You're not allowed to wear socks to bed, so as a result you're being punished! Take your clothes off!"

She made me take my shirt, and pants, and shoes and socks off, as usual. This time she did not give me a *shirttail* shirt.

I had to go bare-chested this time. The only thing I got to leave on was my underwear, period. That meant I did not get to wear shoes, socks, pants, a shirt, or even a *shirttail* shirt. I didn't get to wear pajamas, either.

She then said, "Because of what you just did, you can just sit in front of this closet door in your underwear, Indian Style, now!"

I did what Scarlett said and took everything off except my underwear and sat in front of the closet door, as she demanded.

Another time, Scarlet had a soap box meeting where she cut everybody down for everything she could. Scarlet put some people in *shirttail shirts after she made them take everything off except their underwear* to humiliate them. Others she just condemned verbally. At a couple of the soap box meetings Scarlet told me to take my clothes off right there. She made me sit in front of everybody, Indian Style, in only my underwear again.

One day after Scarlet condemned me several times I was standing outside on the side walk complaining to Jamie about her. Jamie was another patient.

I said, "Scarlet is a thing of rags!"

Scarlet caught me talking about her. She grabbed my arm and drug me toward the cottage door and threw the door open.

She asked, "Are you talking about me again? Is there something you want to say to me?! Are you trying to cause some kind of trouble?! Get in here!"

She dragged me inside the door and then she said, "Take your clothes off, now!"

Scarlet made me take me shirt and pants and shoes and socks off right in front of her again and handed me a *shirttail* shirt and said, "Put this on!"

After this everyone else walked back in the door and they got to see me in a *shirttail* shirt and underwear only, too.

Scarlett never smiled a day in her life that I ever saw. She was always mad, shifted her weight around about her authoritative position constantly, and demanded you take your clothes off over every little thing you did to make her mad.

When I was outside in the field one day, I saw my favorite nurse at the time; Kara. I hugged her several times because I was excited to see her. After I went back into the Cottage for a few minutes, Ryan called me into the office. I didn't know why.

I couldn't figure out what on earth I was supposed to have done wrong. When I walked in the office, Ryan had Kara in there with him. I looked at them both frantically, because I knew I must be in trouble for something, but I didn't know what.

After standing there bewildered for a minute Ryan said, "Brian. Take your clothes off!"

Ryan made me take my shirt and my pants and my shoes and socks off, right in front of her. All I got to wear was the underwear around my waist after I undressed myself.

Kara got to see me stand in front of her in only my underwear. Kara acted like she got a big kick out of it that I had to take my clothes off in front of her.

She stood there looking at me with a smile on her face like it pleased her for me to be forced to let her see me undressed against my will. She was very pleased that I felt humiliated in front of her and felt defenseless against her and Ryan. She acted like she was enjoying herself for being responsible for this whole fiasco and she looked at me degradingly as I stood there in front of her in only my underwear acting like she loved every minute of it.

Ryan then handed me a *shirttail* shirt and said, "Put this on!"

After I put the *shirttail* shirt on, I only had a *shirttail* shirt and underwear on.

Ryan laughed at me and said, "Well Kara! Look what we have here!"

Kara stood there in delight with a smile on her face acting like she thought, "It looks like we showed him! I wonder what he thinks of himself now!"

I think she thought it was funny and felt like Ryan doing this was helping her get back at me for being different.

Ryan was also delighted that Kara got to see me in only my underwear. He thought it was funny I had to let her look at me with no clothes on whether I liked it or not and got a big power kick out of the whole thing.

Kara stared at me with a cheap grin on her face while Ryan, lectured me in front of her for the next thirty minutes. She acted like she was practically congratulating herself for putting me in a position where I would be forced to take my clothes off in front of her because it made her feel big and proud to be able to do this to me.

To her it was like a slap in my face on her part and she loved every minute of it. I felt like she was looking at me like, "See if he ever does this again. I bet he doesn't feel too hot about himself after what I just did to him. Let's see what he thinks of himself now."

Making me let this lady see me in only my underwear and shirt tail shirt made Ryan feel very powerful.

He grinned at me and acted like he was congratulating himself for being able to do this to me. He wanted to embarrass me and humiliate me as much as he could.

Ryan hoped I would be incredibly embarrassed in front of her, and I was. He wanted to make me feel low and he did. This made Ryan feel like he had control, and could make me feel inferior to both him and Kara. He acted like this made him feel very powerful to do this to me. He was trying to make me feel degraded. He wanted to embarrass the tar out of me to get back at me for being different and he did. He knew I was embarrassed to death and this just made him feel as happy as a lark. This made him feel very big of himself and he loved every minute of it. He was proud he was able to put me in this position so I would be afraid of him and Kara and feel embarrassed to death and inferior to them. He acted like he was having the moment of his life and he loved it.

One time, Ryan's mother, Liz was volunteering to help them take care of the other patients. She only did that in about three or four instances at the most. I know for sure of two times. This lady was trying to explain something to me and I didn't get it what she was saying to me. I finally got it what she was talking about and said, "Oh!" Liz got all worked up and got mad at me and said, "No! Did you say know to me! You don't ever tell me no!" Liz grabbed me by the ear and drug me across the room and told me "Don't you ever say no to me!" I said, "I didn't say no, I said oh. I didn't get it and I finally got it." She didn't act like she was paying attention to what I was saying and acted mad anyway. So, she kept dragging me by the ear across the room and kept on griping at me anyway. Liz was a "serious trended" female by the way. She most definitely was not a chipper person and never smiled a day in her life either.

At other times, Ryan and Rico took me in their office, and lecture me together. They did everything they could to twist my words around about everything and called me a liar. They accused me of several untrue things, continuing to call me a liar.

When I tried to defend myself in certain instances they would get offended when I got warm on their trail. If I started getting too close to being able to prove I was right about something they would say, "You're lying. Don't tell me it's the way you're saying it is. You know it's the way we say it is." And I would say, "No, that's not true. 'It was this way.' Or 'This is what I really said', or, 'This is what really happened." they would say, "Take your clothes off!" and I had to take my clothes off right there in front of them in their office. After this they lectured me some more to punish me for standing up for myself after they had me undressed and tried to make me feel lower than ever in front of them and made me feel inferior of them.

I don't stand up for myself at all now and even then I wasn't very good at it, but when I did stand up for myself, I got slammed for it, because every time it meant I had to take my clothes off or I would be forcibly stripped of all my clothes. Either way, I had no clothes on except my underwear when it was over with, it was just a choice thing, either I take them off myself or they will take them off for me. Either way, I wind up with no clothes on in the end.

Rico began saying things like, "I'm going to tell your family this…and I'm going to tell your friends that… and their going to believe me."

A month or two later, a gardening lady had the patients go help her till a garden in the field behind the cottage. I enjoyed it but I got mud all over my shoes and didn't know how to get it all off. I didn't know what to do so I went to the rock (or brick) wall by the back door of the cottage and smacked my muddy shoes against it. I wanted to get the mud off so I wouldn't get the floor dirty. I only had the one pair of shoes.

Then Ryan caught me and said, "Destruction! Two Hundred Points! You'll have to do the following list of cleaning jobs to work your points off because you did this!"

Ryan made me scrub the bathtub and clean the floor in the second bathroom with nothing but an old toothbrush.

I was only four foot, seven inches tall and when I tried to reach the shower head while I was in there it seemed very high above my head and was hard to reach. The rest of it was normal, but felt tedious. My shortness was also an advantage to them considering they were all around five foot, nine inches when I was only four foot seven inches at the time. They figured they could use my shortness as a tool to make me feel more inferior and more helpless towards them. They knew I felt like I could not stop them if they ever made me do something I didn't want to do. They felt like this gave them even more power to make me obey them. They used this to control me as much as possible. So when they tried to make me feel inferior, they did a tremendously good job of it. It's easy to feel powerless against a person in authority that's 14 to 15 inches taller than you when they tell you to take your clothes off. How are you supposed to stop them anyway? You can't. I felt defeated, and felt like I had to do whatever they said and they knew this, and acted like they felt like it gave them a power kick.

I was in their office one day when they said to each other, "Well, this guy's scared of us! If he doesn't do something we like, all we have to do is make him take his clothes off in front of everybody, and he won't dare do anything we don't like, because he'll be so humiliated, he won't dare do anything we don't want him to do!"

My feeling inferior to him is how Ryan got by with making me undress myself in front of everybody all the time.

One day all I did was make a joke about the song Ebony and Ivory and said, "That sounds like Ivory soap!"

Ryan said, "Oh brother!"

I kept on making that kind of jokes, and after two or three more he said, "Brian, take your clothes off."

I said, "No! No! Please! Don't make me do it!"

He said, "Okay, but if you don't quit. I'm going to. So, if you don't quit, you will have to take your clothes off."

Then, Ryan said, "You know you're acting just like a retarded person. You are so bad off; you are acting just like them. I think I'm going to have to put you in the State School."

I said, "No! No! Please don't put me in there!"

Ryan said, "Well, with the way you go on about things, and how goofy you act, it's really not beneficial that you be here if you're going to be this way. If this doesn't change, I may have to put you in the State School."

It's too bad I can't remember what some of the other things I joked about back then were. If I could you would be able to see just how silly it was that Ryan did this to me. A few years ago, I saw a list of names at some place I was at and noticed someone's last name was Foxhound. I got a big kick out of it and said, "Is that like the Fox and the Hound?" That would have aggravated him to death. Last year, we were singing a song in church and I noticed it was written by Ruby Kitchen. I said, "You've got to be kidding me! Hey look at this! It says Ruby Kitchen wrote this song! Does she know Janie Living Room?" That would have driven him nuts too. I also saw two people's names in a set of files I had to put away twenty two years ago at a small town hospital when I worked as a file clerk. I said, "Jerry Christmas! You've got to be kidding me? Did they really call somebody Jerry Christmas?" Then, I noticed there was a file for Merry Green.

I said, "I think Jerry Christmas and Merry Green need to get together if you know what I mean, especially since her name is spelled M-E-R-R-Y!" If I told Ryan this he'd flip. I'd sure get the shirt tail punishment then.

Sometimes I think it would be funny if I figured out a way to contact Ryan just to aggravate him and retell him all my jokes he doesn't like and then when he acts good and aggravated say, "What's the matter Ryan, aggravated? You can't make me take my clothes off in front of everybody now! I don't live there anymore! Sorry! I figured you wanted to give me the shirt tail punishment but you can't do that to me now because I don't live there anymore! Sorry about that!"

There were other times at the institute Ryan and Rico would both come after me for things that were stupid. They just dug up reasons to give me trouble about just so they would have an excuse to punish me for something.

Ryan would take me off by himself, and have a talk with me saying things like, "It's going to be a long time till you get out of here. It's going to be December before you can leave."

A few months later, he would do it again, "It's going to be a long time before you get out of here. It's going to be next June before you get out of here."

A couple of weeks after that he would say, "I'm afraid we're not doing very well right now. It's going to be a long time before you get out of here. It's going to be the next December before you get out of here, and maybe, the June after that."

Ryan knew this made me feel hopeless. He would drive this in the ground to make me feel like there was no escape.

Rico made me watch Halloween, Friday the 13th, and Psycho movies. All against my will and it freaked me out.

When he saw I was scared he said, "It's all fake Brian! It's fake! Get over it! You need to be a man! You're acting silly Brian! Get over it!"

Both summers Ryan and Rico took the kids in the cottage to Six Flags.

That may be exciting to some people but it's not exciting to me. I'm afraid of heights. They knew this and made me ride the roller coasters there anyway.

They made me ride the Judge Roy Scream and the Twister all against my will yet again. Even after I begged them not to make me ride them, they still made me ride the roller coasters. I was so scared! I was screaming frantically, in pure fear. They both laughed about it.

They sat next to me and every time a big drop came they would teasingly say, "Here we go!"

They both got a big kick out of it.

They made me ride all the roller coasters against my will.

One of the rides dropped straight down. Another ride was like a river raft that constantly went up and down in a jerky swerve motion. They scared me out of my wits, and got a kick out of the whole thing. When we left for the day I was glad to get out of there.

In the fall of my first year there, Ryan and Rico also made me walk into a Haunted House once again against my will. They showed these insane acting sprit-like people were all over the place. They would jump out at you in the dark to scare you to death. One of them had a chain saw. It scared me for sure, and I didn't like it one bit.

Years later, some girl I went to class with said that the very motel they had made into the Haunted House they made me walk through was actually shut down. She said there were reports that people were getting killed and that some really wild stuff was going on in there. I found this out eleven years later when I went back to take some extra classes to try to finish my Medical Assisting Degree which I never finished.

Big City Hospitals Don't Like Cowards   Brian Evans

Years later I heard a report on one of my trips to Abilene that a kid
was worried about their seat on the Judge Roy Scream at Six Flags,
and the park person said they would be fine. That same kid got
thrown off the roller coaster, and died. Now, Six Flags is getting
sued for this incident, on the same roller coaster Rico got such a
kick out of making me ride against my will.

One day Derrick, another patient, pushed me in the back bathroom
at night in the dark. He tried to force me to say "Bloody Mary" in
the mirror 5 times to make her appear. I kept refusing but I still
felt trapped.

He kept saying, "Do it! Do it! Do it!"

One time, he did this when the room was dark, and said something
like, "The spirits are coming after you tonight! You're going to go
to Hell!"

I kept saying, "No! No! No! That can't be!"

At the Rose Park Swimming Pool, Kyle, another patient, tried to
push my head under water for long lengths of time one day three or
four times in a row.

Kyle laughed when he did it and said things to me like, "What are
you going to do about it? Try to stop me! You can't pull yourself
back up because you're not strong enough! Can you?"

At the YMCA swimming pool, Kyle caught me in the dressing
room after I went swimming. I was trying to change out of my
swimming suit back into my regular clothes.

There wasn't a private place to change. You had to dress yourself
at the benches in front of the lockers. This made Kyle really
happy, because now he could plan an attack.

Kyle waited restlessly for me to take my swimming suit off. As
soon as he caught me without my swimming suit on, he grabbed
my bag my clothes were in before I could put them on.

He stepped back with it and ran backwards with it while I stood there completely naked in front of him and held it up in the air, proud that he had taken it. I was completely nude.

He said, "Come and get it if you can!" and laughed hysterically.

I immediately yelled at him and said, "Give me my bag back, Kyle A.!"

An adult *male* that was not from the institute that was bigger and taller than I was walked in at the same time and stood there watching and said, "What did you call him?"

I said, "I called him Kyle A! That's his name!"

His last name had two syllables, and the first syllable sounded like a cuss word. I was completely nude when Kyle grabbed my bag and I struggled to get it back. He then got a wet towel, and swirled it up into several swirls, he wrapped it tight, and hit me with it in the legs several times. Then he hit me in the stomach and then my legs again.

I tried to back away from him and kept yelling, "Stop! Stop! Stop it Kyle A.!"

He kept going and started hitting me with it in the chest and the arms as well, and then my legs again.

He kept saying, "Are you going to stop me? I got you now! You can't do anything about it now! I got you right where I want you! What's the matter! You scared?! Come on! Come on!"

And he would be hitting me with the towel Smack! Smack! Smack! Smack! Smack! He kept moving back and forth in front of me as I backed away from him.

He continued hitting me with the towel in motion as he moved back and forth in steps. The man that walked in the room did not do a thing about it and let him at it.

I think he even walked out of the room before he was done with me. After Kyle finally had a lot of fun whipping me several times by snapping a rolled up wet towel at me, he finally stopped. He still made it difficult to get my bag back. He kept moving it away from me every time I got close to getting it back. I was covered in red whelps after I had endured him whipping me with a wet towel for like fifteen minutes. I finally got the bag with my clothes back. I had a very hard time getting dressed because the whelps stung so badly. Not one person ever did a single thing about me getting bullied by this boy.

One time at the institute Kyle threw small rocks and gravel at me several times and laughed about it. He was constantly trying to start something, and trying to sway the others too.

One day at Wilderness Institute, the staff members had another one of their Soap Box meetings with their patients. They usually griped out all the boys but this time for once I was not one of their guinea pigs. They gave four boys the *shirttail* punishment which meant they had to take all their clothes off except their underwear and put the shirt tail shirt on like I did. I was spared this time even if three or four other boys did get the *shirttail* punishment.

I think the second three or four boys were complaining about it and saying, "What did we get this for?"

I wasn't sure either.

The staff warned them not to back talk them, or they would be in even worse trouble. These boys decided to be clever and tried to do that very thing. I know for sure Kyle was one of them. I think the others may have been Wayne, who also tended to give me a lot of trouble, Bo, and one other guy; Shay.

When these boys challenged the staff, Billy was the last staff member I would have expected to do something like this, told these boys "Okay. That's it! Take your shirt off!"

Ryan was in there with him. I really suspect he was probably behind Billy doing this. This was not like Billy, but it was like Ryan to do something like this. Then the boys kept aggravating Billy and Ryan on purpose to get back at them.

Billy told Kyle and his three rebelling partners, "Okay. You want to play rough here?! We can take care of this. You're getting the towel! See this towel here! Take your underwear off, and put this towel on! You can just sit there in nothing but a towel, if you think your so hot stuff!"

I expected Ryan or Rico to come up with something like that, but it was Billy that told them to do this. Billy was normally nice to me. He was a friend of mine there, but I never thought he would have done something like this. I wouldn't have put it past Ryan to do this though, and he was standing right behind him. I think Ryan put him up to it.

One day, Kyle was given the *shirttail* punishment by Rico and he refused and said, "No!"

Rico said, "You better watch out or you're going to be in trouble! If you don't take your clothes off then we will take them off for you!"

Kyle said, "Catch me catch me if you can!"

He ran out the door fully dressed into the field beside the cottage. Rico ran out the door chasing him all over the field. Rico finally caught him, and pulled his shirt off right out in front of everybody. There wasn't much of anybody outside the cottage in the field at the time so he had a free run and he obviously had lots of fun making Rico chase him. After his shirt was taken off he got away again. Rico chased him some more until he finally caught him. This time Rico grabbed his arm and dragged him back into the cottage. Rico tackled him down and swiftly jerked Kyle's pants off and then pulled his shoes and socks off.

After that Rico said, "Well! It looks like I caught you after all Kyle! So much for trying to running off! It looks like I got you anyway!"

Another day Michael was given the *shirttail* punishment by Rico.

Michael said, "No! I won't do it! You can't make me!"

Rico said, "Oh we can make you! If you don't take your clothes off we'll pin you down and we'll take them off for you so you might as well do what we say!"

Michael still said "No!"

Rico grabbed Michael and he started spazzing out, acting crazy on him.

Even though Rico pinned him down he still tried to wrestle with him to stop him from doing anything. Because of his size Michael couldn't stop him.

Rico called Ryan in there and said, "You get the shirt! I'll get the pants!"

Ryan pulled his shirt off and then Rico pulled his shoes, socks and pants off and let him go. They picked up his clothes and locked them in their office while they were at it after they got him undressed. This isn't the first time they did this.

They actually gave me this punishment 10 times more often than all the others. All the other patients may have gotten the *shirttail* about 10 times per person the whole time I was in there, but I got it about 50 times or more, maybe even a hundred.

One day RJ got in trouble with Rico.

Rico said, "Take your clothes off!"

RJ said, "No!"

Rico said, "No! Did you say no to me?! You take your clothes off now or I'll take them off of you myself!"

RJ refused. Rico grabbed him and tackled him to the ground. Ryan pulled RJ's shirt off while Rico swiftly jerked RJ's pants off after he had pulled his shoes and socks off. Like Michael he was also stripped down to his underwear only and Rico and Ryan took the *shirttail* shirt and shoved it over his head and violently forced it down his chest.

One other time, there was an older boy, about 15 years of age that decided to run away from the institution in hopes to escape. After a search was done to find the boy and he got caught somewhere down the road and was brought back to the institution, Ryan made this boy take all his clothes off except his underwear and handed him a shirt tail shirt and said, "Put this on!" and the boy undressed himself as he was told and put the shirt tail shirt on after he was down to only his underwear.

Ryan then took a big huge laundry bag, and went through this guy's dresser drawers and took all of his clothes out of the dresser and put them in this bag. After this Ryan said, "I'm putting this boy in West Wing! This boy will not be able to wear any clothes for a whole week and will have to run around here in front of everybody in his shirt tail shirt and underwear only for a week! This was his punishment for running away!"

One day Jamie and I were sitting on the couch and Shay was leaning in the floor in front of the couch. Shay started complaining about something he was unhappy about.

Ryan said, "Hey Jamie. Look what I have here. I have a book from Mr. Wilderness that says that any time a patient acts out of line I am supposed to give him this *shirttail* punishment and make them take their clothes off. Let's show Shay what happens to people like him when they wine."

Ryan then got one of his *shirttail* shirts out and handed it to Shay and bragged about it and said, "Here Shay. This is what you get for wining! I hope you like it! Take your clothes off!"

Ryan made Shay take his shirt and pants and shoes and socks off and then pushed the *shirttail* shirt over his head and forced it down his chest and acted like he was delighted about it.

Rico caught Bo sucking his thumb one day and got sarcastic with him.

He said, "If you don't quit sucking your thumb, I'm going to make you suck your toe!"

Another day, I walked back from the Counselor's office from across the parking lot and noticed there was a water hose in the back window of the middle room where water poured out into the floor of the middle room when I walked into the door of the Cottage.

Rico spotted me coming in and said, "You went and took a water hose and turned it on and put it in this window to pour water in this room. It's all over the floor. Why did you do this?"

I said, "I didn't do that. How could I do that? I just now walked back from the counselor's office to come in here? How could I do it? I don't even know where the water hose is at?"

Rico said, "You're lying."

I think Rico did this himself.

He took four of us to the back room and said, "Someone defecated in here. Who did this?" I told him, "It wasn't me. I don't know who did it."

Rico said, "I figured you didn't do it, but I'm going to find out who did. Was it one of you other three boys? I'm going to search and ask around until I find out who did this. Be honest. Did any of you do this or not?"

They all three said, "We didn't do it. We don't know who did it but it wasn't any of us."

Rico said, "We'll see about this."

Jamie said, "Are you going to give whoever did this the shirt tail punishment?"

Rico said, "No. I don't know what I'm going to do. The *shirttail* punishment wouldn't be the appropriate punishment in this case. I'll have to think of something else. I don't know what but I'll have to think of something, I just haven't figured out what yet."

Tony got with the other boys and said, "Guys. I don't know who did this, but I'm going to take the rap for you so when ever Rico questions everyone you just take an out and I'm going to tell him I did it."

Rico then had a Soap Box meeting with the rest of the boys and said, "Someone defecated in the back room and I need to know who did this? Is anyone willing to fess up? You need to just straighten up and tell me who you are. It would be better if you just told me. If you did do this I'm going to find out who did this anyway, so you might as well fess up now because I will find out who did this before this is over with."

Every boy said it was not them. Rico finally said, "Anybody. I'm giving you a chance so fess up now."

Tony said, "I did it."

Rico said, "Tony, I really don't think you did this. You have a tendency to always take the rap for everybody else. Did you really do this or not?"

72

Tony said, "Yes. I did this. It was me."

Rico said, "Are you sure? You're not just taking the rap for someone else again are you?"

Tony said, "No. I really did it. I know it was stupid but I just did it anyway. I don't know what I was thinking. I just did."

Rico said, "Okay but I'm still not sure about this. I still don't think you did it. I don't know who did but if you say so, okay."
I think Ryan and Rico set up the whole thing on purpose. They were just looking for an excuse to get a bunch of boys in trouble for no reason just so they could punish them for something stupid that no one ever really did. I think Ryan and Rico did it and not the boys.

One time, Ryan gave Ray the *shirttail* punishment and went further with it than normal.

Ryan told Ray, "Take your clothes off!"

Ryan made Ray take his shirt and pants and shoes and socks off, just like he always made me do. Ray then put on the *shirttail* shirt after Ryan handed it to him when he was down to only his underwear. He then tried to be sarcastic toward Ryan to get back at him.

Then Ryan said, "Take your shirt off!"

Now Ray only had his underwear on. Ray kept on annoying Ryan.

Then Ryan said, "Take your underwear off and put on the towel! Wear this around your waist!"

Ray did what he said and took his underwear off and put the towel around his waist. Now the only thing he was wearing was a towel. Ray had no stitch of clothing on whatsoever except for the towel around his waist. He still thought he had one over on Ryan. He continued acting sarcastic toward Ryan to offend him even further.

When Ray provoked Ryan again, Ryan grabbed him by the arm and drug him to the door to exit out of the Cottage building. Ryan also got all the other boys together while he was at it.

He said, "Boys. I need you to line up next to the door behind Ray. I am going to take Ray over to the next building in his towel down the sidewalk and I need you to follow me."

After exiting out the door of the Cottage we walked down the sidewalk with Ray in his towel only from the Cottage to the South Wing building. We walked in the door of the South Wing Building and past the office and dining room area to the hallway the older boys lived in. At the corner of the office hall and the hall the boys lived in there was a sound proof room with a metal door. This door had a small rectangular window in the top of it where anybody could go to it and look in the room from the hall.

When we got to the sound proof room, we all watched as Ryan opened the door and proceeded to go in with Ray. Ryan had a hold of Ray's arm as he proceeded to walk in the door. As Ryan opened the door he swung Ray in a twirling fashion at the entrance of the room. Ryan flung the door open, grabbed Ray, and ripped his towel off his waist as he swung him into the room.

Ryan then stood Ray in the middle of the room making him face everyone while all the boys watched from outside the door. All of them saw every inch of his body uncovered including his peepee. Nothing was hid from anyone. He was then made to sit nude in the middle of the room like this Indian style. Ryan made sure every staff person and boy in the institute saw every inch of Ray's body so he could really humiliate him.

Ryan made Ray continue facing everybody with no clothes on whatsoever so they could see everything as he lectured him in front of everyone for the next 30 minutes. Then Ryan shut the door behind him. Every boy and every staff member that passed by to see Ray completely nude so that nothing would be hid from anybody and everybody would see every inch of him uncovered. That's what Ryan wanted.

Now even the *male* and *female* staff workers of the South Wing could go to the window of the sound proof room and see him nude if they wanted to. Every boy that lived in the South Wing could also look in the window and see him nude. Even the kitchen people who were mostly *females* could go to the window of the door and see him nude if they walked by. The counselors from the counseling building across the parking lot could also see him nude if they wanted to. Since the workers from the counselor's office sometimes came over to the wings to check things out they could have went to the window of the sound proof room and had a peak at the boy in the nude also. That was the whole plan. Nothing was hid from anybody anywhere. That was what Ryan wanted. He wanted to humiliate the daylights out of Ray so he would never want to challenge his authority ever again. After this by the way, Ray never challenged Ryan ever again. This was Ryan's sole purpose for doing this to Ray.

After Ryan was finished talking to Ray he commented, "Anyone that challenges the staff to the ump degree as this boy did will be next! And they will be completely humiliated as this boy was and be deeply regretful they ever rebelled against the staff! If you don't want this to happen to you, you'd better straighten up or this will happen to you!"

That means if any other boy would have challenged the staff they would have been stripped down to the nude also and everyone would have seen every inch of them including their peepee also.

Not only am I telling the truth about this having happened, but if I would have put Ray's real name in this book and he would have found out about it he probably would have said, "Did you have to tell the whole world he did this to me?"

Since I didn't use his real name no one would ever know who he really was by reading this book because I gave the guy this happened to a fictional name as well as the name of the person that did this to him.

After this, Ryan and Rico started making me take my shirt and pants and shoes and socks off in front of them again for their *shirttail* punishment they gave me. They did this to me several times over to humiliate me. They delighted themselves in doing this to making me undress myself in front of them and practically congratulated each other for it because they knew it embarrassed me. They knew making me stand undressed in front of them made me feel powerless against them and it made them feel powerful to have me in this position and they loved every minute of it when they did this to me. Doing this to me made these men feel very powerful. They would make false accusations against me, and called me a liar about everything. I tried to defend myself, but they were too clever for me. These men kept calling me a liar, twisting my words around and I was unable to defend myself. If I could not remember all the details of a specific situation I struggled to remember to tell them in defense of something, Rico would say, "You can't remember, can you? That's because it never happened."

One time I was worried if I said the wrong thing, they might decide to do something crazy just to make them selves feel powerful.

This was because they loved to humiliate me, and they enjoyed making me scared. I thought, *"I don't see anything on a shelf above the desk, but, I wonder if there going to give me a shot if I don't do something they say, or if I say something they don't like."* They never did but I was still afraid they'd do something crazy.

When I tried to defend myself about a subject Rico would say, "I wouldn't try to push us too far if I were you. We have ways of making you cooperate with us and we can make your life miserable if you try to contradict us so I wouldn't even try!"

Rico would sometimes say, "We're in charge over you and we can do whatever we want to do to you if we don't like something you do so I think it would be best if you cooperated with us because we have ways of making you do what we want and there's not a thing you can do about it!"

In some instances Rico would say, "I wouldn't go tell anybody we said this or we did this if I were you because we are over you and we can make you pay for anything you say about us. You don't want to chance it. I'd be careful if I were you!"

At times Rico said, "Nobody is going to listen to you because we are able to talk a lot better than you can about things and there's no way they'll hear your side when we're done with them. When they talk to us about these issues they'll believe us! There's no way to win, because they will believe us over you any day. So you might as well not even try because we can talk better than you can and we will win."

It would have not been unlike them to say "Okay. Since you think you're so clever you can just take everything off and stand there completely naked in front of us." They never made me take my underwear off, like I feared they would.

Every time I tried to say, "That's not the way it happened. What happened was this." Rico would say, "You're lying. You lie even when you don't have to lie. Admit it. It's this other way isn't it?"

I would say, "I'm telling you it's not, what happened was this!" Rico would say, "You're lying."

If I kept on enough times he would say, "I'd be careful if I were you. If you push us too far there are things we can do to you that will make your life miserable and there's not a thing you can do about it so I wouldn't push it if I were you."

They threatened me and said, "There are ways we can make you do what we want, so don't push it."

I took that to mean, "You try to defend yourself too hard and you will not be wearing your underwear either in a minute! Then you'll be completely naked in front of us! What do you think of that?!"

Rico began saying things like, "I'm going to tell your friends this, and I'm going to tell your family that and their going to believe me!"

By the way this is the way Rico tended to talk too. If you think they wouldn't make me stand in the nude in front of them, guess again. You read about what they did to Ray, when he tried to challenge their authority. I guarantee you if I would have not been obedient to their wishes and not let them con me into admitting to something that wasn't true, they would have made me take my underwear off and would have made me stand in front of them completely naked and then proceeded to degrade me even more. This is what these two men did when other patients challenged them, so why wouldn't they do this to me? I already feared they would do this to me. They never went that far, but were only one article of clothing away from getting me that naked. The fact that I admitted I liked it there in the beginning and them knowing that I was so self conscious of my body made me their favorite target. None of the staff and only two of the other boys even liked me. So I was very lonely. I always got more embarrassed by the *shirttail* punishments they gave me. I felt more powerless and hopeless against them than any other boy they did this to. Having that knowledge made these guys want to do this to me all the more, and the possibility they might force me to get even more naked than I already was to get back at me was a very great possibility.

I feared they would do this to someone if they challenged them, and come to find out I was right when I saw what they did to Ray. They actually did it to him, so why wouldn't they do it to me? They continually inferred that if I didn't watch my step, they were going to do worse things to me than they already did.
What else do you think they would have meant? "We're going to make you strip down all the more if you don't do what we say, or, Hey I think we may have a shot over there. Why don't we stick him with a needle and see how that makes him fare when he gets scared?"

This is not a joke. These men were those kinds of people. I think they were a couple of narcissists my self.

They never went this far in either way with me, but believe you me if I had not been cautious in watching what I said to these men they would have done something like this. I don't remember them ever giving anybody a shot but they may have once. They did make other boys strip the rest of the way down as you read about with Ray. That was how they handled excess back talking.

So you see they didn't go this far with me but I was afraid of them and always reluctantly went along with them. I tried to defend myself to a certain degree but they were too clever for me. I didn't stand a chance against these guys.

I think I even remember these men saying something to the affect of, "Well, we already have this guy down to his underwear, and he's obviously embarrassed to death already, and he's scared to death of us. So as long as he still feels low and doesn't challenge us too bad then I guess we'll just leave him like this. If he complains then we'll just gripe back at him but if he gives us too much trouble then we've got plenty we can do to humiliate him and scare him. If he challenges us too far, we'll just make him take his shirt tail shirt and underwear off in front of us, and he can stand there in front of us completely humiliated. Or, we might be able to scare him with a needle if we wanted to. He's scared of shots. But for right now since he's just cooperating with us to the most extent we'll just leave him in his *shirttail* shirt and underwear. I think he's too scared of us to do anything we don't want now."

Because of my fear of needles, I was given shot therapy at the counseling building across the street to help me with my fear of needles. The guy there would get me used to a needle. He would get me used to seeing it and feeling it, without poking it into me.

He finally did a slight poke a couple of times with a shot, not a blood test. And the shots he was using had very small needles also.

He was working his way up to the bigger sized needles as he got me used to the smaller ones, but wanted to use small ones first, not big ones.

Ryan was getting antsy at the cottage because I was not ready to do a blood test yet. Ryan tried to desensitize me to having a blood test with a long needle himself, and kept rubbing it against my arm without poking me, but he was making me nervous. At first, Ryan was just being gentle, and kind of easy with it. Then Ryan lost his patience when I was so shook up over it.

Ryan said, "This is stupid Brian! You ought to be able to handle this! I shouldn't have to do this. All the other boys do this and they barely feel a thing, and they act like it's no big deal to them but you still act like your scared, and you think it's going to hurt you. You need to get over this! This is stupid Brian! Grow up! Your being silly Brian! It's not a big deal. It doesn't hurt! You just think it does because it's all in your head!"

Then Denny said, "You shouldn't be afraid of this unless you had something really horrible happen. I had one done once and it hurt me because it caused this to happen to me. If it didn't cause something major to happen to you, you shouldn't be afraid of it, because it doesn't hurt anybody Most people don't worry about it unless they have a very good reason. If you had a reason, I could understand but you don't have a reason, and I did, so it shouldn't be a problem, because you didn't have anything like what I've had happen to you. You just need to get over it!"

Denny didn't know about me being tortured at Tragedy Air Force Base Hospital and it didn't occur to me to tell him about it either. Some of the other boys there were making some of these same comments. A few days later, I had to have a blood test at the office across the street, and it took five men to hold me down to get it done.

For a while, because of my bad eating habits Ryan kept spoon feeding me several times in the kitchen when we went for meals.

I would try to drown out the food with my tea by drinking it down like crazy. Rico was usually at the table with me.

One day at the cottage, after being spoon fed against my will for a long time, Rico said, "If you don't start eating right we're going to have to get you an IV! I'm going to make you get an IV if you don't start eating right! What do you think of that? I know you don't want that and don't like that idea! See what you think of that! You're going to be getting an IV! So you better start eating right if you don't want an IV or that's what you're going to get! Take that for size!"

The first few months I was there, every time I smiled Jamie, another patient, would say "Mary Kay!"

Some of the other boys started saying the same thing. Other boys would say, "Oh, goodnight! He has that look on his face again! How stupid?!"

Jamie and a few others would say, "You're so goofy" whenever I tried to say something to be funny. Some boys would act like, "Oh brother. Here we go again. Brian's gone off on his little tangent again. What's he going to come up with this time?"

They also made fun of me for having short legged pants and said, "Why do you have pant legs that stop at the top of your socks? High waters! He's wearing high waters! What's wrong with you? Why don't you get pants the right length? They're supposed to go down to your shoes."

After I was there a few months, they finally got a few nicer staff in there. There was a lady named Jenny that came in that was really nice that I really liked. There was also another lady that came in around the same time as her. As much as I liked the second new lady, I think she was only there two or three times.

After that she was gone. She didn't stay very long and I was really disappointed after she quit working there.

Then, they got a guy named Jed I really liked for a new staff person. After that, they got Denny.

These were our new staff people, which were a big improvement to Ryan, Rico, and Scarlett. Ryan and Rico were still there, but, just not as often.

This lady, Jenny, a chipper acting female staff I liked, was sitting on the couch one day.

Jamie, one of the other boys, caught her sitting on the couch by the window barefooted. She had her shoes and socks on when I first saw her so I think either Jamie took her shoes and socks off or she did herself. Jamie started petting her feet when he caught her barefoot. She really enjoyed it, and he got my attention.

Jamie said, "Try this. I think you'll really like it. This is neat." So then, I pet her bare feet from the top of her feet just above the ankles to her toes. I pet her feet like you would pet a cat on its back. I really liked it. It actually felt similar to what it feels like to pet a cat. I liked the way it felt on my hands, and the lady really enjoyed it. It was really soft and it helped me to calm my nerves. It made her really happy and she acted like she thought I was sweet because I did this for her. The next time I saw her, I couldn't resist. I took her shoes and socks off when she sat on the couch by the window, and started petting the tops of her feet from the top of her feet just above the ankles to her toes. I did this over and over again. Every time I saw this lady I took her shoes and socks off and pet her feet several times, over and over again. I liked the way it felt on my hands because of the softness that helped calm my nerves. It made her feel really happy, because it was like getting a massage, only I was petting her feet like you pet a cat or a dog instead of actually massaging them.

Many times I would sit by Jenny on the couch and lean my head on her shoulder. I was relieved to have her there instead of Scarlet.

One day, Ryan was looking at me from across the room when I sat on the couch with Jenny. When he saw me he kept looking at me like he was trying to find an excuse to make me take my clothes off in front of everyone in the room but was reluctant to do so.

What's funny is, as much as Ryan, the staff member always wanted to make me take my clothes off in front of everybody, and do the shirttail punishment in front of everybody, he was reluctant to do that to me in front of Jenny. He acted like, "I would, but I better not because she might get me in trouble if I do" so he decided not to.

I thought, "Hah! He won't make me take my clothes off in front of her! I'm safe with this lady!" I think he was afraid Jenny would take my side.

Ryan acted like he made sure not to do much of anything around this lady to me he would normally do.

I got the feeling Jenny didn't not approve of the way Ryan, the staff member treated me, and Ryan was afraid if he said or did anything to me he normally would have done to punish me, this lady might turn on him, and get him in trouble, so he made sure to keep it cool when she was around.

Some people I've told this to have said, "That's because she was a woman."

Really?

Ryan didn't care if he made me take my clothes off in front of Kara or Scarlett, and they're ladies, but he didn't dare do this in front of this lady.

I think this lady may have had a talk with him behind my back while I wasn't looking telling him he'd better not mess with me or she was going to get him into trouble. I don't know that for a fact. I just know it's awful funny that he didn't have any trouble making me take my clothes off in front of everybody if Kara or Scarlett were around, but if Jenny was around he looked at her like he was afraid to try anything because he was afraid she'd get him in trouble.

I wonder why? Why her and not Kara or Scarlett?

I think it's because Jenny told him he'd better not mess with me when I wasn't looking to see her talking to him in private or she gave him a look, one. And, the way he acted like, "I'd like to find an excuse to make him take his clothes off in front of everybody to punish him for being different, but I better not" makes me think she gave him the look and he backed off. If you noticed, he looked at me acting like he was thinking it, then looked at her, and then acted like he'd better not. So, I think she let him know someway that if he ever messed with me in front of her that she would turn him in for it.

Jed also tended to take my side on a lot of things. I think Jed believed I was telling the truth about a lot of things Rico tried to call me a liar for, and the same went with Ryan and he sympathized about that. I think he also thought they were a little too hard on the goofy thing. I think he thought I was a little goofy but not as bad as Ryan was making it sound. I told him I thought he was a nice guy.

Jed, the new staff guy said, "Oh man. Why does everybody think I'm nice? I'm not nice. I'm just fair."

Once in a while though, Jed would go along with one of Ryan's crazy ideas because months later he would make a comment like "I think we ought to put you on a roller coaster bare footed to make you better. Then we can kill two birds with one stone. I think that's what you need."

The reason Jed said this is because he thought it was making me a man to make me go on a roller coaster because he knew I was afraid of roller coasters, and he knew it embarrassed me to go bare footed in public. He thought if he made me do both, he'd really make something out of me.

Denny came along, and he always had a feeling something was wrong. He tried to talk to me about things that were bothering me. He even started out believing me about what was going on with the other staff that bothered me.

He used to say, "What's the beef?"

I would tell him, and he would try to make me feel better.

The problem is, one day Ryan, the staff member was commenting things about me to him in front of me, and complaining about certain things, trying to convince Denny that it was all me, that I just needed to get my stuff straight.

From then on, when I told Denny something, he would say, "Well, I don't know. I think it's probably just this….and about that over there…I think it's probably just that…and what I really think is… and I think you just need to get your thinking straight and get your act together because I think your just this……"

This varied from conversation to conversation, but I felt like I was getting the Soap Box treatment every time I talked to him. I couldn't get him to understand me about anything any more. He always wanted to take Ryan's side on everything.

One day, Ryan called me, Jamie, Roland and Derrick out into the lobby, and stood us in the back entry section of the living room between the living room closet and the office. He then made a comment about something, and accused us all of something we never did. I can't remember what it was he accused us of, but it was ridiculous, and he said, "Because these four boys are in trouble for this thing (whatever he was talking about) I'm giving these boys the *shirttail* punishment. Take your clothes off!"

I was like, "What?! We didn't do anything! What is this for?"

Jamie said, "We better do what he says. Come on. Just take them off. I don't know what his problem his but we better not try to do anything. Just do what he says."

Me, and all three of the other boys had to take our clothes off.

This meant we had to take our shirts, pants, shoes and socks off in front of everybody and push them to the side in the floor.

Big City Hospitals Don't Like Cowards   Brian Evans

Then he handed us all a *shirttail* shirt and said, "Put this on."

Ryan, the staff member started giving *shirttail* punishments to everybody on a regular basis, especially me.

He would just say *"Shirttail!"*

At any moment when you didn't expect it he would say this and you had to take your clothes off on the spot. Then he made you put the *shirttail* shirt on.

Every time he did this, I had to run in front of everybody in a *shirttail* shirt and the underwear around my waist only. So did everybody else he ever did this to. I had to stay undressed like this all day long, and everyone got to see me in my underwear, every time he did this. These other boys did too. Ryan acted like it gave him powers kick to do this to everybody because he loved to embarrass the tar out of everybody in front of everybody. I was Ryan's favorite victim to do this to. He did this to me 10 times more often that all the other boys, even when he started to get more carried away with them.

It got to were he would say things to people like Jamie and Sean, "If you don't quit doing this you're going to get the Brian Evans punishment?"

Jamie looks at him questionably and asked, "What's the Brian Evans punishment? I'm afraid to ask?"

He acted like he knew it was another name for the *shirttail* punishment because I had been given the shirt tail punishment so many times that Ryan and Rico started making a nick name out of it and calling it the Brian Evans punishment.

The way they tried to make you take your clothes off in front of everybody every time you did the least little thing they didn't like, they ought to rename this place Wilderness Psychiatric "Take your clothes off" Institute instead of Wilderness Psychiatric Institute or "Wilderness Strip You Naked Institute".

86

One time Rico decided to embarrass me in front of the counselor because he knew he was coming to the Cottage.

He said, "Brian. Take your shoes and socks off." He knew I was embarrassed of my feet so he did this on purpose. He did this several times just to make me feel horribly embarrassed. When Davey, the Counselor came in, Rico said, "Hey Davey! Look! Brian's barefoot!"

He really embarrassed me and I felt completely humiliated because of it. Of course, Rico got a laugh out of the whole thing.

I still have a slight problem with this now but I'm better than I used to be. I've gotten to where sometimes I'll actually get the nerve to show my bare feet to a nurse I'm comfortable with if I think I need to.

I feel weird if everybody sees my feet uncovered because I have a shyness problem and feel like it makes me look goofy to go barefoot in front of people and it still embarrasses me in most instances. I did manage to finally give in without clamming up for a test I had done about a year ago where I was required to go barefoot for the test, but I normally would have been very timid about it.

What's funny is, I get easily embarrassed about my own feet but when it comes to other ladies I'm friends with out there I feel like I'm going to bust if they don't take their shoes and socks off and put on a pair of open toe sandals or flip flips because I feel like I've just got to see their toes because looking at their feet and being able to see their toes is like looking at flowers to me and it drives me crazy when I'm not able to see them. When ladies wear those slip on shoes they tend to wear with no socks on it drives me nuts and I feel like I'm just going to fidget all over the place because I'm just dying to see their toes and wish they would take them off. I wasn't like that till I was 14 years old.

Before that, I couldn't stand to see people's feet and demanded everybody put their shoes back on.

But since Age 14, I can't stand for ladies to wear shoes or socks and I can't stand for their toes to be covered because it drives me crazy when their not uncovered for me to be able to see them. I feel like I've got to be able to see their toes or I'm going to go bananas.

I feel like begging them to take their slip on shoes off or change into a pair of open toe sandals or flip flops one, but I'm afraid if I do they'll get the wrong idea.

I don't really mean anything bad by it at all. I'm just that way because it's just some sort of autistic quirk I have that can't be relieved unless I see their toes uncovered. It makes me feel better when they go ahead and take their slip on shoes off and let me see their toes or put on a pair of flip flops or open toe sandals to wear. They're more pleasant to be around when they do. I already find it pleasing to be around ladies I like when I'm with them but when they remove their shoes and socks and let me see their toes their even more pleasing to be with. I may seem nervous the first few times they do because I want to see their toes so bad I feel like I have to stare intently but after they let me see them a few times I feel like I don't have to struggle to see them as much and it helps me to be able to relax when I see their toes uncovered. It's kind of strange. I wasn't like that before I was 14 years old but I've been that way ever since. You'll see what caused me to be that way a few pages from now. Something would happen to throw me into some kind of shock and I would be this way from then on. You'll see when you got there.

My favorite way for ladies to be is barefoot, and that means with their toes completely exposed as well. I don't mean to make anyone uncomfortable because of this. That's just the way I am and I mean nothing bad by it at all. I'm like a little friendly puppy dog that when it sees a lady go barefoot it thinks, "Oh Goody! Feet!" and runs up to them to go play with their feet because they can't help themselves.

I'm also like a little kid that might think the same thing or do the same thing because it looks neat to them and they just can't help but play with someone's feet or a baby that touches their feet and then giggles because it love's their feet. Every time a lady decides to go barefoot I think, "I want to see! I want to see!" and when I do get to see their feet I think "Alright! They're barefoot!" Their feet are like flowers to me and their toes are like the petals on the flowers.

So, if you're a lady that likes to go barefoot in slip on shoes, please have mercy on me and take them off and put on a pair of open toe sandals or flip flops. Thank you. I apologize if this makes anyone uncomfortable. It just drives me crazy and I need to be able to see your toes as often as possible.

Most of my lady friends already go barefoot 90 percent of the time anyway and the ones that know I'm like this don't really care because they know I don't mean anything by it. And if you're someone that would like to make fun of me for this, please don't embarrass me. Thanks. Anyway, back to the story.

One day I went to school my English teacher sent a tube of tooth paste and a toothbrush home with me, like they did all the other students, while I was living at this institute. Not knowing what to do with the toothpaste and toothbrush I just put it in the drawer of my dresser in my bedroom.

When Ryan, the staff member found out I put it in my drawer he said, "Destruction! 200 points!" He made me clean the bathrooms, dust the furniture, and scrub the floors. He even made gave me an old, worn out toothbrush and made me scrub the bathtub and the walls the regular way with towels and cleaning agents and maybe scrubbers. He was real technical with it to make it really hard. Plus don't forget I was only four foot seven inches tall when he made me do this.

The showerhead was high above my head and hard to reach because I was short. I was also skinny as a rail and only 90 pounds.

The following April I had a growth spurt and reached a height of 5 foot 1 inch but that was a few months away.

School had just started when this incident occurred. I was in this institution at the same point in time as I went to the 7th grade. It was the best school year I ever had.

 In 4th, 5th, and 6th grades they had me in half Regular classes and half Special Ed classes.

In the 7th grade I was in all Special Ed classes. My all Special Ed classes school year was the most wonderful year I ever had at school.

 I had a wonderful Special Ed English teacher and my ex-girlfriend that I went with at school was at the same time I lived at the institution. I loved all my teachers and classes and peers that year considering they were all Special Ed people. That year school was my refuge. While I lived in this horrible institution I would get an escape from it by going to school every time I went there.
This was highly unusual because before this I always hated school, but this year I loved school. The institution I was in was so horrible it felt like the school was a paradise.

I actually told both my special Ed English teacher and my ex-girlfriend I had in her class that these people were giving me these *shirttail* punishments.

They made me take my clothes off in front of everybody in the cottage I lived in on a consistent basis to punish me for being different. They did this to embarrass me and accuse me of things that were not true. They both thought it was terrible but did not know what to do. All they could do was encourage me when they saw me at school.

In April, my ex-girlfriend in the 7th grade told me her mother said she was going to send her to live with an aunt in Oklahoma City. I fretted for a while over it, and she comforted me.

One day I called her house from the institute and her stepmother said she wasn't there.

I went back to class the next day and she said, "I was there, but they wouldn't let me talk to you. They lied to you. I really was there."

Since that, I did not trust her family to tell the truth about anything.

However I began to think, *"Oh, she's not going anywhere, because she never said anything else about it."*
That June, I met her at the Rose Park Swimming Pool, and then again at Skate Ways skating rink. The last time I saw her I thought her mother was upset with me.

Then when I saw her at the skating rink she said, "This is my mother."

I was shocked, because I thought, *"Wow! Her mother's really nice! She must have changed her mind about me!"*
My ex-girlfriend skated the night away with me in excitement, and taught me how to skate and keep my balance.

After that night, I thought surely I would see her again but I never did. The next time we went to Skate Ways skating rink it hit me what my girlfriend said about going to live with an aunt in Oklahoma City.

I suddenly panicked, and thought, *"No! She's gone!"*

It wouldn't be till years later that I found out the woman my girlfriend was with was not the mother she was referring to not liking me. That was her real mother who did like me that I saw at the skating rink, not the one causing all the trouble.

Her stepmother was the one who didn't like me, and that was who was giving us all the problems all this time.

She didn't tell me it was her stepmother that didn't like me. It would have made sense if she would have told me that before.

I kept trying to call the girl and her family said, "She's not here! She doesn't live here!"

Rico latched on to this and said, "She don't want you anymore!"

I said, "That's not true! Her family is lying!"

That second time at the skating rink, Rico and Ryan complained about my rolling my tongue in my mouth from side to side, and said I looked retarded.

Then he pointed out another girl, and it was even someone I would have liked, but I said, "No! I don't want another girl! I want my girlfriend back!"

Then this Mexican bully got behind me when I finally decided to go back out and skate and tried to push me into a girl, and I had trouble keeping my balance because of it. Rico then accused me of pushing another girl.

I said, "That's not true! I didn't push that girl! This Mexican guy got behind me and he tried to push me into her!"

I remember running into a couple more bullies on the way out. When I left we tried to find my shoes and I couldn't find them. Someone I told I couldn't find them thought they were stolen.

Rico and some of the other patients, like Kyle and Wayne, and Roland and Jamie said, "Thanks to Brian, we can't go back to the skating rink because we've been kicked out of there for a month!"

I told them, "It's not my fault! I'm telling you, I didn't push that girl. A Mexican guy got behind me and he tried to push me into her. I didn't do anything."

We went back to the Cottage at the Institute, and Rico got us apples and milk. He kept trying to get me to admit that I pushed that girl, when I did not.

A little bit later Rico took me in his office and said, "You pushed that girl at the skating rink. Now thanks to you we can't go back for a month."

I said, "I'm telling you I didn't do it. This Mexican got behind me and tried to push me into her. I had nothing to do with it. It's not my fault!"

He said, "You're lying."

I said, "No, I'm not lying."

Rico said, "Come on Brian. You lie even when you don't have to lie. Admit it. You did it."

I said, "I'm telling you I didn't do it!"

This went on and on and on. He did everything he could to twist my words around until he could get me to admit to something I never did wrong.

Another time, we were out playing flag football and I think it was starting to get dark and Davey tried to scare me and make me think the demons were after me.

Several times before and after the skating rink incident Wayne would stick his finger in my chest and say "You!"

He would accuse me of things that weren't true or try to twist things around I said to make it what he thought I said so he could complain about something.

Kyle kept giving me problems as usual at the institute off and on. In several different instances, the kids in the back room tried to scare me at night time.

They said the demons were coming after me to get me and that I was going to Hell. They chased me around the South Wing Building in the dark once and tried to scare me.

Rico was trying to get us to watch more movies like Psycho, Halloween, and Friday the 13th again. This is also about when Jed came up with the comment about the roller coaster thing I told you earlier. Denny was giving me trouble all over the place and kept griping at me. Rico and Ryan, the two staff members were acting like I was going to be there a long time again.

Before the summer I had written my girlfriend a note. I asked her to take me out of there and take me to her place but I changed my mind and threw it in the trash. Rico took it out of the trash and complained about it.

He said, "Are you trying to make an escape? You really think you can get out of here?"

Now my girlfriend was not there anymore. I couldn't get a hold of her or find her either one. My favorite staff member Jane had left and no longer worked there. The other lady I liked also quit long before Jenny left so she wasn't there anymore either. Ryan and Rico were there more often again. Scarlet; the staff member even came back again.

Now Jenny was not there to stop Ryan from making me take my clothes off in front of everybody anymore and he had free reign over me again as well as Rico and Scarlet.

Ryan would still do this during the time Jenny was there if she was not working a certain day, but if she was he refrained from doing this to me because he was afraid Jane would get me in trouble.

94

Scarlet was bragging, "I was in the army and I'm tough and I'm not going to put up with anything. So if anybody causes any trouble I'm going to make their life miserable. I've been in the army, and I know how they handle things, and I can be just like them if you don't cooperate with me, so you'd best not mess with me! I'm not taking any flack from anybody! So, if anybody has anything to say to me they'd better watch their step!"

It was shortly after the incident when Jed made the comment about the roller coaster which I wound up riding again a second year in a row, thanks to Ryan and Rico.

It was more Rico's idea that they force me to ride them than Ryan's but both of these men got a kick out of it again, as usual.

When we went to Possum Kingdom one time an older boy from the South Wing named Jake tried to commit a homosexual act with me, and I told on him. Jake found out and threatened me.

He said, "You better not be telling anybody I did this if you know what was good for you! I have a certain kind of knife I can use on you if you give me any more trouble, so if you know what's best for you, you'd better not mess with me!"

After I told Rico what this boy did he made me apologize to him outside. Jake was standing next to Bobby, and Rico insisted that Bobby did it and not Jake.

I said, "No! That's not true! Bobby didn't do it! Jake did!"

Rico was getting really hostile about it and said, "You need to apologize to Jake now! You know Bobby did it! You're just sticking up for him! You can't tell me that Jake did this! I demand that you apologize to Jake now!"

I couldn't believe a staff member of the institution, who was supposed to protect me was taking up for the guy that did it and demanding I say that it was the guy standing next to him that did it instead of him. The whole thing was really ridiculous. I thought the whole thing was absurd.

Rico kept saying, "You can't tell me Bobby didn't do this. Why didn't you apologize to that boy? You know Bobby did it!"

I said, "It wasn't Bobby. It was Jake. I'm telling the truth!"

Rico said, "You're lying! You can't tell me that Jake did this. You know as well as I do that Bobby did it! Now you go back and tell Jake you're sorry!"

I kept saying, "No!"

Rico kept saying, "Why?"

I said, "Because it was Jake that did it, not Bobby!"

Rico said, "You're lying!"

I said, "I'm telling the truth! Jake did it! Not Bobby!"

Rico said, "You're going to have to do something about you're attitude! You lie about things even when you don't have to lie! We're going to have to do something about your stubbornness! I'm not going to keep putting up with this type of thing, so you'd better get your act straight! We'll see what comes of this when I'm done with you! I can't believe you didn't apologize to that boy! You're in real hot water now! You'd better watch your step or I'm really going to get you back! So watch it!"

Everything was getting really terrible, and I had no one to turn to and no where to go. I felt trapped.

I was out in the field one day and I thought, "There's only one way out of this mess. God! God can get me out of here!"

96

I immediately asked my mother to take me to the associate pastor
at our church to tell me how to get saved.

The associate pastor showed me Revelation 3:20 and said,
"Behold, I stand at the door and knock. If any man opens the door
I will sup with him and he will sup with me."

He told me if I confessed my sins to God and believed that Jesus
died on the cross for me and asked him to come into my heart I
would be saved.

I was amazed after this! All of a sudden I was sane! I was in my
right mind! I wasn't wild anymore!

Because my mother wanted to make sure I was really saved first
before she took me out of the institution, she left me in to be sure.
She wanted to see if I could get a blood test first.
I was able to get one but it was not easy. She also wanted me to go
to the dentist and handle having my teeth drilled too.

I now had a new dentist, Dr. Baca and thankfully we found out he
gave the gas to his patients before he drilled. When he gave me
the gas first it worked out well and I was fine. My mother still left
me in the institution just a little bit longer after that but was getting
close to taking me out. She knew it was not my tendency to lie and
when these two men, Rico and Ryan were continually accusing me
of lying, that they were either making it up or they were teaching
me to lie, one of the two, because it was not my tendency to lie.

Because of this, she wanted to take me out right there. She wanted
to be sure I was really saved so waited to see if there was still a
change in my behavior before she took me out.

I kept telling Rico and the others "My mother is going to discharge
me."

Rico kept saying, "You'll be back in six months!"

That July, one month after Jenny left, Ryan actually took the cottage boys to my church. This was the first time I was out where there were other people I know I like around in the public at my church where Ryan and Rico took me.

The youth were having a movie in the gym upstairs. I did not even know what was about to happen or how I was going to feel when I opened the door to the gym that day. I was just glad to be there. When I opened the door, I suddenly saw the first girl at the bottom of the stairs I liked wearing open toe sandals and got excited and thought, "Alright Feet!" I had never felt this way about anybody's feet before except for Jenny's feet at the institution. I suddenly felt like I was desperate to see the feet and toes of every girl in sight I could and I didn't even know why I felt that way or why this was urgent to me all of a sudden. It was never urgent to me before.

Before I met Jenny, I always demanded ladies and girls put their shoes back on when they uncovered their feet and left them bare.

Now I suddenly felt like I desperately had to see their feet and their toes or I was going to bust. I felt like I needed to be able to see the feet and toes of every lady and girl I possibly could and it was urgent I got to see their feet and their toes. This had never happened to me before and I couldn't figure out why this was so urgent to me all of a sudden. I didn't even know why it was so urgent all of a sudden that I got to see their feet and their toes but it was. I couldn't figure out what was going on. It was very rare for these guys to take anyone to church too.

I actually walked up stairs in the gym urgently trying to see the feet and the toes of the first girl I saw wearing sandals. Then, I skipped up the stairs to the next girl gazing down at her feet and toes. Then, I skipped the rest of the way up the stairs and saw another girl in open toe sandals and gazed down at her feet and toes. Then I skipped around the upstairs entry, turning the corner into the room where the movie would be desperate to see which other girls were showing their feet and their toes.

I was overjoyed when I found to my amazement that several of the girls seated to watch the movie were wearing open toe sandals and I got to see all their feet and toes and felt relieved.

This had never happened to me ever before. As a matter of fact, I didn't even go in there hoping to see girls in their bare feet when I first walked in the door. It wasn't until I spotted the very first girl in her bare feet on the stair case that I got excited and felt like I had to dash up the stairs from one girl to the next to see who was barefooted and who wasn't. It was just an automatic reaction I had to being able to see a girl in their bare feet that I never had before. This never mattered to me before this. But for some reason, on this day, it was urgent I got to see every girl's feet and toes. When I did, I was incredibly relieved. I felt like I was about to rejoice and celebrate.

It was like consciously I was thinking, "Alright! Feet!" but subconsciously I was thinking "They'll protect me! Ryan won't get me when their around!" That's the way I felt. My emotions had now gone from "Scat your feet!" to "Please! I've got to see your toes! It's driving me crazy!"

So, from that day forward, I had to see every lady's and girl's feet and toes or I was going to bust and this has been a problem since.

I think what happened is, was, Jenny was my "protection" against Ryan. Jenny has now left the institution. The "protection" is now gone.

Now, these girls I was desperate to see the feet and toes of became my "protection" against Ryan because I did not leave the institution till the following October.

At that stage in my life, the girls always had to protect me from the boys and the men. My female peers and female teachers constantly had to protect me in school from other boys and male teachers all throughout my Elementary and Junior High School years. I was also short for my age.

I was only 14 years old and I was only 5'1" on the day this happened. When I went into the institution at 13 I was only 4'7".

I didn't even reach 5'3" till several months later when I turned 15 in March of the following year.

What has had me confused all these years is, I got to see Jenny beginning in April of 1983 when I petted her feet and my ex-girlfriend was still around for a couple more months before she disappeared and there were still two months of school left where I got to see all kinds of girls in class so why did it not bother me when I didn't get to see my ex-girlfriend's feet and toes or any of my female classmates' feet and toes when they all wore shoes and socks at school?

You would have thought this urge for me to see every girl's feet and toes would have started then but it didn't.
I never got to see my ex-girl friend wear open toe sandals or any of the other female classmates wear sandals. All of them wore tennis shoes and socks every time I saw them. No one ever wore sandals or showed their toes in class. They always wore shoes and socks.

Even more strange, I actually got to see my ex-girlfriend's feet and toes at Rose Park Swimming Pool in June 1983 when we went swimming together.

Why did I not feel like I had to stare intently at her feet and toes then?

I liked her feet and her toes and thought they were very pretty but I didn't feel like I was going to just bust if I didn't see them.

I even saw my ex-girlfriend again at Skateways Skating Rink before she disappeared and she was wearing tennis shoes and socks again then and it didn't bother me that I didn't get to see her feet and her toes after I saw her feet and her toes the week before.

I didn't feel like I was going to just bust if I didn't see my girl friend take her shoes and socks off again and see her toes.

100

It wasn't going to bother me then if I didn't get to see them again and I liked what they looked like and even thought they were pretty.

Why did it not bother me when I saw my ex-girlfriend that I didn't get to see her feet and her toes when I saw her at the Skating Rink after seeing her feet and toes uncovered at Rose Park Swimming Pool the week before and even liking what they looked like and thinking they were pretty?

The next time I went there my ex-girlfriend was gone. Now my ex-girlfriend would be lost forever and be nowhere to find.

Then, two weeks later, Jenny, the lady I petted the feet of, left the institution.

All this had me confused until I remembered this true story of what happened when I went to the gym at the church Ryan and Rico took me to the following July. I always remembered the part about seeing the movie I saw and what it entailed but I had forgotten about this scenario with feeling like it was urgent I got to see the feet and toes of every girl I saw on the stair case in the gym after seeing the first girl at the bottom of the stair case in open toe sandals and when I remembered this happened and realized this was the first time I ever had this problem because it had never been urgent for me to see the feet and toes of every girl I ever saw before this day this happened, then, it hit me. So, this is what caused me to be like this.

It took me decades to figure out what caused me to be this way myself and I just figured it out last September.

When I suddenly realized all this and put all this together I came to the following conclusion:

I think I was "traumatically shocked" into being this way, because get this, before I met this lady, I demanded that every girl or lady I saw barefoot put their shoes back on and cover their feet and now I feel like I have to beg every girl and lady to take their shoes and socks off and let me see their feet and their toes. Strange isn't it? I think this is what caused this to happen. It's almost like "the barefooted lady saved the day".

So, if you're someone who likes to go barefoot in flip flops or sandals and you see me staring at your feet, please do not be alarmed. I just like to be able to see every lady's feet and toes I can because they look like pretty flowers to me. I mean nothing amiss by this.

And, if you are someone who likes to go barefoot but wears closed toe shoes, don't be surprised if I look at you nervously, looking down at your feet longingly acting like something is wrong.

When I do this it is because I like ladies' feet and I want to be able to see your toes and you are hiding your toes causing me not to be able to see what looks like the petals of the flowers. I'm like a kid in a candy store that thinks, "I want to see! I want to see!"

So, please don't see me as an adult male acting like this but as a child in a man's body acting like this. And if I ever ask to see please do not scold me for this because in reality it is a child inside of a man's body that is thinking this and acting this way. So please do not be offended by this. It is just my autism. My friends already know I'm this way. I just wanted my nurses to know this too so they would know what was going on.

Seeing a ladies' feet without being able to see their toes is like not being able to see the petals of the flowers in a flower garden, the blooms that make the flowers pretty.

Their feet are like flowers to me and their toes are like the petals on the flowers, the blooms on the flowers that make the flowers pretty.

Without being able to see their toes it's like seeing the stem of the flowers without the petals or the blooms that make them pretty.

When I get to see their toes then I get to see the part that makes their feet pretty to look at.

I'm kind of like Rain man is with his camera when I look at ladies feet.

If you notice, Rain man nervously takes his camera when he is in the car with his brother and points the think out the window taking pictures of everything in sight like he can't get enough pictures of what he sees and doesn't want to miss anything.

I feel like I've got to look and look and look and stare at a ladies' feet and toes as much as I can so I can get relief from not having been able to see their toes when I do see them so I can relax. For some reason, it's incredibly urgent I get to see their toes and this is actually an automatic reaction with me just as it is with Rain man and his camera.

Now, being able to see a ladies' feet with their toes uncovered is like my being able to have bright colors on the walls or have the furniture a certain way or have pretty trinkets all over my coffee table and shelves throughout the house and being able to have pretty stuff I like all over the walls to make me feel boxed in so I don't feel agoraphobic.

I have the same reaction to being able to see their feet as I do to being able to have the walls a certain color, have the furniture arranged a certain way, or have the house decorated for Christmas with trinkets all over the house and a decorated Christmas tree next to the couch.

Ladies feet are like flowers to me and being able to see them is almost like being able to see another pretty ornament on a Christmas tree I put up.

It's really strange, but it's just an additional autistic quirk I have with a nervous thing behind it where it drives me nuts not to be able to see their toes, just like it drives me nuts not to have the furniture arranged a certain way, or the walls a certain color, or the house decorated for Christmas.

Not being able to have all this stuff this way makes me a nervous wreck. And, for some reason, I'm the same way with not being able to see a lady's toes. That makes me a nervous wreck too.

If I don't get to see their toes I feel like it makes me a nervous wreck, but when they remove their shoes and socks and let me see their toes then I feel relieved. It's really strange but it's true and it's not my fault. I'm just that way. I mean no harm at all by any of it. I'm just that way because of my Autism and it's just a nervous thing I struggle with all the time. That's just the way it is. It's not anything against anybody else. I'm just that way because of my Autism.

Anyway back to the story.

After I got upstairs and sat down to watch the movie they were having, there was a guy on this movie that was asked to give up rock music by his pastor. In this movie, the guy thought his pastor was crazy but gave in anyway.

At the end of the week, after struggling with the whole thing, the boy went up in front of the church on the movie, and said, "I want everybody to know that rock music is wrong and I hereby give up rock music!"

He took the record at the pulpit and broke it and said, "I'm not going to listen to this stuff anymore and I'm not going to let anyone else listen to it either!"

I felt convicted at that moment and immediately decided to give up rock music. When I got back to the institute and told the other boys what I did. I was now against rock music, they all got mad.

I was in the living room area of the cottage and they were making fun of me.

Davey, another patient, grabbed my arm and raised it in the air saying, "Let's lift up our hands in praises to God! I want to Rock!"

Some of the boys in the back room tried to scare me again and told me I was going to Hell because the demons were coming to get me.

I was panicking saying, "No, no! They can't!"

Other than that I was doing a whole lot better regardless of what was happening around me and the people in the counselor's office there were really impressed.

I went to the counselor's office and they said, "You seem to be doing really well now! Do you think we are helping you?"

I said, "No! I think it was God that helped me! No one did anything! God is the one that made me better!"

The counselor then said, "Well, I guess there's nothing more we can do for you, then!"

He acted like I was a hopeless cause.

On October 24, 1983 my mother discharged me from the Institute after putting me in there on June 1, 1982.

The staff did not let me go and were not about to let me go.

My mother took me out herself because she was the one that put me in there so she got to take me out whenever she pleased. She discharged me herself on October 24, 1983 four months after I was saved.

This institution currently has a "D" rating with the Better Business Bureau.

Although the name I gave this place is fictional, the real name of this institution is similar to the fake name I gave it.
Plus this institution has changed names and hands since I was there. At the time I was there it was only a rehab center/nursing home for mentally disturbed boys who had general emotional problems including things like fighting, back talking, etc.

The new institution at the same facility with a different name is now an inpatient drug rehab. I have also seen the reviews of their patients about this facility and they are downright horrible.

The staff members at this institution seem to have moved from using fear and humiliation to straighten out their clients, as they claim, to using violence and bickering, and even more controlling. This facility should be shut down for doing what it is doing to its current set of patients. I have not been there for years, nor am I in there now. I am only speaking on behalf of those who are currently in there in their dealings with the staff that work there now, those who went there when I was there, and on behalf of myself for the time I spent there from June 1, 1982 to October 24, 1983.

All other chapters in this book are about "medical hospital facilities and doctors offices". Please note that. This is the only chapter about a mental health facility. All other chapters in this book are about "medical facilities where everyone in the public receives "physical medical care".

Some people take one thing I say and run with it and assume that every chapter in the book is about a mental institution just because one chapter, Chapter 3 is about a mental institution.

This is the "only" chapter about a mental institution in the whole book.

I repeat, "All other chapters in this book are at a "medical facility", not a psychiatric ward.

106

When you consider the trouble I had with *male*s and serious trended females at this institution as well as all the trouble I had with *male* nurses and serious trended female nurses at the military hospital, and one more thing not even covered at this point, the fact that I always got jumped by other boys in Elementary and Junior High school, and *male* teachers treated me like dirt, and kicked me around like a dog, just like the boys did.

Put all this together, and you can see why I would never want a *male* nurse, or therapist, ever again, after seeing what happened in all of these above mentioned situations where I was persecuted, humiliated, and condemned by all *male* figures in almost every setting of my life.

We're talking *male* nurses in the Medical Field, *male* nurses in the Mental Health Field, *male* teachers in school that were domineering, and hateful boys that wanted to pick fights and jump me all the time.

Why would I want a *male* anything in a hospital setting after this?

So when you read about the Speech Pathology Department incident in the chapter about the Director who got the wrong idea, and thought I was after the women because I asked for a *female* therapist, and not a *male*, remember what you read here in the past two chapters, and it will make you see just why I would make such a request. I never want a *male* nurse ever again.

I insist that only happy go lucky *female* nurses be my nurses in every place.

That includes the doctor's office, hospital – every department, nursing home (if it ever takes place), home health, physical therapy, speech therapy, cardiac rehabilitation or any other rehabilitation, surgery center, any of it, happy go lucky *bubbly acting female*s only.

These happy go lucky, chipper acting, cheery female nurses also need to be willing to give me hugs, and rub my head to calm me down and hold my hand through all needle sticks and invasive procedures.

That includes any IVs, shots, blood tests, biopsies, tube insertions, catheter insertions, blades, scalpels or anything else scary and I need to be completely put to sleep for all invasive procedures as well as any catheter insertions (heart or urinary).

You give me these people and meet my list of needs and we are good to go.

If any one every refrains from any of these and gives me a male nurse, serious trended female nurse, or refuses to put me to sleep for invasive procedures, or doesn't give me chipper acting female nurses willing to meet my childlike needs or they themselves refuse to do this for me and I will not be sticking around, so please meet my list of needs and all will be well.

Please do not refuse to meet my needs because you read these stories and others to come about being "forcibly stripped of all my clothes" to force my cooperation by "serious trended female nurses". They did it, not the chipper ones, and I am not telling inappropriate stories about nakedness to make you have to think about naked people.

If you think I am making this up, ask my mother. She knows because she was there when it happened. I will not allow nurses to refuse to meet my needs because they think I told inappropriate stories about naked people in this book.

I only told these stories to stress how horrible the "male doctors and nurses" and "serious trended female nurses" treated me.

If you refuse to meet my needs because of this, I will not stick around.

I want "chipper acting, cheery female nurses" only. I want hugs from all of them.

I want them to rub my head to calm me down and hold my hand during needle sticks. I want to be able to put Lidocaine/Prilocaine 2.5% cream on 1 hour before the needle stick. And, I need knocked out completely for all invasive procedures. You do this, and we're good. You don't do this and there's no deal.

Please read the rest of this book as you will see the further persecutions I faced from Junior High through High School at the military hospital, and the persecutions I faced from any "serious trended female nurse" at all other medical facilities I ever went to in my lifetime afterwards all the way to the present time. The "chipper acting, cheery female nurses" were always nice to me, always hugged me, always comforted me, and always rubbed my head to calm me down and held my hand through needle sticks. And that's the way I plan to have it now, forever, from now on. No one else. No other way. "Chipper acting female nurses" only comforting me in the way I need comforted and not another way they come up with themselves.

My needs are my needs and they are genuine legitimate needs.

I have a need to have all this done this way and this is what I am comfortable with and this is what I need you to do.

Nothing else will work.

You will do it my way or not at all.

You don't and I won't be sticking around. Thank you.

Please continue to read this book and discover the lifetime nightmares I faced with "male doctors and nurses" and "serious trended female nurses" and the good experiences I had with the "chipper acting female nurses" that made things better. The remainder of this book begins on the next page and goes all the way to the end at the back cover.

Chapter Four
New Dentist That Caters to Cowards

After my mother sent me to the Institution when I was 13 years old, she was looking for a better dentist that would give me the gas. Before I got out of the institution one of the things she wanted me to do was to be able to go to the dentist office without having a fit. When I got there we were shocked to find out that this dentist gave the gas and we were relieved.

He had a sign in his office that said, "We Cater to Cowards." And I was really happy about it and really liked the people there.

I got this really friendly lady for a Dental Assistant to help keep me calm while my new dentist did his procedure on me. They finally did the gas after he was through checking in my mouth with an instrument for cavities and stuff and looking for the tooth he needed to fix and x-rayed it. From this point on, I had many wonderful dental experiences because the lady hygienists were always nice to me and always gave me the gas to numb my mouth before the dentist drilled.

I was really happy I found these people and everything was wonderful at the dentist's office from that point on.

Chapter Five
Male Nurses at Tragedy AFB Hospital in Texas
Part II
Nightmare at Tragedy AFB Hospital Continues

One time in the 8th grade, two bullies had rammed my head into a brick wall. I had to go to the Emergency Room. The doctor saw me in a private room around the corner from the Emergency Room. He acted like he did not care a thing about my pain. My mother tried to get him to be easy with me because I was scared of needles and oversensitive to pain.

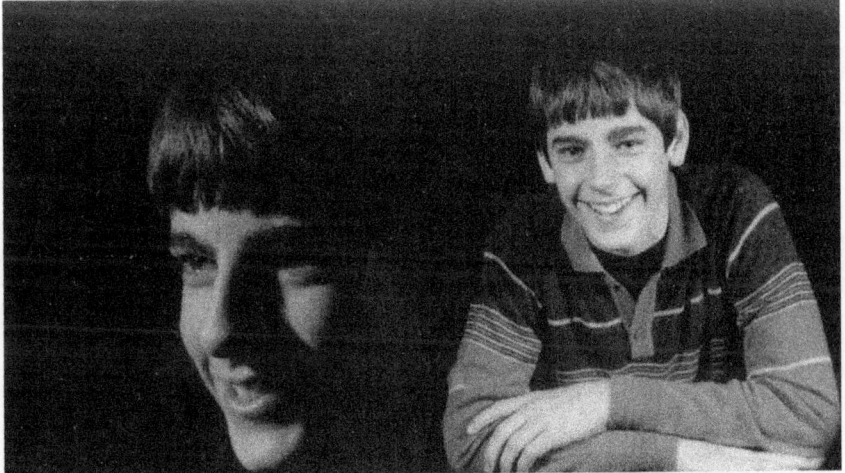

As he proceeded to get his injection to stick it in my wound in my head he told my mother, "Well he's going to have to bite the bullet! I can't have him giving me any trouble! He's just going to have to take it like a man!"

Then he immediately put in stitches! If the shot was some sort of anesthetic he didn't even wait for it to work so it was of no use. Of course I screamed because not only was I scared to death but it hurt!

He complained, "Do we have a baby in here! I think we have a baby in here! What a baby! Come on you, cooperate with me! You need to take it like a man! Don't be giving me any trouble! You're just nothing but a big baby! What a cry baby!"
My mother could not believe his unsympathetic attitude.

In the eleventh grade, I did fine with a TB Tine Test but then when I was asked to do a Tetanus shot. I was so afraid I backed out. My Dad got upset about this when he found out, and my mother decided to try again the next day. She took me up there, and some guy lined up about five different happy go lucky ladies that looked around 30 years of age. I was about 17 years old at the time.

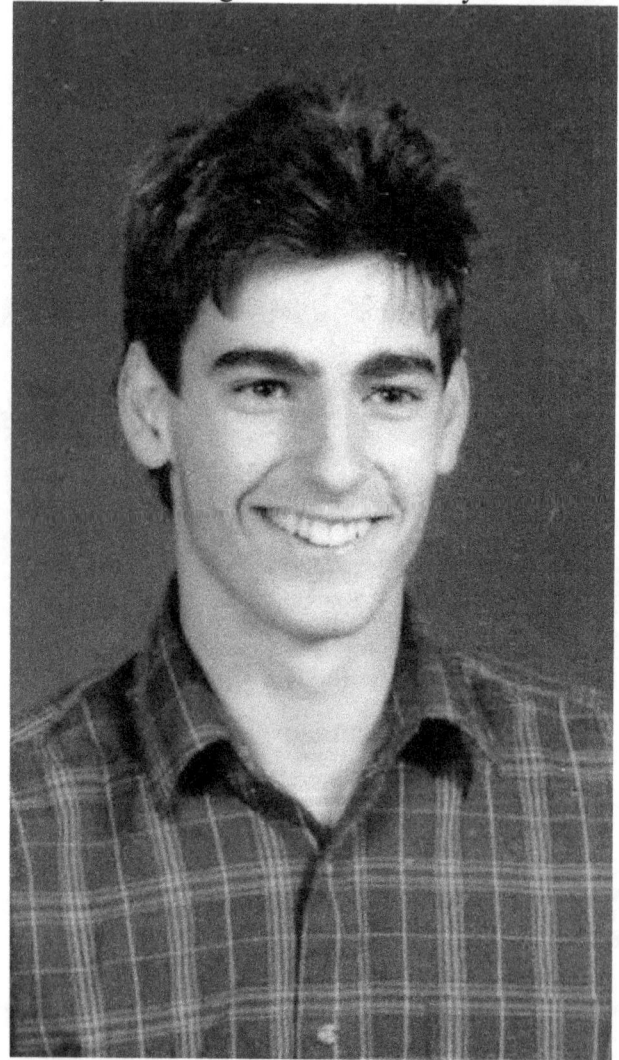

They said, "I have all these ladies right here that can do your Tetanus shot. You just tell me which one you want and I'll give you whoever you want."

I looked and looked at all of them, not able to decide who I wanted, and thought, *"I like them all!"*

I looked and looked again, and scanned them all over, and finally chose one and said, "That one! I'll do it for her!"

The guy said, "Okay then, if you want that one then that's who you'll get. Will you do it for her?"

I said, "Yes."

I got hesitant because I was scared and nearly backed out.

Then I asked, "Can you do it in the hip? I'm scared of having it done in the arm. It really hurts."

The lady said, "Sure. We can do that. No problem!"

I managed to get the shot, and made the school and my mother happy. This was still not the last thing, even more things transpired later as you will see in another chapter.

Chapter Six
Septoplasty at an ENT Office
And
The Ladies that Helped Me with My Fear of Needles

One time I was out applying for manual labor jobs and tried to get a job as a Pharmacy Clerk at a tiny grocery store in town down the block from where I lived.

The lady that was over the pharmacy clerks told me, "If you will take a Pharmacology Class and a Computer Business One class I will give you a job."

So I went to the junior college in town and took these two classes just in order to get this cashier job I wanted in the pharmacy. When I went to this college to take my Pharmacology class, Christy and Janet were very impressed.

They asked, "Are you going to major in Medical Assisting?"

I said, "Oh, no. I'm not about to major in Medical Assisting. I have a fear of needles."

They said, "But you're so good at this. Please. We'll make a deal with you. If you take a major in Medical Assisting we will help you with your fear of needles. There are only two classes that require the students to stick each other with needles and everything else is clerical. You can be a clerical Medical Assistant or a Clinical Medical Assistant. Will you do it for us? If you agree to take a major in Medical Assisting we'll give you shot therapy. It will be okay. I think you should. You're really good. Is it a deal?"

I said, "Yes."

So I majored in it and made A's and B's in almost everything. I made an A in Medical Terminology.

We had to take suffixes and prefixes and be able to memorize them, spell them, pronounce them, and tact them together into bigger words. My teacher, Velvet Schrader and my classmates were really impressed. Judy Parson taught my Medical Transcription class. She was my favorite teacher. I did well on most of my medical transcription assignments when the doctor spoke well. I made a B in her class. She did everything she could to help me get a job. She got me a temporary job at the Apple Hospital for a month.

Four years later I got to work there again for a year. I did well in my Computer/Business I class. The times I did get stuck my teacher was really helpful to me. I took Anatomy and Physiology with Bonny Dobson who also taught my Pharmacology class. I was very good at naming the body parts, and learning their structure and function and made a B. Marilyn Francis was my Medical Administrative teacher and was very nice to me. I also had instances in her class where I would get stumped over silly things. She helped me when I got stuck and got me back on track. This is the lady that told her students that if a patient came to them that they had to do whatever they asked them to do in order to comfort them through a needle stick.

During the semester she kept noticing I had nose bleeds that started out of nowhere. I always had trouble getting them stopped. I couldn't figure out what was going on. I had this same problem when I was a kid. It hadn't happened since. Now it was starting all over again.

She came to me several times and said, "Do you have this problem very often? Does this happen a lot?"

I told her, "It used to happen a lot when I was a kid, but then it stopped. Now it started again."

One day she said, "I'm really concerned. I think you need to check this out. You know Christy and Janet don't you?"

I said, "Yes."

She said, "And they've always been really nice to you too, right."

I admitted, "Yes."

She said, "I think they can help you. It just so happens that Christy and Janet work for an ENT named Dr. Coffee. I really think you need to go to him and they can help you because they work for him. If you make an appointment to see him I'm sure they'll be there for you and they can help you. I really think you need to be seen. This is really concerning. I want you to be okay. So make an appointment with Dr. Coffee if you can and they can help you because they know you and they understand."

So I made an appointment with Dr. Coffee as she asked. He found out I had a deviated septum and decided to do a Septoplasty surgery at his office and cauterize the bleeding while he was at it.

Christy said, "We can do the IV awake if you think you can do it because you're doing really well lately but if you think you won't be able to handle it we can give you the gas first. We can put the IV in right before you fall asleep and you won't feel the pain. You'll just feel the pressure, whatever you decide."

 I said, "Well, I'd almost be tempted to try it since you guys got me to do so well but I think I'd probably better let you do the gas first. I don't think I can handle it."

She said, "Okay. We can do that. If you change your mind you let us know."

I went with the gas first.

She said, "You'll have to wear a hospital gown and you may feel a little naked. We don't normally let people wear their socks but you can wear them if you want."

I said, "I guess I'll wear them."

I was embarrassed. I almost went without my socks because I knew that's what they wanted but I feared I'd get even more embarrassed so I kept them on.

I was pleased they were willing to help me with the IV. They helped with the procedure after I was put to sleep. They gave me the gas first before the IV and they still stuck the IV in before I feel asleep. I felt a great pressure from the IV that almost felt painful. I could feel the intense pressure of the IV more than the actual normal pain because I had already been well numbed out with the gas a few minutes before they even stuck it in. I grunted and almost jumped. I was glad I decided to do the gas first instead of the IV. If I would have felt that IV like I felt the pressure of them sticking me with it, I would have screamed to high heaven. The whole place would have heard me because it would have hurt so badly it would have been absolutely excruciating. Those things are sharp and hard. An IV to me feels like having a butcher knife stuck in me, especially a standard sized IV like the one they used. I was so glad I decided to do the gas first when I felt that. I don't think I would have been able to handle it. I started daydreaming about things a little. I looked around at Christy and Janet feeling pleased about how sweet they were being to me. Then I fell asleep. They said I did well. I was really happy with the way it went.

It was very rare back then to have that wonderful experience at a doctor's office, especially for a surgery, but this guy was nice and so were these two nurse ladies I liked. It was very nice.

Chapter Seven
Male Nurses at Tragedy AFB Hospital in Texas
Part III
Nightmare Experience at Tragedy AFB Strikes Again

The last time I went to this hospital that I saw in my records was at age 21. I believe that is when I had my very last visit as a patient there.

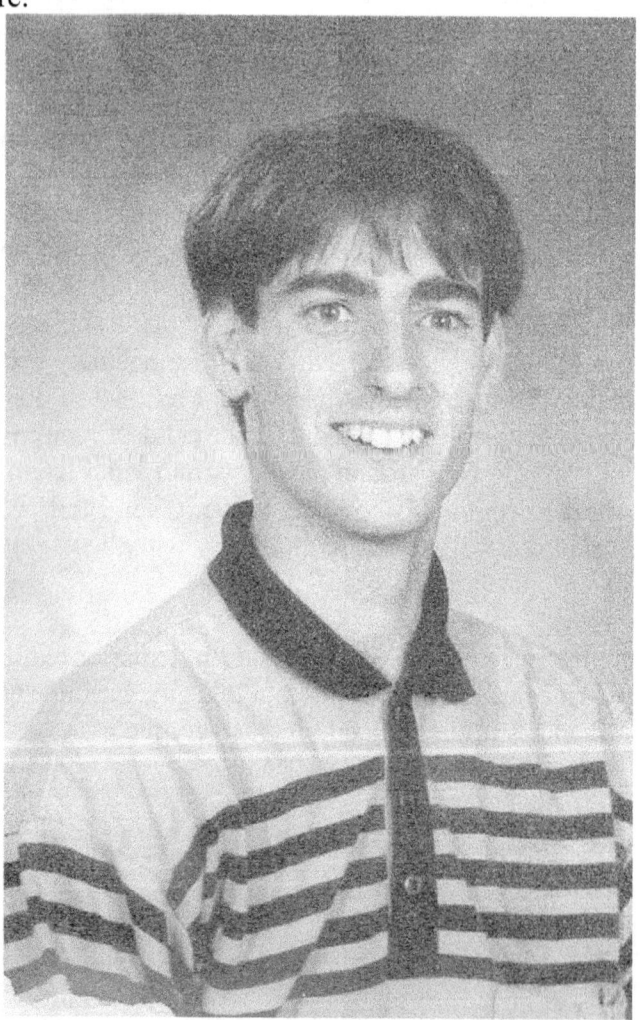

My mother was in the hospital for three or four days in a row after having bladder tuck surgery in 1990.

One day, I went to visit her in her room. I went back down the hall toward the elevators probably to get a drink or snack or lunch or something. When I came back down the hall toward her room I saw the door open to another room with a baby in it that was crying immensely and it had an EKG connected to it that was going absolutely buzzurk. Its pulse was so high; I knew something was terribly wrong. I was so overwhelmed with emotion over this baby's suffering that I walked two or three steps past the room and then suddenly passed out. I think I must have had a panic attack because of my helpless emotions over wishing I could do something for the baby. A male nurse saw me pass out in the hall, of the second floor and caught me.

He got me back up and said, "Are you okay?"

Even though I was frantic I said, "Yeah, I think so? That baby was crying like crazy in there and the EKG was going absolutely buzzurk. I was really worried about the baby!"

I then walked in my mother's room and told her what happened and she said, "You probably just got panicked over the baby and it shocked you. That's probably why you passed out."

The nurse said, "Are you sure your okay? I really think you ought to go to the Emergency Room."

I said, "Oh, I think I'm okay now. I was just worried about the baby."

The nurse asked, "Are you sure? I really think you ought to go get checked out. Why don't you go down the elevator and walk down to the Emergency Room?"

I said, "I don't think their going to believe me now. I'm fine now. Those people never believe me, and if they ever do they get real mean with the needles."

The nurse acted very concerned and said, "I think it will be okay. Just tell them I sent you. I really think you ought to go. Could you go ahead and go?"

I said, "Okay, but their not going to believe me. What am I supposed to tell them anyway?"

The nurse said, "Just tell them you passed out and I saw it and I thought you needed to go down there."

I said, "Okay. I guess I'll go, but I hope I'm not sorry. I really don't like those people down there. They're usually mean."

So I walked back down the hall to the elevator and had to ask directions to the Emergency Room because I was on the opposite side of the hospital from the Emergency Room and there were several long halls I had to go down just to get there.

When I finally got to the Emergency Room, this ugly *male* nurse immediately asked, "What are you doing here?! Why are you here?!"

I said, "I passed out and this nurse upstairs saw me and told me he thought I needed to come down here to see you."

The *male* ER nurse then said, "Yes! But, why are you here? You look fine to me! What in the world did you come down here to bother us for?! You're just fine! What do you want with us?!"

I said, "I'm fine now, yes. I really didn't want to come down here but I did because this nurse asked me to and I really don't want to be here! I passed out in the hallway when I saw a baby in distress and his EKG went buzzurk and I panicked! I really didn't want to come down here anyway! I'm fine now! I was just doing what I was told to make this other nurse happy! I don't know why you are being so hateful! I came here because I was told to!"

120

The *male* ER nurse said, "If you aren't sick and you don't have a good reason to bother us then go home and leave us alone and don't come in here! Let us know when something does happen and then we will take care of it, but as for now, you look fine to me so I don't know why you even bothered to see us about this!"

I said, "Fine! I'll go! I didn't want to come down here anyway! I only came down here because I was asked to because I passed out when I saw that baby stressed out! I thought he was in trouble and he scared me! I'm fine now! I didn't want to come down here in the first place! I'm leaving!"

I walked off and went back upstairs and told my mother, "I knew they would be that way! I hate going down there were those stupid men are at! I hate the Emergency Room! I only went because that nurse wanted me to!"

The nurse that told me to go to the ER asked, "Did you go down there and check it out? What did they say?"

I said, "They didn't like it I went down there. They said I was fine and didn't know what I bothered them for and should only go down there when I am sick because I looked fine to them. I tried to tell them I passed out and you asked me to go down there and that was the only reason I went down there because you thought I needed checked out for having passed out! I knew they would be that way! They're always like that! And when they do take me seriously, watch out buddy, they're going to get rough and I'm not about to go back down there and deal with that again! I've had to put up with this my whole life with them and I'm tired of it! I don't ever want to go down there to those people ever again! I can't stand that Emergency Room! I never wanted to go there in the first place! I knew this would happen! This always happens! Every time they act like this! It never fails! I'll be glad when I'm out of here! I can't wait to go somewhere else to be seen. I hate this place!"

Big City Hospitals Don't Like Cowards   Brian Evans

At age 23, my ID expired for being able to go in there and I went to other places in town from there on out. I was glad to get out of there when I did.

Chapter Eight
Good IVP Test Experience at the Radiology Building

When I started having problems using the bathroom and I went to an Urologist, Dr. Skippy about it he did some prostate tests. He did a Cystoscope and an Urethrogram himself which did not go to well. When he did the Cystoscopy on me he had anchored some piece on me in order to stick his pipe in me.

He said, "Whatever you do don't move or I'll hurt you! Scream all you want, but be still! If you move you will get hurt!

I screamed loudly, "Ahhhh!!!"

He found prostate blockage just as he suspected and sponge kidney but he also wanted to do an Urethrogram in his office just to see what he could find with my bladder and urethra. When he got ready to do the Urethrogram his nurse was in the room waiting for him to show up.

She said, "I hope you really need this, because some people just come in here to have this done to show off just so we will have to see them."

I said, "Oh no! You don't have to worry about that! Believe me! I'm not about to volunteer to do a test like this! You've got to help me! You've got to comfort me, please!"

The lady looked at me like she wanted to believe me but still thought I was half crazy and said, "Alright! I guess I'll help you if you need me to."

The Urologist stuck his pipe in me again and I went, "Ahhhh!!!!"

The nurse didn't know what to think but then acted like, "I guess I'll comfort this guy. Apparently he's not putting on after all. He's scared to death."

When I finally got that test done, he decided to send me to the X-ray Department of the Radiology Associates building where he had previously done the Cystoscopy.

I waited in the waiting room scared to death.

Everyone kept acting like I looked fine to them and grinned at me like they were thinking, "What is he doing here?"

They made me go into a dressing room behind the desk somewhere and change into my hospital gown. When I had to do a test at Dr. Skippy's office, he let me wear my socks. So I was shocked when these people told me everything had to come off including my socks. I walked down the hall behind the desk barefoot in my hospital gown embarrassed to death.

Everybody was staring at me and grinning acting like, "What is he doing here?" This made me very self conscious.

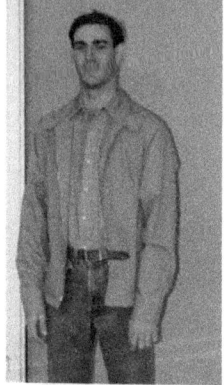

I finally spotted somebody in the hall and said, "Where am I supposed to go? What room do I go in?"

This person said, "You'll go in here." It was about four doors down on the right.

They said, "Just step in here and the lady doing your test will be here in a minute."

Then a very nice lady came in the door and said, "Hi, I'm Lacy. You just sit right in here and I will be back in a few minutes. After quite some time, she finally came back in and noticed I was really nervous and scared.

She said, "I'm going to be doing this IVP test on you on your kidneys. There's going to be an IV, but its okay. I'm going to use a small needle okay. I'm using a baby IV."

She somehow slid the needle in my arm with one arm, and took her other arm, and rubbed my head to calm me down. Then she cooed me like a mother coos her child.

She said, "Its okay. Don't be scared, okay. It's going to be okay. You're going to get through this. You just wait and see. Don't you worry? I'm right here. I won't leave you. I'm right here, if you need me. Just try to stay calm, okay. It's okay. Everything's going to be just fine. Just try to hang on for me, okay. Are you okay? We're going to be just fine. There. There. I'm sorry this hurts. We'll be done in a minute, okay. Just try to hold on, alright. It's alright. It's alright. Just relax, and try to breath. It's okay. You're doing well. We're done now. You did well. Are you alright now? Okay. It's okay. We made it. You're done now. Just relax, and get up easy when you feel like it. Good. Good. I think we're okay now. You can go now."

I believe I gave her a hug hello, and a hug goodbye, too.

It went really well. I was very pleased.

When Dr. Skippy got all the test results back he decided to do surgery but when he found out that I was low income and had indigent health care only, he decided that he wasn't going to do the surgery after all. My dad had gone to Dr. Skippy and said he was not too happy with him anyway and suggested I go to Dr. Filler instead, so I started going to Dr. Filler for my Urologist after this. He believed me about my problem and kept giving me antibiotics, but he would not ever do surgery. I'm not sure he's the type that would have put me to sleep for it either.

I didn't want to have to go through what I went through with Dr. Skippy again. I was glad Dr. Filler never did a Cystoscopy on me. He also kept charging me like $50.00 a visit and I was getting tired of having to pay him that much. There was even a time he was starting to act grumpy so I just quit going to him for a while and just let my family doctor take care of it.

Chapter Nine
Horrible Experience at Small Town Hospital in Texas
The GTT Experience

I was diagnosed with Hyperthyroidism in July 1991 by the family doctor I was going to. A couple of years later, I found out about the Medical Care Mission where low income people could go there to see the doctor and went to them.

Then in 1994 I got a job a small hospital in a smaller town North of where I lived. I began seeing a doctor out there in order to make things easier for the hospital I worked at. I was having my usual thyroid symptoms with my excess energy spells followed by severe fatigue and my eyes were starting to bulge again and I was losing weight believe it or not. I already only weighed 130 pounds at 25 years of age and then I dropped even further to 125 pounds so I decided to ask the doctor if he would do a blood test to check my thyroid and the doctor agreed. Since I have a severe needle phobia and a severe oversensitivity to pain I started to panic when the lab technician started to put the needle in. I was hyperventilating when this nurse walked in to do my blood test. Somehow I was able to calm down a little bit when I saw how compassionate she was but I still screamed and cried in pain. She was still very nice to me anyway. They were not able to find anything thyroid related so they did another blood test to see if I had diabetes. Somehow I was able to make it through yet another blood test.

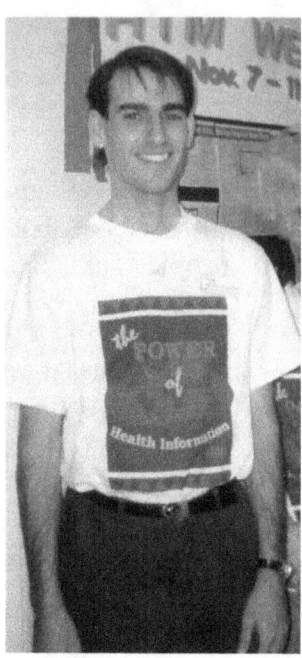

The head nurse Bonnie said, "Brian, your glucose reading was normal but I'm not convinced so we are sending you to the hospital for some more tests."

"What kind of tests?" I asked in panic!

"It's a GTT test. You will have to fast the night before and they will have you drink this sugary substance then do a blood test every hour for eight hours."

"Do I have to?" I begged.

She said, "Yes, we need to figure out why you're losing weight."

Just a few days later, I went to work hungry from having to fast. I was tired from not being able to sleep well at all, because I was terrified of what I was fixing to endure. I was scared to death when I walked into the lab room. I wanted to get it over with so I was there as soon as they were open.

Big City Hospitals Don't Like Cowards   Brian Evans

There was a young nurse Rita, and a much older, rather hefty nurse, Gina.

Rita said, "We need you to drink this, and come back every hour for the next eight hours so we can do blood tests."

I felt like I was about to cry. I was trembling inside I was so scared. I drank the sweet liquid and went to work right down the hall. When I went back in an hour, I was absolutely terrified.

I pleaded, "Please don't hurt me? Can you do it in the right arm because it hurts worse in the left?"

With a short, impatient tone of voice Rita said, "Don't jerk your arm! I know you hate it but we're going to have to stick it in!"

Gina said, "I'll hold his arm!"

When Rita stuck my arm I screamed loudly and cried horrendously. I was in horrible pain.

Rita said, "That don't hurt! Don't tell me that hurt! I don't believe it! You can't tell me that hurt! You better get used to it because you're going to have to come in here again in an hour!"

She showed absolutely no sympathy for me. I had to go right back to work. An hour later I went back to the lab.

"Please still do it in the right arm!" I begged again.

Gina glared at me as she grabbed my hand and jerked my arm straight.

With a smirk on her face Rita said, "I don't know if we're going to do it in the right arm or the left arm!"

She acted like she was getting a kick out of torturing me. I screamed in horrendous pain as the needle went in my arm again.

They ended up doing the blood tests five times in my right arm.

The next time I cried out in fear, "No! Don't do the left! Please! That's even worse!"

Rita said, "We have to! You're going to have to do this. Hold him Gina!"

Gina growled, "Be still already!"

Even though Gina was rather large and I was only 125 pounds she had a very hard time holding my arm. I screamed even louder this time! I almost didn't go back for the last two blood tests. My paralyzing fear of them making me do it all over again is the only reason I went back. The next time it was quite a fiasco. It was impossible for me to just let them do their job.

Rita said, "Brian! You have to let us do this!"

"Not on the left side!" I demanded hugging my left arm close to my body.

Rita yells out, "I think you're going to have to sit on him Gina!"

"No! No!" I pleaded. I let Gina hold my arm but went ballistic as soon as Rita stabbed me with the needle.

Rita said, "You better hope you never wind up in the hospital for anything! They will test your blood all day, every day!"

As soon as the needle was out of my arm I shot out the door as fast as I could. The last time was even more traumatic for me. I was trembling with fear. I wouldn't even get on the bed this time. They chased me into a corner. They each grabbed one of my arms and dragged me to the table.

Rita screamed, "You're going to have to sit on him this time, I know?!"

Gina sat on me, and I could barely breathe, but I still fought for my life. I kicked my feet forward and tucked my left arm behind my back. Gina shoved her chubby hand under me and pulled my arm out straight.

"I've got him! Hurry up!" Gina was out of breath.

Rita said, "Tell your doctor to never send you over here again! We can't take any more of this!"

Rita filled the tubes as fast as possible then said, "Okay, let him go!"

I was hysterical from the whole thing, and everybody was exhausted. I was functioning on pure adrenalin now. The whole thing was horrible. I was scared to death from being traumatized by them taking blood from my left side. I was really hungry because I usually snacked throughout the day, and I hadn't had a thing except for the sugary drink. Not to mention I was exhausted from having to work all day in between, fighting for my life through all the blood tests. I was glad it was over.

They never even found out anything that would explain my weight loss so I had to endure all that torture for nothing. I was put on appetite enhancers after this to increase my appetite. They also recommended I eat a lot of food items with gravy in order to make me gain weight. I ate a lot of chicken fried steak at the time and got the gravy that way.

Chapter Ten
Sweet Dental Hygienist at Oral Surgeon's Office

When I was 25 years old, I had impacted wisdom teeth. My Dentist sent me to an Oral Surgeon that worked in conjunction with him at another office to get them removed.

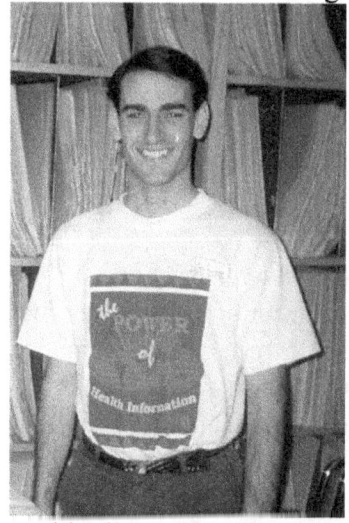

He could tell I was really scared so he said, "I have this really friendly lady here and she will be your dental assistant."

When I got there she noticed I was so scared so she did her best to help me out. Her name was Daisy, and she was very nice to me. She was very compassionate to me because she understood my anxiety.

I was pleading with her, "Please don't hurt me!"

Daisy sweetly said, "I won't, I'm even going to use a baby IV!"

I asked, "You do have the gas don't you?"

She said, "Yes, we have the gas, but I have to put your IV in first. Just lie back in your chair and relax. It's going to be okay."

Daisy gently patted me on the shoulder and rubbed the top of my head like a mother calms her child.

Daisy was super gentle when she inserted the needle, so I wasn't nearly as bothered by it as I normally would have been.

She helped me out of my chair and then escorted me to the operating room.

I was breathing hard and fast because I was scared out of my mind. As soon as I sat in the chair my eyes darted all over the room.

Daisy said, "Lie back and I'll give you the gas now. You'll really like that so don't worry, just relax for me. I know you're scared but it's going to be okay, I promise."

Daisy rubbed the top of my head again, like you comfort a scared child, to comfort me while I was being put to sleep.

After I woke up the dentist said, "You did very well Brian."

I said, "Thanks."

"You're ready to go home now. You need to be on a liquid diet for a few days. Do not drink any hot liquids or you will start bleeding again."

My mother filled my prescription for pain pills at the pharmacy then took me home and put me to bed. The whole experience there went really well.

Chapter Eleven
Bad IVP Test Experience
At The
Main Hospital Radiology

I went to my family doctor in 1994 at the Medical Clinic to tell
him about my problems I was having with my prostate. This doctor
did a manual exam and said this was in fact a problem but he also
wanted me to have an Intravenous Pyelogram of my kidneys at the
hospital radiology department. He wanted to make sure my
kidneys were in good condition while he was at it. He didn't want
to take a chance on that being a problem too, so he ordered this test
at the hospital to see for sure. I hoped they would be as good at the
hospital in 1994 as they were in the Radiology building in 1993,
but I was a little worried about the fact it was in the hospital's
radiology department instead of the clinic's radiology department.
I really liked the lady in the clinics' radiology department, and I
was afraid the people at the main hospital might not be as nice. I
hoped they would be nice but highly doubted it.

I drove to the hospital for my retest that day. After I sat in the
waiting room for three hours, I worried that my mother would be
wondering where in the world I was. I figured she was thinking
I'd be back home by now. Come to find out it was going to
probably take another hour, so I asked if they could get me in for
my test sooner. Back in those days, there were no cell phones and
I had to use the hospital's pay phone to call my mother and kept
having horrible luck catching her or getting through on the phone.
I would have happily waited longer, hoping to get a better
radiologist than what I was about to get, but I had already sat there
for two hours, worried sick my mother would be worried sick
about where I was, thinking the test was already done when I
hadn't even started the test yet. So I asked someone where I was
in line and told them my situation and asked them if there was
someway I could get in earlier so my mother wouldn't have to
worry about where I was.

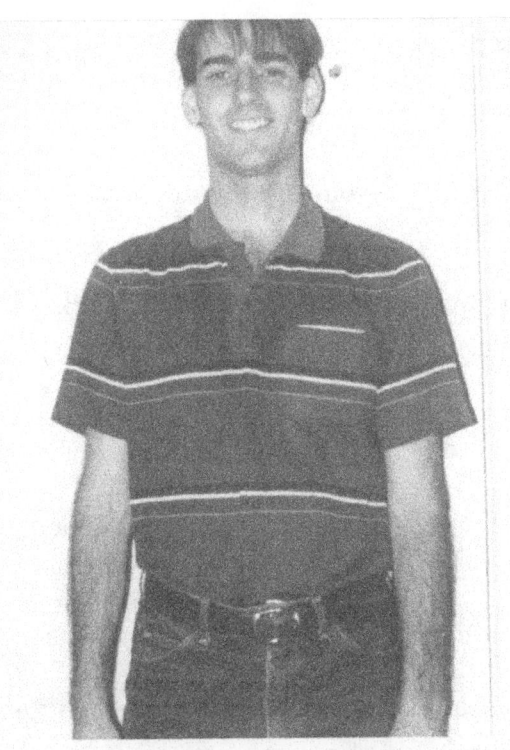

I had no idea what I was about to get myself into. This grumpy acting old lady called for me and took me to a room. I was scared to death of Mrs. Grump! Luckily, a very sweet young girl came into the patient room to tell me about the test and I was relieved. When she told me what it entailed I got scared. I didn't know there were going to be any needles until it was too late. I was hoping she would stick around so she could comfort me when I got scared over the needle stick. I had forgotten I would have to have an IV. She talked like she was going to help, and I was relieved. She was exactly the kind of person I needed to help me get through the test. Then she suddenly walked out of the room, I panicked!

I begged, "Are you coming back?"

The sweet young girl said, "Yeah. I'm coming back. I'll be back in a few minutes. You just let me know when you're changed into your gown and I'll come back in here."

I waited for her to come back, because I thought she just had some sort of errand to run. Then, all of a sudden, Mrs. Grump walked in the door, and I was terrified!

I said, "Do you know where the young girl went that was just in here that was going to help?"

Mrs. Grump said, "She went to lunch! She won't be back for a while! We're going to have to get somebody else!"

I listened to her snap back and forth on the phone, "Can you get someone in here? We need to hurry and get this guy through here!"

A macho looking guy Frank, walked in the door, and I got really nervous.

Mrs. Grump said, "You'll have to have an IV to start the test!"

I was startled, and my heart raced with fear, and I pleaded for mercy.

I begged, "Can the doctor order the gas?"

Mrs. Grump said, "No! The doctor can't order the gas! If you wanted the gas you should have thought of that before you came in here! If you want the gas he'll have to send you in here again, and we'll do it then!"

I said, "I don't know if I can get him to order the gas, but if I can, will you give me the gas first, and then do the test?"

Mrs. Grump said, "No. You'll have to do it a different day?"

She said, "This tech is going to go into the camera room while Frank does the IV!"

Because I was tortured by men with needles at the air force base as a child, I got really nervous, and was horribly frightened.

136

Then she said, "It looks like we're going to have some problems with this guy! You'll have to do what you can!"

I asked, "Is this guy going to do the IV stick?"

She said, "Yes! That other girl went to lunch! We're going to have to go with him!"

I begged, "I don't know if I can handle it or not. Please be gentle. Please don't hurt me."

Mrs. Grump got mad as a fire, and started yelling at me, something tremendous.

She kept snarling the same thing, "Are you going to do it?! Are you going to do it?! Are you going to do it or not?! Are you going to do it or not?!"

I couldn't handle it anymore and blurted out, "Okay! I'll do it!"

Mrs. Grump said, "Stick it in!"

Frank had a smirk on his face as he came at me with the needle, and he rammed it in my arm hard! I was petrified!

He scared me to death and I screamed "Ahhhhh!"

The entire hospital could probably hear me screaming in agony.

Mrs. Grump said, "Take it out! I can't take it anymore!"

I got dressed as fast as I possibly could, and ran out of the hospital shaking up a storm. I was so traumatized by what had just happened I had to sit in my car to calm down enough to drive home. I went and explained what happened to the doctor, and asked if he could reorder the test with the gas this time.

He said, "No. I don't want to bother with it. Have you been to an Urologist? I'm going to set you up with Dr. Filler."

I said, "I've already been to him. I don't want to go to him again. He's expensive and the last time I went there he acted kind of irritated with me."

My doctor said, "Don't worry about it. I'm going to set you up with him anyway. We're going to put you on a charity thing so he'll charge you $10.00 a visit, instead of $50.00."

I said, "Okay."

Dr. Filler gave me the usual antibiotics, and I cleared right up.

Mrs. Grump never smiled. She just acted mad as far the whole time. I just wanted you to know that so you'll get that in your head. She was a "serious trended female nurse". She had a straight face and never smiled and acted mad as a vulture the entire time I was in there, especially after I got scared over the IV. That made her madder than ever. I hope everybody gets this. I repeat, this lady was a "serious trended female nurse" not a chipper one. Remember that, they are the ones that act this way, not the chipper ones.

Chapter Twelve
Horrible Experience with Urologists that Didn't Believe About My Prostate Problem Because I was Young

I had moved to Arkansas in 2000 to get married, I was having Urological problems again. I had trouble finding an Urologist in 2003 that would believe I had a prostate problem. Even though, in Texas, I had already been diagnosed and was being treated for a prostate problem. The first Urologist I went to in this area, Dr. Old, thought I had a bladder control problem.

When I told him about having already been diagnosed with a prostate enlargement he said, "I don't think your two Abilene doctors know what they are talking about. You have to be 50 years old to have a prostate problem. I don't think you have a prostate problem. I think we just need to calm the bladder down."

He gave me bladder control medicine which is what one of my family doctors, Dr. Torah had tried to do years before. I told him how one of my ex-urologists, Dr. Filler in Texas complained when another doctor tried to give me bladder control medicine.

Dr. Filler had said, "No! That's not the way to treat it! That's the wrong medicine! You have a prostate problem and he doesn't need to be giving you that stuff! Don't ever let a doctor give you that stuff! It will shut your bladder down!"

I also told him how my current family doctor, Dr. Sammy I went to at the time thought he was crazy for giving me bladder control meds in the first place.

Dr. Sammy had asked me, "What in the world did this guy ever give you this stuff for?"

Dr. Old, in Arkansas kept giving me bladder control medicine anyway which did nothing but mess me up.

Even my family doctors in this area, Dr. Sammy and Dr. Mark thought he was completely nuts, and he was. My problem got continually worse and I had even more trouble urinating than I already did.

We found an Urologist, Dr. Young that actually believed I had a prostate problem at first in 2004. He even diagnosed me with Prostatitis, stage three. I had a couple more visits with him that went well. I believe Dr. Young either got a hold of my ex-urologist records that misdiagnosed me, or talked to him about it.

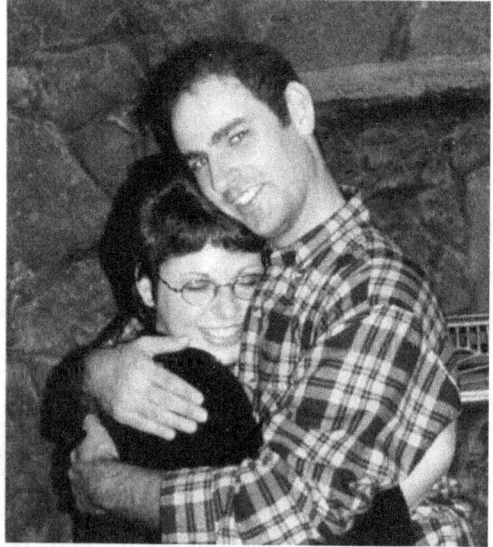

Wouldn't you know, during my next visit Dr. Young decided to give me bladder control medicine?

I tried to explain, "The other Urologist, Dr. Old misdiagnosed me."

Dr. Young said, "He is much older than I am. He must know what he is talking about because he is more knowledgeable about it."

I said, "But that's not the problem."

Dr. Young replied with, "I'll set you up with a therapist to retrain yourself to urinate the right way. I think you may just be having bladder pain."

I was not happy at all about having to go to therapy, but I did it anyway. Of course, since that was not the problem it did not work.

During my follow up visit Dr. Young insisted I had to have an Urodynamics study done. He sent me to another Urologist's office he knew, Dr. Nightmare. I showed up for my Urodynamics study scared to death because I had no idea about what I would have to go through. The nurse Hilda was a "serious trended female nurse."

The nurse Hilda said, "Brian, you have to be awake for this study in order to follow our instructions, okay?"

Bertha said my eyes got real big, and I yelped.

I frantically said to this nurse, "I don't think I can handle it!"

I was scared to death. My heart was racing with fear.

Hilda said, "We will use catheters instead of the pipes we normally use to make it easier for you."

I said, "I don't know. I still think it's going to hurt really badly. I really think you need to knock me out."

Hilda said, "We have to do it awake. We can't put you out for this. We have to keep you awake so you can answer our questions. You're going to have to decide. Are you willing to take the test awake or do we need to reschedule?"

She did not understand.

I panicked and said, "I'll go ahead and take the test to get this over with, but I can't guarantee you that I will be able to handle it, because it really hurts to do this kind of thing. I'm really sensitive that way. It really hurts! I may not be able to handle it."

I looked desperately at the assistant Macy and begged her, "You have got to help me through this!"

She did not understand.

At first, she was not very comforting to me. She acted like I was just trying to get inappropriate attention. I tried really hard but the pain was so excruciating I screamed very loudly.

Then when the assistant, Macy saw that the experience was so overbearing to me she put her hand on my shoulder and tried to encourage me, "Come on! Come on! Just a little bit longer we're almost there! Just half way to go!"

Macy was all shook up. She acted like she could hardly handle it. Finally she gave in and tried to comfort me. I think it shocked her when she saw just how traumatic the pain was for me. It was a horrible experience. She saw for herself that I wasn't being inappropriate. It was that bad.

After what seemed like forever Hilda, the nurse trying to insert the catheter said in pure frustration, "I'm Sorry, I'm going to have to quit. I'm hurting him too much!" Hilda never smiled.

I looked over to the assistant, Macy. Her eyes were filled with tears. She was so overcome by the horrible pain I was experiencing. She was trying really hard not to cry. I could tell she was trying to hold back the tears. They were not able to complete the procedure. Macy finally understood too late.

When we started home, I had horrible sharp, shooting pains in the urethra. The next time I went to the bathroom I bled like crazy because of the test I just had. We had to go to my family doctor, Dr. Mark at the time to get some kind of medicine to fix it. He gave me AZO standard for bladder spasms until it cleared up.

The next Urologist, Dr. Jonathon also gave us trouble. He said, "There's no way any 35-year-old is going to have a prostate problem! No way!"

Dr. Jonathan demanded we get the records from Dr. Old, the Urologist who wanted to treat me for bladder control. He wanted to know what he had to say about it. Dr. Jonathon's nurse, Stacy showed me to my room. I looked nervously at the catheters in that office.

Stacy said, "They're probably going to do a Cystoscopy on you and they may use these catheters, but it will only be catheters they do it with. You won't have to worry about any pipes. They may even decide to catherize you with them."

I asked Stacy full of panic, "You're not going to stick me with one of those things are you? Please don't make me do it!"

Stacy said, "Not today but we may do it on your next visit depending on what the doctor decides. Right now you're just doing your initial evaluation but he's probably going to make you have one done if he thinks you need to when you come back. We need to make you a follow up appointment, and I hate to say this, but you probably will have to do it then."

I wrote to Dr. Jonathon and complained that two of my Abilene Urologists found a prostate problem long before I even moved to Arkansas and I wanted my money back.

He wrote me back in disagreement but said, "I disagree with your decision and I agree with your other Urologist, but since someone else has told you that what your saying is right and you want your money back I'm sending it to you here. Here's the check."

This Urologist was in Missouri, the other Urologists who did not believe me were in Arkansas.

We tried Dr. Bullhorn next and he didn't believe me about my prostate problem either. He thought there must just be some kind of blockage in the urethra itself. He decided he was going to do a Cystoscopy on me with one of those pipe things.

Bertha told him that he needed to put me to sleep, and the man just said, "I'm not going to put him to sleep just for a quick test check with a Cystoscope. He'll just have to try to do his best to take it."

She said, "He's going to scream if you do it without putting him asleep. Just don't quit when he screams. Keep trying I don't want him to have to do it again. You may never get another chance."

The doctor said, "I will."

The nurse, Janice had me change into a hospital gown and had me lay on a patient bed. She tilted the head of the bed up at an angle. They started rubbing me with a swab and I got real nervous.

She said, "We haven't started yet."

I think I remember she, and two or three other nurses had to hold me down. I had to put my feet into the kickstands at the end of the bed. Then Dr. Bullhorn started at me with the pipe.

He barely touched me and I screamed, "AHH!" and I jerked.

Janice said, "He hasn't even gone in yet. He barely touched you." She was very upset. She didn't understand my pain.

 Dr. Bullhorn barely pushed the pipe in there about a half an inch or so and I screamed horrendously, "AHHHHHH!", "AHHHHH!", "AHHHH!" in excruciating pain.

I was in so much pain I kicked so hard the kickstands went flying and landed in the floor. We tried to tell them I couldn't handle it awake. I had gone ballistic on these people, and now they were upset.

Janice said, "If he thinks he can handle this awake better the next time, you can bring him back in a week. If not, then don't bother coming back! We'll give him one more chance, but he'd better get his act together and behave himself and let us do this or we're not going to do it again! You decide!"

Chapter Thirteen
Tribulation Regional Medical Center
Part I: The PreOp Experience

In November 2004, the Urologist I went to decided to do an Urethrogram. Only this time he would use anesthesia at the hospital, which was right across the street. Bertha tried to tell him how badly I handled IV's. We warned him the best we could but he didn't completely understand. We did talk the hospital into doing the gas, but they insisted they were going to do the IV first. We bugged the lab about this, and they had me talk to a nurse on the phone, after they finished doing my blood test I was required to have. When I have to have a blood test it feels like being stuck with a steak knife. This time, I went in the lab an old lady helped me out. It comforted me to have a granny type nurse with lots of compassion to help me get through it. The second time I had to get a blood test, when I went in for surgery, a nice young girl did the blood test, and she was good.

They still asked her if she needed more help but she said, "No. I think I've got it. It's okay."

I wanted to give her a hug afterwards, but I was afraid she wouldn't understand so I skipped it, but it really depressed me not to give her a hug. They gave me a nurse to talk to on the phone. The nurse tried to console me, but I was so scared I still persisted with insisting I have the gas first.

She finally said, "Okay. I'm not going to say that it's not going to hurt, but I will assure you that the IV person will try as hard as they can not to hurt you. They will be as gentle as possible."

I finally figured out they weren't going to give in on this one so it was no use to keep after them about it. Three days later I went to the pre-op for anesthesia to be put to sleep for the Urethrogram x-ray and VCUG x-ray. I met this IV-helper nurse, Lori that was really nice. Being in a hospital is even scarier to me than it is for your average person, even the average child.

I told my IV helper how scared I was, and she got all pumped up, and said reassuringly, "Don't you worry! We're going to get you through this! You're going to be okay!"

I asked, "Do you think you can handle someone like me?"

Lori said, "Yeah. That's no problem! We can handle this! We can get you through this! You'll see! You're going to be alright!"

When it was time to go Lori said, "Come on, and come with me, and I'll show you were to go! It's okay! You're going to be alright! You'll see! It's going to be okay!"

I always need my nurses to be upbeat and positive like she was. It really freaks me out when their not positive and upbeat. I did a lot better for this nurse than I normally would have.

Lori helped me to my room and said, "Now come in here and change into this gown and let me know when you are ready."

I changed into my gown and when I was ready I called her back into the room. Lori came back into the room. The IV-sticker, Carley came in after her. They got on each side of the bed next to the sides of my arms. They stood next to the railing real close like they were trying to trap me in case I gave them any problems. Lori and Carley acted like they weren't about to let me go anywhere. Lori was there to hold my hand when Carley stuck me with the IV. I looked back and forth at both of them in panic. I particularly looked at Lori in fear, hoping for sympathy.

I started frantically asking questions and looked over at Lori like a child looks at their mother and said, "Is the anesthesiologist going to come in?"

Lori paused for a second. Then she went outside of the room and stood in front of a table leaning against it. She looked straight at me from there, and at the same time another IV helper nurse, Jenny came in.

Carley, the IV sticker nurse said, "Mind if we have a substitute?"

I said, "I guess not."

I actually really did mind, and wished I would have told her to stick with the lady that originally stood by me. She was the one I wanted. She was the one I liked. She was the one I was comfortable with. Having her would be like having a mother nurse there to comfort me. Lori was probably actually around 30 years old when I was 35 ½ but she still had the motherly qualities in a nurse I was looking for and was like a buddy and a mother to me at the same time.

Even though, I went with the new IV helper, Jenny, I was still wishing I would have stuck with Lori. She was the one I really wanted to help me, and it really hurt my feelings bad that she wasn't the one that helped me, after all. She got me all wound up over the idea of her being the one. Now they give me a different one I didn't even really care for. I just didn't know what to say. I was really terrified. My security blanket nurse I was comforted by just left the room. Carley began to feel of my arm, and I looked at her frantically.

She said, "Just looking for a spot. I'm not putting it in yet."

Then I looked at Jenny, who I wasn't as comfortable with.

The nurse said, "Switch sides!"

They switched sides. Then, they switched back. After that, the nurse felt my arm again.

She said, "Now look over there at her and hold her hand and I'm going to stick it in right now!"

I looked at the second helper, Jenny, frantically. I screamed the instant the nurse stuck the IV in my arm. I screamed and hyperventilated the whole time. I was really loud too when I screamed.

Being stuck with the IV was the most excruciating pain I'd ever experienced in my entire life. I felt like I had just been stabbed with a butcher knife, it was so bad. I was crying and hyperventilating, even after I got stuck. I was desperate for the anesthesiologist to get there. I thought he'd never get there.

Then the nurse said, "Here, why don't we give you some oxygen? I think it might help. I think you really need it right now. Now breathe this and try to relax."

When I get stuck with an IV it feels like I am being stuck with a butcher knife. I was given the oxygen, and it helped a little, but I was still frantic. The anesthesiologist finally came in to give me the gas several minutes later. The original helper, Lori observed the whole thing from the table outside the room. I was very sad she wasn't the one that helped me after all. I was extremely depressed because of it. I felt like I would have done better with her. It was very traumatic for me. When the anesthesiologist put me to sleep they did an Urethrogram and a VCUG.

I woke up in the x-ray room and two nurses asked me to try to urinate through the tube into the catheter bag.

They said, "It's really going to hurt but we need you to try anyway."

I tried to urinate several times but I was unable to go. Then they said they would remove the catheter and have me try to go in a plastic urinal.

They said, "Okay. We're going to take it out now. You ready?"

I said, "Okay." They took me by surprise, and removed it quickly.

Then, I tried to go in the plastic urinal with no luck.

After that they said, "Now hold on to me and we're going to take you to the bathroom."

I tried going several times standing up with no luck.

They said, "Do you think it would help if you sat down?"

I said, "I don't know, but I'll try."

I was doing everything I could to do what they wanted to the best of my ability, and didn't want to disappoint them, but I failed anyway. I was hoping something would work, but I still had no luck, so they just gave up. They decided to help me get back on the table, and a guy came and took me to the recovery room. I was terrified.

I thought, *"Please, not a guy."* I needed the comfort and nurturing of a *female* nurse to help me in my situation with all my pain. I didn't know if the guys always pushed the patients out of there into the recovery room or if the ladies ever pushed anybody. I preferred a lady nurse wheel me in there and that is what I needed. I was upset, because they gave me a man, anyway. Luckily he just moved me from one room to another and dropped me off for a different set of *female* nurses to take care of me. That would have been really been bad if I would have been stuck with him and needles would have been involved. That would not have gone well at all. I told the recovery room nurse what happened and she said that was unusual because most people were able to go after the dye was pumped into them.

The nurse said, "You are the first one in seven years to every have this problem."

I had to wait forty-five minutes in the recovery room for the doctor to come after already waiting twenty minutes in the x-ray room trying to use the bathroom but not being able to go. I really needed to go bad in there but I couldn't.

The recovery room nurse brought me a plastic urinal to urinate just in case. I still wasn't able to go. I finally saw the doctor who told me I retained abnormally large amounts of urine and said I had an overactive sphincter and that was part of the reason I couldn't go.

The sphincter kept closing shut when I had to go to the bathroom and it was preventing me from being able to go. I was glad to have a name for my problem.

Bertha was in the recovery room with me. She held my hand and rubbed the top of my head while they took the IV out. It was huge, and really long.

I was thinking, *"No wonder it hurt me so bad! That thing is huge! It was the biggest IV I'd ever seen."*

Finally, I said, "Is there a bathroom in here?"

A nurse told me where the bathroom was. I went in there and had trouble at first, but then I went like a race horse and it was as if the whole thing never happened.

I thought, *"Finally, I finally got to go."*

After this I got dressed and another nurse wheel-chaired me to the car. The doctor scheduled me to come back in a month.

Chapter Fourteen
Tribulation Regional Hospital
Part II: The Surgery Experience

I continued to have so many problems urinating I had to go back to him in three weeks

Bertha told him, "We're tired of medicine and we want to have a surgery to fix the problem."

I tried to talk him into a TURP, but he decided to do a TURVN (Trans-urethral Resection of the Vesicular Neck [bladder neck] to create an opening into the bladder). The doctor scheduled this operation for December 13th of 2004.

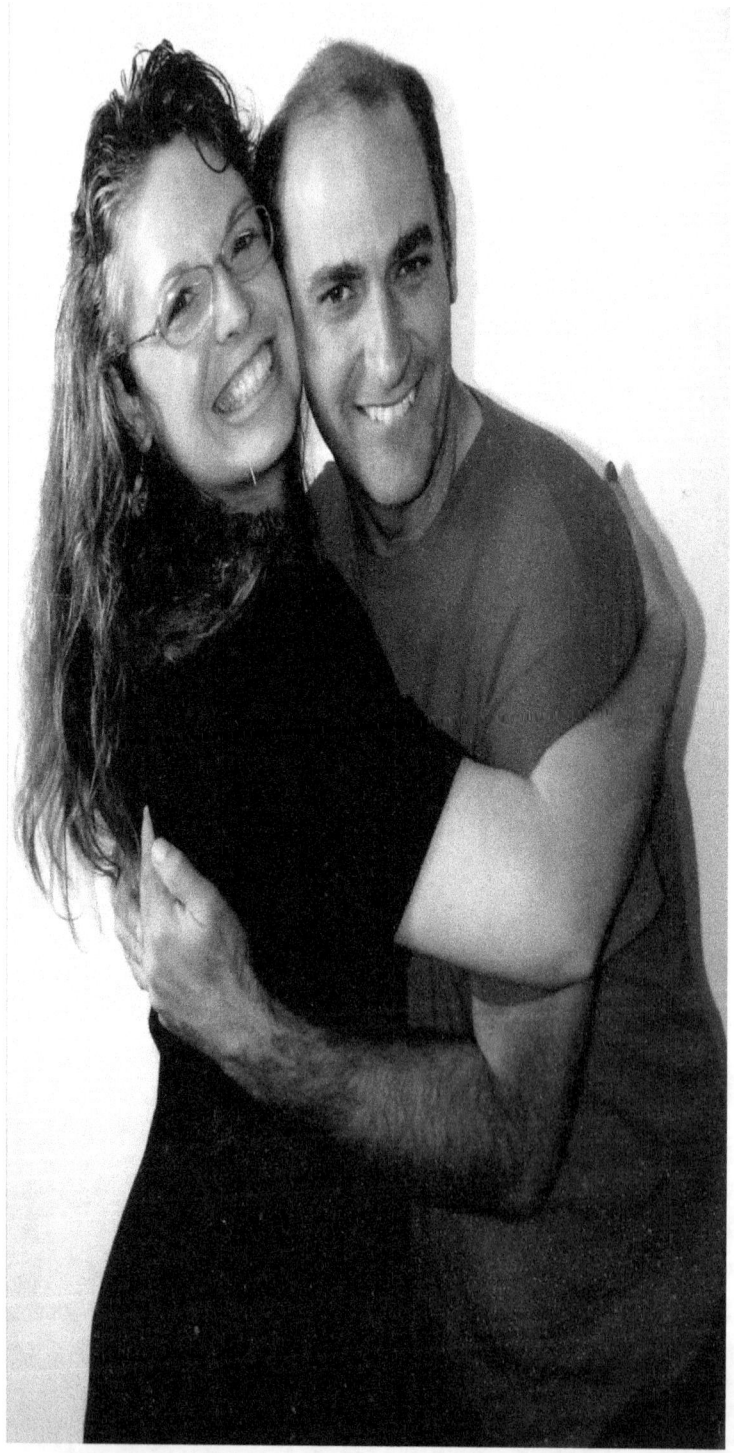

When I arrived at the hospital, I told the anesthesiologist to tell my doctor if he finds something and he sees prostate blockage, remove it. He said he would tell the doctor.

When I first got to the PreOp waiting room I saw my favorite IV helper, Lori. I was so excited she even gave me a hug. I felt I had to go to the bathroom several times before my appointment even though I was not allowed any liquids after midnight. I was unable to empty my bladder completely. I apologized to her and told her I couldn't help it. I asked her for a hug and she gave me one.

When it was time she said, "Do you remember how to get back there?"

I said, "Kind of, but you might want to show me anyway."

So she took me back there then told me she had to go to a meeting so I'd have to have a substitute. This kind of upset me even though she said Bertha could go in there with me this time because they were short on help. I wanted her to stay and be my IV helper again. She did such a good job encouraging me last time, even though, in the end she just watched from outside. I almost begged her to stay but I didn't say anything. She was working at the waiting room desk that day so I figured she had to be there.

Bertha comforted me through the stick this time, but I really need someone who works there to do the comforting so I have one of "them" on my side. They didn't even let Bertha go back there with me the first time. Now I was used to the idea of having to let a nurse do everything for me. In the past if I needed comfort, it was always a nurse that did it, after all that is what to nurse means, to comfort. It was never a friend or relative who did this for me so I was still disappointed when I didn't get a nurse to comfort me through the procedure. I really wanted Lori to do it. I screamed loudly when the substitute nurse stuck me with the IV. All the nurses turned and looked at me grimly.

Since the anesthesiologist set in part of the time with me, I asked over and over, "There isn't any chance you'd give me the gas first, is there?"

The anesthesiologist just kept saying, "No."

They waited for a few minutes, after I had been stuck, then finally they gave me the gas.

After my surgery, I had to wait several minutes before I could get a room upstairs. While I was in the recovery room they told me the doctor did find prostate blockage in the bladder neck, so he did a TURP, a TURVN, and a Sphincterotomy. This made me very happy. I finally proved I was right, and they did the surgery I needed to correct it. Now I had a name for my problem.

Chapter Fifteen
Tribulation Regional Hospital
Part III: The Third Floor West Scenario

When I went into the Inpatient Care Department on 3rd floor west, the two nurses I had on the very first day were nice to me.

One of them Jennifer told me, "You will not be able to do the things you are normally able to do in the morning. You will be weak from the surgery."

"I take a bath every morning. Will I be able to take a bath?" I asked.

Jennifer explained, "There are no tubs and no showers. You will have to ask for a sponge bath, and your day nurse will take care of this for you. If you do not ask for one, you will not get one, because they will only do it if you ask."

At three in the morning, a nice young lab girl Tara came into my room to give me a blood test.

Tara cheerfully stated, "I need to do a blood test."

I replied with, "Can you do it in my right arm? It hurts me even worse in his left arm."

Tara said, "I'll try but you have your IV in the right arm."

She looked but was unable to find a good spot.

She gave up and said in a defeated tone of voice, "I'm sorry; I'm going to have to do it in your left arm."

She stuck the needle in a place that no one's ever done it before. Instead of going to the direct middle of my left arm, she went to the corner just above the mid arm to the left. She was very gentle with her stick, and I was really amazed.

I barely felt it, and in that arm I would normally be in excruciating pain. Tara was very good at taking blood tests and she was very friendly too. I really liked her because of this.

In the morning, the Charge nurse Tracy came in my room first and I remembered what Jennifer had told me so I immediately said, "I take a bath every morning. Can I have a sponge bath?"

She replied, "Yes, but it will be a couple hours." She talked like she was really busy.

I said, "Okay."

I waited for three hours for Tracy to give me a sponge bath, and I was getting worried that she may have forgotten me.

I pressed the call button, and asked, "Can Tracy please give me a sponge bath?"

The nurses' station said, "It will be a little while. She has other things she has to take care of first. Then she can come in there."

I said, "Okay."

I was just doing what Jennifer told me to do the night before. I just thought that was what I was supposed to do if I wanted a bath the next morning, or I wouldn't get one. I didn't mean anything bad by it. Immediately after talking to the nurse's station, this RN, Paulina came into the room in a rage. I suspected that Tracy may have sent her in my room to give me a sponge bath because of the way she came in like clockwork after I asked for Tracy to give me a sponge bath.

Paulina said, "You know you could do this yourself if you wanted to?! All you would have to do is get out of bed and jump into that chair over there and you could do all this yourself! You don't have to have us give you a bath! You can do it yourself!"

Actually there was a big sign on the wall in big black bold print that said, "**DO NOT GET OUT OF BED! A NURSE WILL COME AND ASSIST YOU!**" Paulina had no idea about my oversensitivity to pain and she wouldn't have cared if she did. Paulina was obviously mad. She angrily tried to get me out of bed but kept having trouble with it. She couldn't do it herself because my catheter had me in excruciating pain so bad to the point that I could barely move. I felt almost like an invalid. I think I almost was.

The nurse's aide Maude walked in the door and Paulina said in pure frustration, "Come help me with him! I'm having a hard time getting him out of bed!"

Being in horrific pain, Paulina should have realized I would not have been able to do it myself. I was absolutely terrified of this lady because of the way she acted. She was very mean and had no compassion at all. Paulina and Maude both tried to help me out of bed but because of the pain I was having from the catheter I had in me after surgery. I could barely move.

Maude nicely instructed me, "Now try to set up in bed. We've got to try to make it now."

While going through several steps, I was screaming in pain in the process.

Maude asked Paulina, "Why is it hurting him so much?"

Paulina said very bitterly, "I don't know!?"

Bertha said she was thinking, *"I know what's wrong. It wouldn't have been half the traumatic experience if you had not acted all put out with him. You should have been compassionate with him not irritated by having to do your job. That's what you are being paid for, is it not?"*

Maude kept on trying to encourage me, "Now try to swing your legs over. We need to try to make it now. Now try to get down. Take your time. Be careful now."

Since Maude was nicer and much more compassionate with me, I felt better about trying to get out of bed for her than for Paulina. No matter how hard I was trying I still had a lot of trouble moving around in the bed because I was in such an invalid like state that I could barely move. They had to move me around in the bed in steps just to get me turned around and sat up before they even had me step off the bed. When I placed my feet on the floor, I was groaning in agony just to get down off the bed.

Maude said, "Good. We finally got you stood up. Now we need to get you to the chair."

Paulina scared me even worse when she said abrasively, "You better hope you're able to do all this stuff yourself! If you're not, you'll never get out of here because I'm not going to let you go until you can prove to me you can! You're going to be here a long time if you don't so you better hope you can!"

I could only take baby steps to the chair because I was in so much pain and it took me a while to get over there just to get set down and they even had to help me into the chair.

Then the Paulina said, "See, you could have done it yourself if you wanted to! All you had to do is get in this chair and bathe yourself! You didn't need us!"

Maude then said, "Now remove your gown. You can get your top and I can get your legs."

After they finished my sponge bath, I thought Maude was going to help me back to bed but she just left me in the chair. Thankfully they helped me put on a clean gown or I would have froze to death.

Paulina suddenly abrasively blurted out as she stomped out the door, "I'm going to come back in here, and I'm going to drag you out of that bed, later! I'm going to make you walk down that hall and I'm not going to tell you when!"

I begged her in fear, "Please, can we just do it now?"

Bertha said my eyes were huge. I was filled with panic.

Paulina said, "Hold on. I have to go down the hall real quick. Let me go find out. I'll be back in a minute."

Maude left a couple of minutes later.

I waited for 20 minutes for Paulina to come back and take me for a walk. She never came back. Because she was furious by the way Paulina had treated me, Bertha was going to talk to the Charge nurse, Tracy. She was going to tell her all about how awful her nurse, Paulina treated me, and how she had lied to me. Paulina should have at least told me the truth. Bertha wanted her to know just how uncompassionate her employees were to me. She finally came in and talked to us.

I told Tracy, "Paulina said I could have given myself a bath if I wanted to."

All the Charge nurse, Tracy could say was, "Yeah, I know. You probably could have. It just would have been very painful."

I thought, *"What's wrong with you? Don't you have any compassion at all? Don't you feel at all sorry for me for what this woman did to me? Why do you have to be so cruel?"*

I wondered if Tracey knew about the big sign saying, "**DO NOT GET OUT OF BED! A NURSE WILL COME AND ASSIST YOU!**"

Bertha thought the same thing and nearly came out of her skin. Tracy had no idea how traumatic the whole ordeal was for me. Later that day, Paulina, Tracy, and Maude came in to adjust my catheter. I felt like they were trying to torture me. They took forever, and jerked my catheter all over the place, and it hurt really badly. It was so excruciating, I could hardly handle it.

I started screaming, "AHHH! AHHH! AHHH! AHHH!"

Every time they touched my catheter, I was in excruciating pain because of it. I reached out for Tracy's hand in desperation for mercy and sympathy. She stepped back and jerked away from me. She started working with my catheter all over again like she was happy to torture me some more.

I reached for Paulina's hand and she stepped back and jerked her hand away too. Then, I desperately reached out for Maude's hand and she jerked her hand away as well. I was shocked and didn't know what to do because I was desperately reaching for their hand one at a time for comfort. I was in agonizing pain and all they did was jerk their hands away. For some reason all three of them kept messing with my catheter for several more minutes without having any sympathy whatsoever for my feelings. They also did not care about my oversensitivity to pain. I needed a little compassion, but instead everyone around me shunned me. They all acted like they were having a ball torturing me.

Tracy kept making suggestive comments in a derogatory way that really scared me.

Tracy said, "You know. If they pull your catheter out and you're still unable to go they'll have to reinsert it when they take it out on the third day."

I begged, "Please if they have to reinsert it please make them send me to PreOp to put me back to sleep to do it. I can't handle it awake. Please don't make me do it awake."

160

Tracy said, "It depends. They may decide to send you to PreOp like you ask, but they may not either. If they decide they want you to do it awake you'll have to do it awake."

I begged some more, "Please, please, please don't make me do it. Don't make me do it."

Tracy said, "If you can't go, and they decide they have to reinsert it, if they want you to do it awake then you'll have to do it awake. You'll just have to let them do it awake, and you'll just have to take it."

Tracy acted like she was getting a kick out of it, like she was trying to scare me.

Then, Tracy said, "You know. They usually have to take the IV out every three days. So you know if you have to stay in here longer that they're going to take that one out and make you redo it again don't you?"

I pleaded, "Please, don't. Please, please. Don't make me do it. Don't make me do it."

Tracy said, "If you're here longer, they'll have to take it out, and they will have to reinsert it. You know you're going to have to just let them do it, and just take it if you do, don't you? I'm sure it will be very painful, but you'll have to do it anyway. We don't really know you're going home in three days; you may still be here with as much trouble as you're having. We'll have to see. But if you are here longer then they'll have to reinsert it, and you'll just have to take it. Sorry."

She acted like she was just getting a big kick out of the whole thing and was trying to scare me, because she knew it scared me. She acted like she would have loved to have the honor to pull the catheter out and jerk it and reinsert it all over again just to torture me so she could have fun hurting me. She strongly inferred I would be there longer than three days.

She acted like she also hoped I'd be in there longer so she could take my IV out, and shove it back in as hard as she could, just to here me scream, too.

I don't know what her problem was, but she acted like she was just dying for me to have to stay in their longer, just so she could do all this to me, just to scare me, and have fun doing it. She acted like she got some kind of kick out of going along with that crazy Paulina lady who threatened to keep me in the hospital forever and never let me go. I don't think Tracy wanted to let me go, either. They did everything in their knowhow from that point on to stop it from happening too so they could enjoy the show.

That night, Irene, the nurse I was comfortable with finally came in and I was relieved. I had such a traumatic day that I fell asleep easily. Bertha was exhausted as well, as soon as her head hit the pillow she was sound asleep. At three in the morning, I suddenly woke up and started crying really hard because I was petrified from the traumatic experience with the nurses, especially over them jerking their hands back when he reached out for their comfort.

Irene heard me and rushed into my room!

Frantically she asked me, "Are you alright?"

I was crying horrendously and said, "No. I did what Jennifer told me to do. Tracy, Maude, and Paulina tortured me by moving my catheter around later in the day, and they wouldn't even hold my hand to help me get through it! If I just hadn't asked for a sponge bath this whole thing would have never happened!"

Irene said, "Now don't you think you did anything wrong! You've done nothing except be kind and polite ever since you've been here. I've got nothing but good reports about you!"

Irene went to the side of my bed.

She gently caressed the top of my head just like a mother would her child, for nearly two hours till I went back to sleep. This is exactly what I needed, because I was extremely upset, and could hardly handle my situation.

Irene said, "Brian, I think you get to go home today, I'll take your catheter out for you."

I panicked and told her, "Tracy and Paulina said if they took it out too soon they would have to put it right back in! I begged her to put me under the gas if they did!"

She said, 'Only if the doctor orders it, we will. If not, we're just going to reinsert it if you are still unable to go."

Irene agreed with Tracy and Paulina, but tried to encourage me, anyway.

She said, "They will not let you go home till you are able to go to the bathroom without it, but as long as you can go to the bathroom you are scheduled to go home today. I think it will be okay to take it out."

This really got me worried, because I didn't know if I would be able to go or not. Irene removed my catheter 15 minutes before the day nurses came in. I could move then, but I still had the IV in my arm. Bertha handed me a cup of ice water and told me to drink as much of it as possible so I could go to the bathroom. I had to do this so I would be able to go home.

I said, "Okay."

I walked out of the bathroom with a big smile on my face, "I went to the bathroom pretty easily, but there was a lot of blood in it?"

Bertha said, "I know, I heard. Did you notice there is a shower in the bathroom?"

I said, "Shower? They had a shower in there? The girl that worked that evening we first got here said there were no showers. She said that there were no tubs and no showers and if I wanted a bath I'd have to ask a nurse for a sponge bath or I wouldn't get one."

Bertha said, "Yeah. There's one in the bathroom and I just used it this morning."

I immediately called the nurse's station, "I don't know how to move my IV without hurting myself so I can take a shower."

The nurse said, "Shower? Not without a nurse's assistant you're not! Besides, you have to unclip the thing in the middle of your IV first, and your nurse would have to show you how to do it!"

Maude checked with the nurse's station to see if it was okay for me to take a shower. The doctor was supposed to be there that morning but he never showed up. At 3:00pm I was starting to get worried so I walked to the nurse's station to find out what the problem was.

Bertha asked the nurse, "Brian was able to use the bathroom already, early this morning; do you know why his doctor has not released him yet?"

She desperately pleaded with the first person she saw.

The nurse replied, "Oh yeah, we found out it would be 5:30pm before the doctor is able to get here."

Bertha wondered how long they knew that, and didn't bother to tell us. I was wondering the same thing. I was getting very impatient. Maude never came back to tell me if I could take a shower. Since I was able to walk without my catheter in, I decided to walk down to the nurse's station in my hospital gown with my IV still connected to my right arm, to see if they would let me shower yet. The minute I got to the edge of the nurse's station Tracy turned her back to me, and just died laughing.

164

I felt like she was laughing at me. Then all the nurses turned their heads around at me and laughed hysterically. The nurses looked like they were staring at me trying to make me feel self conscious and humiliated. They did this by looking at me in a way where they tried to make me feel weird that I didn't have any clothes on except for my hospital gown. Because of my self-consciousness this made me very uncomfortable.

I felt like I was the laughing stock of the nurse's station, like they were thinking, *"Look at the little cry baby in nothing but a hospital gown coming to talk to us!"*

I felt like I was their slave. It felt like it made them powerful to make me have to plead with them in only a hospital gown for whatever I wanted. They all acted like they thought it was funny I only had a gown on.

I felt like they thought, *"Look what we have here! This guy has to come to us undressed in nothing but a hospital gown and plead with us and beg us for anything he wishes for us to do for him and we have him right where we want him! He's not going anywhere, because we're not about to let him go! We're going to make sure it takes as long as possible for him to leave so he has to beg for everything he wants from us in agony and never be able to go home! How delightful can it get! This guy feels inferior to us and has to adhere to all our wishes and we have him trapped in here forever! This guy isn't going anywhere!"*

All the nurses acted like they thought it was funny, turning around and laughing at me after Tracy got their attention as I walked toward the nurse's station. They acted like they had control over me and I was like an ant to them.

Maude walked me back to my room and I asked her, "Were they making fun of me?"

Maude said, "No, it wasn't about you. It was about somebody else but I'd rather not repeat what they said."

Big City Hospitals Don't Like Cowards   Brian Evans

When we got back to the hospital room, they took my IV out. Then Maude and I went into the bathroom.

I said, "Since I got the IV out now, if you want me to I can take my own bath this time."

Maude said, "No. I can't let you do that. You're not allowed to take a bath by yourself. I need to help you. I need you to disrobe for me. You need to take off your gown right now in front of me and I'm going to stand right here. I need you to step in the shower while I watch to make sure I don't need to assist you. I need to help you into the shower and stand here until you're done. When you're done let me know and I'll help you out. Then I can help you get dressed."

So she made me remove my gown. Then she helped me into the shower, regardless of the fact I was able to walk. It really bothered me they had been complaining about having to give me a bath themselves the other day. Now that I was willing to take one myself they insisted on helping me. Now that I didn't have an IV or a catheter I was more than capable to do everything without their help.

If they had not complained about it previously, it would not have bothered me and I would have thought, *"Okay. If that's what they need to me to do, I'll do it."*

They griped about having to bathe me three days earlier and hatefully told me, "You could have done this yourself if you wanted to!"

I thought it was crazy that when I was an invalid state they griped about having to bathe me themselves, and now that I could do it myself, I wasn't allowed to bathe myself.

I thought, *"If the reason these three nurses were upset about giving me a bath themselves the first time is because they didn't want to see me get undressed in front of them then why when I was willing to do it myself, three days later, did they insist I was not going to take my own shower and force me to get undressed in front of them?"*

It just doesn't make sense to me. I felt like I was being scolded for being naughty for asking for a sponge bath the first time because they didn't want to see me naked. Three days later I was getting scolded for offering to take my own bath. Plus they made me get naked in front of them anyway. It was crazy, even though I was able to; I was not allowed to take a bath myself.

After the doctor discharged me, I went to the nurse's station to get my papers filled out and signed.

A man with a really ugly look on his face rudely asked, "What do you want?! Is there something I can help you with?!"

I said, "I just want to do my paperwork to get discharged."

Men make me very uneasy anyway. As a child men were nothing but mean to me in the hospital setting, so this made me very nervous.

Then, a *female* nurse said, in a rude tone of voice, "Can I help you?!"

I said, "I'm waiting for the charge nurse to fill out my paperwork so I can go home."

When we finally got to leave the hospital, a lady tried to insist on rolling me out in a wheelchair. I wanted to walk so I could go tell my favorite PreOp nurse, Lori goodbye. I was hoping she was at her desk, but when we walked up to the desk she wasn't there?

"Is Lori available?" I asked the lady sitting there.

She replied with, "No she is busy in the operating room. You can leave her a note. I will be sure she gets it."

Everyone at the desk acted very happy to see me.

As we were walking toward the exit one of them sweetly said, "We hope you get to feeling better."

I was glad to get out of there so I could get away from those three ladies that gave me so much trouble. I was afraid of them. They acted like they thought I was their prisoner. They acted like they got some kind of power kick out of torturing me, and threatening to torture me. Suggesting I may have to go through certain traumas all over again like reinserting the catheter, or reinserting the IV just to scare me, they acted like it made them feel powerful. They acted like they enjoyed scaring me and hurting me. They seemed to enjoy making me think I was going to have to go through the whole thing all over again. They acted like they couldn't wait to have the opportunity to make me have do to the IV and catheter insertion all over again so they could have the honor of being the ones to hurt me so they could hear me scream and laugh their heads off about it. I was glad it was over.

Maude and Paulina never smiled. Paulina came in the room in a rage from the very start and acted mad as fire at me every time I saw her and acted hateful toward me with every word and move she made. Maude was also derogatory toward me but not as bad as Paulina. Tracy did smile, but she also acted cocky, and had a controlling personality. She had some sort of twisted mindset that made her find pleasure in hurting others that were less than she was from a physical standpoint. Anything she could do to inflict pain or scare me into thinking she would do to inflict pain she thought was funny and acted like it was a thrill for her to do this to me. This lady was strange. Maude and Paulina were both "serious trended female nurses" and Tracy was a "vibrant, but cunning female nurse who found pleasure in bringing hurt to those who feared her. It's kind of like Nellie Olson on Little House on the Prairie but with a little more modern day laid back personality behind it.

Nellie can be very smiling, but she can be very cunning and very mischievous and also finds pleasure in hurting others. This was the mindset of this lady's, the same as Nellie's but in a different way.

Chapter Sixteen
Tribulation Regional Hospital
Part IV: The Phone Call to the Inpatient Speech Pathologist

It had been years since I took speech therapy in Abilene, Texas but since I was having such a hard time getting doctors to listen to me, I decided to look into getting speech therapy again.

Since I liked the people at the hospital I tried to find one there. I took it upon my self to call and find a speech therapist I would like, because Bertha was gone a lot volunteering at the Free Store.

I asked for a *female* therapist. I was not at all comfortable with having a man do therapy on me. Bertha said she thought she should have called herself, because I'm got good at getting through to people. I tend to get taken wrong, because they don't understand what's going on. They don't understand why I need what I need, or even what I'm talking about. She didn't know that I had autism yet. She just knew I had autistic tendencies just from seeing my disability records. We didn't know I had actual full blown Autism.

I called the hospital, "Can I talk to the speech therapy department?"

They transferred my call, "Speech Therapy, how may I help you?"

I told the person I had taken Speech Language Therapy before when I lived in Abilene and I wanted to take it again.

I told this lady that answered the phone, "I'd like you to do the same thing and see how much further I can get!"

This lady that answered the phone said, "Are you an inpatient?"

I said, "No, I'm an outpatient, but I was hoping you'd be able to give me therapy yourself since you are a therapist yourself aren't you?"

The lady said, "I'm just an inpatient therapist. If you are outpatient you would have to call the people at the other building."

I asked the lady if she could tell me what their number was and she was reluctant to tell me. I got this feeling she didn't think they'd be as friendly over there.

She asked me, "What is it exactly that you need?"

I said, "Well, I'm not too bad off anymore and it's very hard to tell that I even have a communication problem. You might talk to me about one thing and I might have all the right words and sound like I've got it all together. Then you could ask me to explain something different that I'm not as familiar with or put me on the spot about something and I don't have a clue what to say. People can't figure out what I'm talking about. I can even have a serious medical problem with something and not be able to get through to my doctors because no matter how hard I try to convince them something is wrong they want to believe it is something else. When they find out I'm right and their wrong, it's too late by the time they do something about it."

The lady said, "Well, I don't know. You seem to communicate fine to me."

I said, "Yeah, I know. Most people think that because I have been so educated to death to the point that you can't even tell I've even got a problem. But get around me a while and then you start to notice and think something's not right. You figure it out long after you thought I was fine, and then you get disappointed. I also have a sequencing problem and I have a problem with problem solving. That's not math. I don't mean math. I mean I don't know what to do in an emergency situation. Or any unusual situation I find myself in? I'm totally stumped and clueless. If you could just give me one of those IQ tests with a Language Barrier, and I don't mean an easy one, I mean a tough one, because I'd probably pass an easy one with flying colors, but started getting tough with the Language Barrier section of the test and ask tough questions and try to get me to figure it all out and I'm sunk.

People don't realize all this, and they think that because most of what I say is well intended, and that I communicate well with them most of the time, that if they just got me in the right situation, I would be totally blown away about something they never even dreamed I'd have a problem with. It's that bad. I just need you to give me a chance. You've got to believe me. I'm telling the truth.

I also told her, "You think I sound pretty self-explanatory yourself when I talk to the doctor? Most other people do too, and they think what I say sounds convincing, but go try to tell the doctor the same statements and your walking in a whole other ball park and I don't have the alternative language skills to be able to get around them, or state things in a way that they themselves would understand or that would be convincing to them, because they are hard to convince unlike some other people out there. People just don't realize that, and if I don't get this problem fixed, I'm had."

After I had called her several times, almost daily for a week or so, she finally told me, "We only do inpatient therapy so you will have to talk to somebody at the building across from the hospital."

I had a horrible time getting their phone number, but I finally got it. They acted almost as if they didn't want to give it to me, for some reason. Bertha even admits that most of the time I communicate real well, but sometimes I get in sticky situations and don't know what to say, or how to handle things. Sometimes I have days where you wonder what on earth I am talking about.

Bertha said she imagined the hospital probably already warned the therapist's office across the street about how persistent I was after they gave me the phone number.

I called the number I was given and asked, "Who do you have that can give me speech therapy?"

The secretary that answered the phone said, "We have a lady and a man."

As soon as she answered my question, I got a bad feeling about both of them.

I asked, "Can I have the lady therapist?"

The secretary at the outpatient Speech Language therapy building got all defensive and said, "It depends on their schedule; you'll get which ever one is available."

I only asked if I could have the *female* because I had been treated so badly by men in the medical field as a child so men scare me.

Chapter Seventeen
Tribulation Regional Hospital
Part V: Meeting the Secretary at the Speech Pathology Building

Bertha decided to go to the building of the speech therapist with me when we went to my next urology appointment. We both thought it would put an end to any misconceptions about my wanting a *female* therapist if my wife was with me. I wanted to meet the therapists to see which one I would be more comfortable with.

When we saw the secretary there I asked, "Can we meet the therapists?"

"Do you have an appointment?" she asked.

Bertha said, "No we just need to meet the therapists to see which one my husband is comfortable taking therapy from."

"You need to have an appointment to see a therapist?" She was getting very irritated with Bertha.

Bertha tried to explain, "My husband has autistic tendencies. He needs to be comfortable with his therapist."

I frantically asked, "Can I have the lady therapist? I prefer the lady therapist I talked to on the phone, but since she only does inpatient therapy I want the lady outpatient therapist, not the man!"

The secretary acted funny again and said, "The person at the hospital only does inpatient therapy. We do all the outpatient therapy; you will get either one of them. Whoever is available?"

Bertha said, "Brian is on disability but isn't going to get Medicare till June. Do we need to make an appointment to meet them?"

The secretary said, "I can leave the therapists a note. They will check their schedule to see when they can meet with you."
I thought we finally got through to her what we were after.

Bertha said if she just knew what was about to happen, she would have explained why I wanted a *female* therapist.

The next morning, Bertha called the outpatient speech therapy number and left a message, "Can you please call me back so I can explain my husband to you?"

Bertha didn't want to sit by the phone all day, so after a few minutes she decided to go to the Free Store, where she volunteered for a couple of hours to go through donations.

The phone rang so I answered the phone in my usual way with a very loud, "Hi!"

In a sarcastic, very abrasive tone of voice, the person on the phone stated, "I'm the Director of Speech Pathology; I have a note here that you would like to meet with my Speech Pathologists! My Speech Pathologists cannot meet with you! I keep them busy, and they don't have time to talk to you! I suggest you call back in June!"

I didn't know what to think. It was obvious that the Director of Speech Pathology was furious with me, because he said all this in a very domineering dictatorial tone of voice, yelling at me. The way they acted, reminded me of a horrible experience from my childhood, I immediately felt very defensive. I started writing letters to all the therapists to defend myself. I liked the Inpatient Speech-Language Pathologist the best, and I begged her to do my therapy, whether she only did inpatient patients or not. I told her I was afraid of the people at the other building where they did the outpatient therapy services. I gave her lists of all my autistic tendencies, sequencing problems, communication problems, problem solving problems and whatever else I could think of, as well as difficulties I had with my Language Learning abilities from birth until present.

Little did this lady know that the head of the department at the ACU Speech and Hearing Clinic I went to in Abilene that was so nice to me actually asked for all this information at her clinic.

175

She told me to give her every problem I could remember having from birth to the present. I told this lady it was so important that I got her, because she was the one that I was the most comfortable with. I told her if she could go over this Director's head to get it fixed where she could be the one, that I would really like that. I also told her how my ex-therapists would comfort and console me when something had me really down or something tragic happened, etc. I'm not sure what this lady's reaction was, but I get the feeling she probably took the whole thing wrong.

I told the outpatient therapy lady in the letter I wrote her that I had six *female* clinicians one at a time at ACU Speech and Hearing Center in Abilene, and I didn't know what the problem was. I said they were perfectly fine with me, and if she would just give me a chance, I thought she would too. I started defending myself to her as well about my character, because I thought this man probably made her think something bad about me. I think I also told the inpatient therapist about the six ex-language clinicians I had in Abilene, and how they were fine with me. But you would think, with all that, they would have figured out I wasn't someone they had to worry about. Instead I think it made them think all the more I was someone to worry about when all I was doing was defending myself against their Director of Speech Language Pathology.

Next thing I know, I get a call from this Director of Speech-Language Pathology again saying, "I have here letters to all of my Speech Pathologists! My Speech Pathologists cannot meet with you! I would like to ask that you not write any of my Speech Pathologists. Can you do that for me? You can contact us in June when you get your Medicare then, and by the way, you're therapist will be Dan when you come!"

Then I thought, *"Oh no! What if this Director of Speech Pathology finds out about my favorite IV helper, Lori? If he lies to her about me because he thinks I'm after the women she might think of me what those college girls thought of me after my Opera Trainers got a hold of me!"*

I wrote Lori a letter begging her not to say, think, and do what some college girls had said and done to me. This was because I was afraid if this Director made her think I was after the women, and just trying to get inappropriate attention from her, she would believe him and begin to act just like these people did. I did not think to explain in the letter where I was getting all my strange sounding statements from. It did not occur to me to tell her that he was the reason I feared she would think all these things about me.

Chapter Eighteen
Tribulation Regional Hospital
Part VI: The Misunderstanding about the Letter
To Lori, the IV Helper

I had a bizarre experience in college where everybody got the wrong idea about me because I was taught to walk, talk and act like someone out of the 1800's from my previous opera instructors. Ever since I was trained to look like them, I was treated like a freak by all my peers. It was my fear that if the Director of Speech Language Pathology lied to Lori about my character and expressed his false opinion about me based on his own lame assumptions that Lori would get the wrong idea about me.

I feared if she believed his lies about me she would say and do the same things the girls I went to college said and did to me based on the body language I learned off of my opera instructors.

I feared all the things they thought about me that were untrue of me would also become her thoughts of what I was like.

This would have been a false view of my character, but I feared she would believe it anyway.

Before those opera people got a hold of me, nobody thought I was crazy and nobody was afraid of me.

Everybody I knew actually just thought I was retarded before that. I liked it better when they thought I was retarded. I'd rather be thought of as a retard than a freak.

I wish I would have never found out I had the voice, then I would have never met those opera people and no one would have ever thought I was crazy.

 I wouldn't have ever gone to college either because that was the only reason I originally went.

The voice professor, I took private lessons from, wanted me to go to college because he thought I would get somewhere with my voice talent.

Then someone told him I was retarded and he changed his mind. If

I hadn't have found out I had the voice and just left everything alone I just would have been considered retarded as usual and everything would have gone a lot better. Then something like this would have never happened. Since I moved to Arkansas nobody up here ever thought those things either.

But like the girl on the "Princess Diaries" movie that was ridiculed by her peers for looking different because of her training to look like a princess instead of a normal everyday person I feared I would be falsely accused of things for looking different too. This girl was made fun of by all her peers and treated like some kind of weirdo and even got cut down verbally by some of her ex-friends because of what these people made her look like. I thought the girl was kind of snooty my self, but still people treated her different after her training. Her friends were even snootier than she was. They thought she was strange. Some of the people she thought were her friends even started playing dirty jokes on her to get back at her for being different. She wound up having a nightmare of a day of the opposites situation at the school she attended all because she was told in the movie by her grandmother that she was really the Princess of Geneva unknown to her. This really stressed her out and even ruined her reputation with people around her. Her grandmother taught her how to carry her body around like these sophisticated, royal acting people that no one in modern day society acts like. Thanks to her training she was thought of as weird because of the way she carried herself. Everyone around her acted like they wondered what was wrong with her. She sure did act weird all of a sudden.

All her peers thought, *"What got into her? What a weirdo?"*

She carried her body around like royalty because that's the way these people taught her to carry her body around.

There were major changes in her body mechanics and body language and she was ridiculed for it.

This is what these opera people did to me. That's why my peers regarded me as a freak from that day forward. Because they did the same thing to me that they did to this girl. This is the reason they made all the accusatory remarks toward me with sexual connotations to them, and also remarks inferring I was a villain that was going to attack somebody, based on my body language. This is what they were complaining about. That body language they continued to pick at me about, every last thing they brought to my attention and everybody else's was their body language. It was the same body language the girl on this movie was taught to have. It looked weird on her and she was treated like a freak.

Ever since I was taught to look and act like they taught this girl to look and act, all the *chipper acting* girls that normally would have thought I was the nicest guy in the world turned on me.

They thought I was a criminal because my body language matched that of the body language of the members of the Metropolitan Opera.

There were usually a couple of serious trended girls with a disgruntled personality that would start making accusations against me based on my body language. They would try to convince the *chipper acting* girls I was some kind of freak based on their "so called" presented facts.

These "so called" facts were based on my body language and not actual facts. These *chipper acting* girls would latch on to what these disgruntled girls said and believe it.

What's worse is that they would pick guys that they thought were slick for their boyfriends, or macho guys that wanted to shift their weight around I would not have wanted to meet in my back alley. They would act like they were afraid of me and these macho guys would protect them from someone like me.

I thought, *"What on earth?!" What is going on here? Why is everybody acting so funny? What's wrong with everybody?"*

These girls may have thought they were safe with them and not safe with me, but let me tell you something. I ran into guys that acted just like these boys before when I was in elementary and junior high school and they were bullies. I actually experienced boys with the same personalities as them jump other boys in back alleys and beat them up at elementary schools when I was around them. I was one of their victims. If they thought they were safe with someone like them they had another thing coming.

My thought was, *"How do you know this macho guy will not turn on you? I wouldn't be afraid of me. I'd be afraid of him. I wouldn't trust him if I were you. He's your wife beater type, not me."*

That's what they said, "He has a swelled jaw. He's going to beat up his wife!"

My first private voice instructor taught me to lock my jaw into a certain position and I had trouble with my jaw locking on me ever since.

Before I met him, everyone always said "Are you trying to catch flies?" because I always dropped my jaw before that.

Now my jaw locked up on me tight as a door latch thanks to him. I remember complaining to the youth director of my church that set me up with this guy for private voice lessons that my jaw was tight and it kept getting stuck since I took lessons from this guy.

Now I was being accused of being a wife beater because I had a swelled jaw and I didn't even have a wife. I was still trying to find a girlfriend in desperation back then hoping someone would have me but everyone thought ill will of me because of what these three men made me look like.

I also found out by this time that I had a swelled jaw because I had impacted wisdom teeth that were far past due to come out.

I also found out recently I have TMJ (Temporomandibular Joint Dysfunction). The dentist already suspected it back then.

They also said things like, "Look at the way he smiled at me! Sexual Harassment!"

I was told by one girl that the corner of my lips were not positioned correctly when I smiled that they were one quarter of the way too much this way or three quarters of the way too much that way.

 I was thinking, *"Since when did people decide there was a mathematically correct way to smile? I smiled the same way I always smiled as far as I knew and no one ever complained about it before this. The only thing I can think of is if my opera training made it look different because of all these body language and mechanics things these guys taught me to do all different."*

One girl told me that I smiled with my teeth and I needed to smile like Mary Kay.

I thought, *"I got made fun of as a kid for smiling like Mary Kay. Now I'm being told I need to look like Mary Kay when I smile some other way?"*

I thought, *"What on earth kind of talk is this? This is ridiculous. I never heard anything like this before."*

I'm pretty sure my private voice instructor taught me to smile with my teeth.

They also said, "A man with a low voice is a villain".

Look at the way he walked in the door, "Weird! Look at the way he picked up the coffee pot! Weird!"

My first private voice instructor from 1986 picked up the coffee pot like a robot and taught me to do the same.

He actually taught me to open a door knob to a door like it was a heavy latch to a bank vault.

As far as the "Look the way he walked in the door part went", my private voice instructor taught me to stand tall, put my shoulders back and walk like a beam pole from one end of the room to the next, or from one destination to the next.

So what they were complaining about there was also his fault.

A guy told me once the girls said I looked a little rowdy because of the way I lifted my shoulders up and locked them into place. Guess who's fault that is, you've got it, the choreographer of the very first opera I was in, the stage director.

The stage director of H.M.S. Pinafore in the town's opera made me raise my shoulders up and back and made me lock them in place. He kept saying, "Like this! No! Like this! Like this! Like this!" He kept acting like, "I don't think he'll ever get it right."

I thought I'd never get it down right for this stage director when he asked me to do my shoulders this way. When I did I got stuck that way for years and couldn't seem to get unstuck. I seemed to be locked into that position permanently whether I liked it or not. And, then I got ridiculed for it. I was a freak or a creep because of it. It wasn't my fault. It was the stage director's fault in the first opera I was in from April to July 1987. He's the one that taught me to look like that and I got stuck looking that way from then on.

The choral director was never satisfied with how loud I was regardless of the fact everyone else thought I was plenty loud enough and he kept saying, "Louder! Louder! Sing up man!"

When I walked down the hall and talked to him once, he said, "I can't hear you! Louder! Louder! Speak up man!"

I was also taught by my first private voice instructor and my stage director to stand tall and walk like a beam pole. I was judged severely by my peers for this because it looked weird to them.

The choral director and the stage director and my voice professor, all three expected me to talk at the top of my lungs at all times as loudly and boldly as the people you see on Broadway shows, especially the choral director of H.M.S. Pinafore.

You think I'm weird because I look different? If it has to do with this kind of stuff, guess why. Them!

These three men did a whole list of things to make me look different. Look at the girl on the Princess Diaries movie. What did they do to her? The list goes on and on.

These college girls also said I was self centered and would never do anything for anybody. I may be a little selfish about a few things, but I would do a lot of things for a lot of people if I thought I could.

Now, if I'm too weak to do whatever it is they ask because of my physical limitations I might not.

Plus, while they were complaining about my being someone that would never do anything for anybody I was building up a hope chest in my closet at home for any girl that would marry me.

You call that not doing anything for anybody.

I wanted to make it special and floor the girl that would have me with nice beautiful gifts.

What these people were suggesting was far from the truth.

And, by the way, to the ones of you that did this to me in the summer of 1991 and the spring and fall of 1994 I have this to say to you. I've been married for 15 years and 9 months now and my wife is very mad at you for all the garbage you said about me.

Big City Hospitals Don't Like Cowards   Brian Evans

I never did anything to anybody and I never did anything to you.

As far as the sexual harassment accusations go which were also based on what I was taught to look like she knows the whole thing is ridiculous and thinks you should have left me alone.

And if you insist on prying, I am not a very sexual person. I do have a drive, but I have a very low drive.

Hasn't it ever occurred to any of you girls in Texas that accused me of all this that most mentally disabled people have low sex drives and some mentally disabled people have no sex drive?

I'm not a sex fiend, I'm a sissy. However, I am not gay. I like girly stuff and have the same kind of emotions as most girls do, but I only looked manly because of what these opera people made me look like. I'm not even the guy type. The guys I hung around were the arts and entertainment kind of guys.

If they hadn't have been I would have hung around mostly girls to begin with and would not have looked funny to them because of what a bunch of opera people made me look like.

And, as far as a comment goes a nice Speech-Language Therapist I liked said to me about "I wouldn't tell girls you like to bowl and ask them to bowl with you because girls don't really like sports and just want to have fun doing things like eating out or going on a picnic or shopping or something." I have no problem with what she said but what she didn't know is, bowling is about the only thing I like to do that guys like to do.

I actually liked this therapist. I'm not complaining about them. I'm just complaining about these other girls I told them about that were giving me a hard time. They were very nice and very understanding of me, but I'm just pointing out that this is one thing they didn't get about me.

 I'm really not into guy stuff, it's just that there's not much left to do besides guy stuff in Abilene accept for the eating out which I also like. I do like miniature golf, which guys might like, but other than that, I like walking nature trails, listening to Christmas records, having Christmas and Birthday parties, eating out, having picnics, playing board games, taking pictures (photographs), painting pictures (paintings), and things like going to antique stores, thrift stores, and gift shops like the ones you see in places like Eureka Springs or Branson, or other country towns in Arkansas.

The problem is, they don't have all this in Texas.

You have to live in Arkansas to get this kind of entertainment, and if girls would have known this is how I felt, they would have thought, "Well, I guess he's not so manly after all. He likes what we like, not what guys like."

Then, maybe these girls would have realized I wasn't a threat to anybody if they knew all this. Bowling and Miniature golf were about the only thing you could do in Abilene besides eat out or go to the Mall, and I'm really not that into the mall. I like gift shops. Why don't you girls in Texas that made these accusations against me pick on someone who really does have a high sex drive and leave me alone?

I never did anything to anybody. I just looked like a stupid robot based on what those stupid opera people made me look like because they choreographed me to look like what you were complaining about in 1987 for the opera production of H.M.S. Pinafore.

Ever since this happened no one will leave me alone.

No one ever accused me of these kinds of things before I met these people, ever.

Some of the accusations started as early as 1986 but that was the year I took private voice lessons from a private voice instructor that made me walk, talk and act like some rich statue acting person from the 1800s. Back then I wasn't accused of sexual harassment yet though, I was just accused of being a womanizer because of what I was made to look like by my High School Peers. And, as soon as my private voice instructor got done messing up what I looked like in the way I carried my body around, one girl said, "He's not retarded! He's crazy!"

Do you want to know something interesting about this comment?

Before I was an okay guy in these girls' eyes but they still didn't consider me worthy of having them for a girlfriend because they thought I was retarded.

Even if I just wanted to be friends with them when they thought I was retarded a lot of them kind of acted like, "Why don't you go play with some retarded people? We don't need you here." But, "before I got out of Special Ed" I was "girl's best friend", and if I did want one of them to be my girlfriend, I got them in a minute, but the minute I stepped into the Regular Classroom setting that all ended.

That was bad in itself, but at least they didn't think I was crazy. They just thought I was retarded. They thought I was just a nuisance and I felt like a fish out of water. At least, I didn't have an identity crisis. That didn't start until I took private voice lessons.

And, then it amplified something fierce after I was in the production of H.M.S. Pinafore in 1987 because I had three of these trainers over me that really messed me up and made me look weird to everybody.

When I met this voice instructor is when this all started. After the opera production in 1987, the problem only dramatically amplified itself because I had a whole crew full of people making me look different from everyone else.

These were not the only two years this kind of thing happened. They were just the two years these specific comments were blurted out about me based on my body language.

I was treated strange by everyone since I met my first private voice instructor in 1986 and he taught me to act this way.

I was seen as being even stranger when the stage director of the opera, H.M.S. Pinafore in 1986 to 1987 made me to look so mechanical him self.

Regardless of this, the worst experience I had with this was in 1991 and 1994 and it only got worse from there all the way from 1994 to 1999 until the day I moved to Arkansas in the year 2000.

Then, the whole thing ended and I was treated like a normal human being again.

 I was telling Lori in the letter I wrote her how I grew up with people that had the relational theory of "You pump me up! I pump you up! You pump me up again!"

I don't think I thought to tell her this, but that is the way Special Ed people react to each other both peer to peer and peer to teacher and teacher to peer. One day, I saw a girl I liked at college and I was excited to see her. She got excited back. So then I got excited back, and then she acted like she was mad because she thought I was to forward. The girl I was telling her about did not understand I was trying to get her to pump me up again. You see that's how they did in Special Ed with each other but I forgot to explain that part.

Now you're probably thinking, "That's just not the way it works in the normal world."

Guess who it does work that way with though besides them, the opera people.

You're thinking, "What?"

My answer is, "You got it buddy, and they're that way too."

I told her how I was interested in this one girl, and I also told her that there were some of them I just wanted to be friends with and others I wanted for girl friends.

I told her that one of the girls I said I needed somebody to said, "I don't think I need anybody that needs me."

I told her how estranged I was a girl would say something like that.

I also pointed out to Lori that one of these girls in College said, "Prince Charming come to save the day is not true love."

I also told her a girl I was just trying to be friends with because I needed a friend said, "I'm not your mother! I'm not your hero! I'm not your girlfriend! What do you want from me anyway?"

I was like floored by all of it and I told her that too and begged her not to be like they were being.

It just didn't occur to me to explain that I only thought she would say things to me like they did because I thought the Director of Speech Pathology was going to lie to her about me and make her think crazy things about me that weren't true.

No one ever talked like that to me before I met my opera trainers. Ever since I met them I've never heard the end of it till I came to Arkansas. I even found out some of these girls, mainly the ones that got the other girls stirred up were mixed up in some kind of New Age Cult.

I let these girls give me trouble over and over again without really defending myself not knowing what to do.

One day, when they were inferring I was going to do something to somebody to watch out for me I asked, "Have I ever done anything that would make you think these kinds of things?"

They said, "No, but you might!"

Sometimes they would come up with these crazy phrases about things that didn't sound right. They would have bits of truth to them but it sounded like there were things being thrown in them that weren't true but I couldn't prove it because they were so clever with their speech I had a hard time even completely making out what they were talking about.

When I tried to call them on these things they would say, "They say! They say!"

I would think, *"Who's they? Is this some kind of phrase going around?"*

I suspected either they were just throwing a bunch of catchy phrases around they heard somewhere that weren't exactly accurate or they were getting it from a cult somewhere and I didn't know it. I actually kind of suspected it. It was really crazy.

If you want to know what these people from the Metropolitan Opera look and act like watch one of their shows. You'll see what I'm talking about. Different isn't it?

Do normal everyday people walk, talk, and act like that? No. Did I walk, talk, and act like that? Yes.

Why? Was it because I naturally walked, talked and acted like that? No.

It was because the opera people that trained me to walk, talk and act like some rich person from the 1800s taught me to act like that and I've been treated like a criminal ever since. I was sick and tired of it. I wanted my true identity back. I'm Brian Evans. I'm not them.

I just got stuck looking like them and wound up displaying what they taught me to look like everywhere because I was stuck that way and couldn't figure out for years how to carry myself my own normal way again or even talk like my own self, until the past few years.

This is why I was worried Lori would think what those college girls thought if the Director of Speech Language Pathology lied to her about me.

I feared if I accidentally looked like one of these people that look and act like people from the Metropolitan Opera thanks to my training I would be falsely accused of things that were not true.

This is especially because what these people crammed down my throat to look like doesn't even look right on me. It doesn't really fit my personality; so as a result, it made me look strange to everybody else just to look right to them.

Training me to look right for the opera was like training Gilligan to look like the Skipper on Gilligan's Isle.

They trained me to look somewhat militaristic which is not my personality and I looked like a walking robot and I got condemned for it because it made every college girl in sight think I was some kind of freak.

It wasn't my fault I looked like this. It was theirs.

And now, I would never hear the end of it from then on and the nightmare of my life would continue forever until I moved to Arkansas in the year 2000.

After these girls acted like this toward me at the colleges because of my body language I've had a series of panic attacks ever since. That's why I panicked on Lori.

The letter to Lori was really nothing more than a panic attack. I wanted to save my identity and I wanted to let her know my needs and beg her not to think I'm being inappropriate for asking her to meet them because I feared she'd think the worst of me if the Director of Speech Pathology lied to her about me.

If I did slip up and looked like these opera people again, even for a moment, I feared that all the accusations that were made against me by these college girls based on my body language I learned off of them would be blasted in my face all over again by the nurses the worked with me.

I was especially afraid of my favorite IV helper nurse acting like this, because the Director of Speech Pathology would lie to her and have her convinced I was a bad person and it wouldn't be true. I feared I would be accused of things that weren't true if I even looked like them for just a moment. It was not the Metropolitan Opera that taught me to look like this, but an opera in Abilene Texas, where people looked and acted just like they did. That is why I was afraid my IV helper nurse would think horrible things about me, because of what they made me look like.

Those mannerisms are their mannerisms, not mine. I thought I'd never get their mannerisms down right for their staging of their plays and once I finally did I got stuck that way. Once they got me to look the way they wanted me to look, everyone thought I was a freak, because I looked like them. Every accusation against me was based on my body language, which was technically their body language, not mine.

On top of all this, there were guys that would come to me in private and tell me they thought I was evil because of what my voice sounded like. My singing voice sounds like Christopher Reeve's speaking voice when he plays Superman. One girl came out and told everybody she thought I had a psychological problem because I sounded like Superman. I can't help it if I sound like Superman.

The guys even told me, "You're talking in your singing voice." when I would talk to people.

Girls would see me in the hall speaking and give me dirty looks because of what I sounded like and say, "Ooh."

Because of the way I was taught to look and sound, I didn't know the difference. Plus this is the way I really sounded. It was hard to shift gears and just sound and look like the normal me when I wasn't practicing for an opera or a play. I displayed this same behavior everywhere and looked really strange every where I went. It was not my fault. I was taught to look like that I naturally sounded like Superman after I was trained to sing up and speak up.

I can't help it that I sound like Superman. That's just the way I sound. These college girls considered it to be a crime for me to sound like Christopher Reeves when he plays Superman when I talk. They had it in for me because I sounded like this. Many of my peers in High School and College said, "I hate to say this but you're really evil. I know that's hard for you to comprehend, but you're evil whether you like it or not because of what you sound like when you sing or because you sound like what you sound like when you talk. You're evil whether you like it or not, you just don't know it."

Many college girls hinted to each other that I was a devil because of what my voice sounded like, and even made the comment, "A man with a low voice is a villain!" They acted like they were scared of me because of what my voice sounded like.

These girls would make absurd comments about my voice and then shirk away from me like they were trying to get away from me. I thought I'd never hear the end of it, or look like the real me. I may never be considered to be the real me ever again, and it was their fault I looked this way. These people ruined my life.

A few years ago, me and Bertha went to a lady's house that had a light display and Bertha talked me into singing for this lady with my tapes because she wanted to impress her.

This lady said, "You know what? You sound like Andrea Bocelli!" I thought, "I do!" After she gave me the tape and let me listen to it, I went back to her and said, "You're right! That's really weird! He really does sound like me! I do sound like him!"

But this excited lady was someone up here in Arkansas, those college girls that gave me trouble over the exact same thing were in Abilene, Texas.

When this Director got the wrong idea, I thought, *"Oh no! My Abilene experience I had that was horrible is about to happen all over again because of him!"*

This Director of Speech Pathology reminded me of my 5th grade History teacher who tried to turn my favorite 7th Grade Special Ed English Teacher against me and I thought this man might do the same thing with my favorite IV helper, Lori.

I kept begging Lori not to think all these crazy things they thought and at the same time I also kept begging her to be the one to comfort me through the IV.

I wanted to ask Lori to rub my head to calm me down and hold my hand through the IV stick but I kept going back and forth with it, like…Please do this for me, but you don't have to if you don't want to but please do this for me. I really need this.

I feared if that man in the Speech Language Pathology Department had anything to do with it, Lori would think I had alternative motives for my wanting her to comfort me, but I did not. And it never even occurred to me the first time to tell Lori in this specific letter that he was the reason I was writing all these bizarre sounding statements in the letter.

It was because of him that I thought Abilene, Texas was going to happen all over again. I was scared for my life.

That's why I wrote the letter in the first place. I thought history was going to repeat itself if this Director of Speech Pathology lied to her about me because of what these opera people made me look like years earlier, and the problem that was once resolved by moving to Arkansas and getting away from those weirdo people that thought these things about me would begin again if he got her to think what they thought. She apparently misunderstood the whole thing. She couldn't figure out what in the world was going on, and thought I'd gone absolutely nuts. In reality I was only trying to defend myself because of this man. I kept begging her to be my IV helper again.

I pleaded with her not to let anything she might misinterpret about me get in the way of being the nurse to comfort me through my IV stick, but just give me a chance anyway.

The whole time, all I wanted was for her to rub my head to calm me down and hold my hand every time I went to her PreOp department for a procedure. I wanted her to be there for me for every procedure I would ever have done in the future because she was the one I was comfortable with, and most of the other nurses I met later were not very nice.

Had I not been taught to look different by my opera instructors, I would not have appeared like a freak to these girls at the colleges. Because of this, I repeated some of the accusatory remarks they made toward me.

I suggested she would say the same things these college girls said and do the same things to me they did to me if she believed the director's lies about me. Because of this, I put words in her mouth she never said, and did not explain this is where I got it from. Plus, I begged her continually to be my IV helper again and asked her to rub my head to calm him down through an IV stick, but feared she would not understand if she believed this director's lies.

So because of this I went back and forth with this request and said, "You don't have to do it if you don't want to, but please if you would could you please do this for me. I beg you. I really need you to do this to be able to get through the IV. Please."

All this is what I think made her misunderstand me. After this we got a phone call.

I answered the phone with my loud as usual, "Hi."

A police officer said, "We have letters here to several of the people at the hospital. I'd like to ask that you not write letters to the hospital again could you do that for me?"

I said, "Yes."

There was a police officer that went to the Church we attended so Bertha asked him, "If a police officer called Brian and asked him not to write anymore letters to the hospital do you think it would be okay if I went to the hospital to explain Brian to them?"

He said, "That's a good idea, I think it should be fine."

Since the officer thought it would be fine after my next appointment we went to the hospital to talk to Lori. When we walked up to the desk where she was usually sitting, she was not there.

Bertha asked, "Is there any way we can talk to Lori? It is very important."

The person behind the desk handed her a slip of paper and said, "You can use that phone and dial her extension."

Bertha went to the phone and called the extension she was given and this is what happened.

She said, "Hi, I'm Bertha Evans. Is this Lori? I really need to talk to you about my husband Brian."

Lori said, "It will have to be quick! I only have a minute to talk to you in the waiting room."

Bertha said, "It will take more than a minute."

She said, "I get off at 2:30."

"Okay, we will wait for you to get off work. It's very important we get to talk to you."

Since it was 2:00 I assumed if we waited she'd come and talk to us when she got off work.

At 2:20 here comes a police officer and asked, "What are you doing here?"

"We came to talk to Lori." Bertha answered.

"No, but why did you come here? You drove two hours to come up here just to talk to her. Why are you here?"

Bertha told him again why we were there, "We came to talk to Lori."

The officer asked, "Has someone upset you? Are you mad at somebody? Why are you here?"

The officer frankly stated, "I get a little nervous about things like this."

The officer proceeded to frisk me right there in the waiting area! He acted like he thought I had a weapon or a gun!

Of course he didn't find anything. I don't have guns because they make me very uncomfortable and I don't want to have a thing to do with them either. One thing that will confirm this fact, are the Men's retreats at my church. If I know they are going to do a shooting range or hunt deer or anything like that I always say, "No thanks."

As far as weapons are concerned, this guy was wasting his time there too, because I never carry any weapons, and I would never hurt anyone. I have no weapons. I never do.

As a matter of fact a coworker at Wal-Mart tried to give me a big, fancy light blue pocket knife for a gift during the Christmas gift exchange at work fifteen years ago and I didn't want it and it made me depressed.

When I told Bertha, she said, "You have the receipt don't you? Just trade it in for something else." So I traded it in for a watch. The guy was not very happy with me but I did it anyway because I didn't want a knife. I like girl stuff. I don't care for guy gifts. I like Christmas trinkets and antique girl dolls and candles and flowers and kid movies and all kinds of pretty stuff. I'm not into guy stuff. I like what little kids and girls like to entertain myself.

I enjoy the things a child would enjoy, not a man.

Bertha said my eyes were huge, and she thought my eyes were going to fall out, I was so scared! I didn't know what in the world was going on, but I was very cooperative and did everything just as the officer directed.

She was scared too and I thought they were going to take me to jail. She didn't know what to do. She had no idea what was going on.

I told the policeman, "We can go over the content of the letters if you want to."

Bertha didn't know what letters I meant, because she didn't know I sent all those letters in order to defend myself.

The officer just said, "Oh no. I'm not even going to go over the content!"

She said she was glad the officer did not discuss what was in the letters because she didn't think she'd be able to stick up for me not knowing what was in them. But she knew I was innocent. She has had to explain me to people because I get misunderstood for writing quite often. It's easier for me to write out my feelings than it is to tell someone about them.

She has told me, "No matter what anyone writes, depending on the mindset of the reader, it can be taken many different ways."

I do not have reasoning skills that would have helped me to write the letters in a way that I would not have been taken wrong. If only I would have thought to have her proof read the letters, instead of sending them behind her back, she would have been able to pick out and change the parts that were obviously taken wrong.

The policeman looked at me and said, "The hospital has a stack of letters 14 inches thick that you have written to several different people."

Bertha has pointed out to me that because there have been murderers who did the exact same thing; the hospital was trying to protect its employees. But if they just would have read just one of these letters they would have figured out that I was not a criminal. She wishes we would have known before all this happened that I had autism not just autistic tendencies.

She told the officer, "Brian has an anxiety disorder, and autistic tendencies."

The officer said, "The law doesn't recognize disabilities."

She said, "Brian is autistic, and people with autism are not able to communicate like you and I. Some people with autism can't even talk. Brian can talk, but his method of communication is writing, which is why there were so many. The letters were long, because he shared every detail of his entire life with everyone, and more than once, I'm quite sure."

The officer took us downstairs. While we were walking, Bertha told me to let her do all the talking. We went into a small room where two deputies were sitting there waiting for us. She was so scared. We were outnumbered and the only experience she had with an officer was to get her out of her abusive home as a child. The officer had obviously made up his mind that I was dangerous.

I told him, "I know a policeman in Berryville that knows what kind of person I am. Can I have him explain me to you?"

The officer said, "That won't be necessary. I don't need to talk to him. You were told on the phone not to come to the hospital."

Bertha remembered me telling her that the officer asked me not to write or call the hospital, which I hadn't done; he never said a thing about going to the hospital.

The officer said, "If you are so concerned about which nurse you get, get your doctor talk to the hospital about it. Only a doctor can say who will be your nurse."

After the officer was done getting on to us, he showed us a shortcut out of the hospital. He wouldn't let us talk to anybody.

We were both traumatized by the whole thing. We went to the Urologist's office across the street and I told the doctor what just happened. My own doctor didn't understand why it was so important to me.

We found out later everybody, the Urologist included, thought that I was stalking Lori. I wasn't stalking Lori. I was just begging for mercy.

This whole mess happened on January 5th.

Finally, we had saved up the money to have me tested to see if I had full blown autism, not just the tendencies, but the soonest appointment was January 19th.

On the phone when Bertha called about the cost she was told it was supposed to cost $475.00 because it would take three one hour sessions to diagnose me. I was 35 years and ten months old when I was tested for autism. I took everything. I had all my childhood medical records as well as every report ever made about me by therapists and counselors.

I handed my big stack of records to the psychologist, "These are my childhood records."

"Wow! How did you get them all?" the lady psychiatrist asked.

I answered, "I've been collecting them my entire life."

She took her time and read every one of them. She then gave me an oral test.

She asked me, "Why did they not diagnose you as a child?"

I said, "I don't know?"

Bertha told her, "Brian has a needle phobia and an over sensitivity to pain. He can't help it when he freaks out when there is a needle involved."

She asked, "Have you ever tried Emla?"

Bertha said. "No, what's that?"

The Psychiatrist said, "It's a cream you put on the site they plan to do the stick one hour before the procedure and it will numb the area and make it hurt less."

Bertha said that even though I still scream and cry a lot, I have actually done a whole lot better since I started using the Emla or the generic version, Lidocaine, before getting stuck for procedures.

Big City Hospitals Don't Like Cowards   Brian Evans

This lady psychiatrist said, "It is so obvious from the records and the things you have told me about the present that you don't need to come back. You have autism active."

Thanks to that, instead of paying the $475.00 that we saved, we only had to pay $175.00!

That made 25 years since my mother first thought I had the disorder and nobody ever tested me for it. My mother knew my behavior matched perfectly with an autistic child. When she asked to have me tested they told her that I was too old. People don't grow out of autism. If you are autistic you are always autistic!

Chapter Nineteen
Tribulation Regional Hospital
Part VII: The GI Experience

I had to go to the Urologist about every two weeks.

The urologist said, "Your problem is an overactive sphincter. I think it should get fixed since I made an incision in it."

 Bertha didn't think it would work because I was still having trouble urinating.

The urologist said, "I can't do another sphincterectomy because you would be incontinent and urinate all over yourself."

I replied with, "I don't know what to do but I keep having pencil lead streams and occasional dribbling. You have to do something."

He said, "I am eventually going to have to go in and see what's going on. Give it some time to heal."

After almost six months of not being able to urinate correctly the urologist decided he better do something regardless of the problems I had at the hospital. My Medicare did not start until June 1st so the urologist made me wait until June 7th.

I kept bugging Bertha saying the same thing about Lori and it was driving her up the wall. I was stressed out and complained over and over.

I would desperately say, "I've got to have Lori for my IV helper! I don't want anybody else! I want Lori! They've got to give me Lori! I don't want to go to GI! I want to go to PreOp! They've got to do something! They've got to give me Lori! I don't want a different nurse! I want her!"

The urologist's nurse insisted I would go to the GI department instead of PreOp. She claimed to have talked to Lori in PreOp.

The urologist's nurse said she talked to her and Lori had told her, "If at all possible, if I am working that day, I will be his IV helper. If not the lady in the GI department will do it."

When I got there, I was supposed to ask for Lori to help me, but when I did, they claimed they didn't hear anything about her coming over there. I insisted they call Lori. They finally called her, or pretended to call her.

They said that Lori said she couldn't come over there, because she was too busy with other patients. I was upset I didn't insist they send me to the PreOp department like I did the time before when I had the surgery and wanted to go over there so they would give me the gas. Bertha already figured that Lori wasn't going to come clear to GI to help me. She was right.

When they took me in a room, Bertha noticed a security guard following me everywhere. He stood outside of the room I was in.

The nurse told me, "You can change into your gown, but if you're too embarrassed you can wait a few minutes."

I think they said this because of the letter I sent to Lori about the nurses humiliating me on 3rd floor west.

I changed into my hospital gown and after several minutes this boring IV nurse came in to do my IV. She was not near as good as the original IV sticker, Carley that I liked. I reached out and at least she let me hold her hand for a minute.

She said, "Now let go of my hand okay."

She really hurt my feelings because I really needed her comfort to get through the IV because IVs are hard to handle and I feel pain much louder than everybody else and sticking an IV in me is like being stabbed with a butcher knife.

I asked her, "Can you put it in my right arm?"

She looked for a spot and tried to put the IV in. I screamed very loudly.

Another nurse in the GI department said, "You're going to have to go ahead and put him in the Cysto Suite! I can't take anymore of this screaming! He's scaring the other patients!"

It was a few minutes before they took me to the Cysto Suite.

Bertha talked to the IV nurse out in the hall and said, "You're going to have to put him out! He can't be awake or he'll freak out!"

The nurse said, "He's going to be a little woozy! He won't be completely knocked out!"

Bertha said again, "You're going to have to put him out! You can't let him be awake! He's going to freak out!"

She told Bertha, "He won't remember a thing."

She seemed to be ignoring her.

She told her again, "I'm telling you, he's going to freak out if you don't!"

Bertha was afraid this nurse would not cooperate with her but when she got finished arguing with her she said she would knock me out. She thought it was a miracle they gave in because they were being so particular about it.

I saw the security guard in the hallway and eventually another man went in the hall and started talking to Bertha. I assumed he must have been the Administrator.

They finally took me in the Cysto Suite and the security guard followed me in there. Bertha looked at me like she was worried I'd have to do everything awake.

The doctor finally came in and I said, "Your going to have to put me completely out. I can't handle it if you don't!"

The doctor said, "Okay I'll have them put a little something in your IV."

The doctor and the IV nurse looked at the Security Guard and the doctor said, "We won't be needing you in here."

The security guard actually acted like he thought the whole thing was ridiculous and wondered why he was even there. He went along with it though and never said anything.

After my dilatation was over the Security Guard, the doctor, and the IV nurse all three wheel chaired me to the car.

Bertha said, "I never want to go back to this hospital. They don't deserve another cent of our money!"

They treated me like I was a criminal! I drove Bertha up the wall so much about wanting Lori that she finally decided to put me on some medicine because of my anxiety over this whole situation because it was too incredible a situation for me to handle.

I wrote very long letters to my Urologist about how horrible I was treated at the hospital and insisted people treat me like a normal human being instead of a criminal. Later I got a letter from the Urologist's office stating my letters were offensive and that they wanted me to cease the correspondence immediately. If the Director of Speech Pathology at their hospital, would have minded his own business and let me just explain to people what I needed and let Bertha explain to everybody how I was and stayed out of everything, this whole event would have never took place in the first place. In the letter I received from the Urologist they stated that they were going to schedule me to be seen when there were no other patients scheduled.

They said I caused too many distractions in the waiting room when they tried to get another patient for the doctor.

Bertha took this letter to say basically, "You're no longer welcome here."

I was still having a lot of problems going to the bathroom so we were on a search for an Urologist yet again. We found one Urologist's office that made me an appointment.

We were told, "Sorry. We can't see you till we get the records from your current Urologist."

We made another appointment. When we came back the doctor acted really funny.

The Urologist asked Bertha, "What about all the letters Brian has written?"

Bertha said, "My sweet, dear, autistic husband finally found a nurse that was able to get him through an IV. Brian wrote letters asking her to be his IV helper. The letters were misunderstood."

The Urologist said, "I can't take him because of the stalking letters."

Every other Urologist we tried refused me right away. That's why we didn't immediately sign a medical records release. We were tired of being let down. Bertha was so afraid she was going to become a widow because we just could not find an Urologist. I wrote all these letters in panic because of a past experience similar to the one I currently faced. It freaked me out, and even thought I didn't make it clear what I was talking about. I just didn't want Lori to act like the people in Abilene, Texas. The comments I made were simply repeats of what girls in Abilene said to me when I was younger. If I had not been scared of history repeating itself I would have never written the letters in the first place. (To get a broader understanding of what happened at the colleges in Abilene read Autism Undiagnosed Part Two, Will I Always Be an Outcast?)

Chapter Twenty

New Experience with General Surgeon Who Did an EGD
On Me and Then Introduced Me to A Nicer Urologist
Who Understood My Emotional Needs and Accepted Me

Not only was I having urinary issues but I was also having multiple bowel movements.

My family doctor said, "I think we need to do a colonoscopy."

I said, "Okay."

He said, "I'll set you up a PreOp appointment with a surgeon."

I said, "Okay."

We went into the office for my PreOp visit. He explained exactly what was going to happen. This surgeon was extremely sweet to us both. Bertha literally broke down.

She said, "We can't seem to find an Urologist for Brian and he is having a very hard time going pee. I'm too young to be a widow. I'm really worried because nobody will help him thanks to a horrible experience we had with a hospital. It is very important that Brian gets to have happy go lucky *female* nurses. I don't want to go through that again!"

The surgeon said, "In this case, you need to give him a little more slack. Brian just needs to find a circle of doctors who understand his autism."

When I went for my colonoscopy I asked Bertha to tell the doctor's nurse to see to it that I got all happy go lucky nurses. The nurses all needed to be *female* because I am very uncomfortable with men.

I told the surgeon, "I particularly need the IV sticker to be happy go lucky. I need another nurse that is very happy go lucky to hold my hand and rub my head to calm me down."

Bertha called the hospital and told them herself, even though she had already told the surgeon, she wasn't taking any chances!

Come to find out, all of my nurses were *female* but the person doing the IV was a guy. This made me very nervous.

"I'm really scared!" I told the guy that was going to do my IV.

He thankfully said, "Because of your autism we are just going to go ahead and give you the gas first. We will put the IV in after you fall asleep okay?"

This made me very happy. Before they put me to sleep with the gas I got to see all five of my PreOp nurses. My two favorite ones got to stand next to where my head was. They were all lined up from head to foot.

When the test was over the doctor told me, "You have a stretched out colon and your stomach and colon are both very inflamed. Other than that everything was normal and no major diseases were present."

I said, "Okay."

I was so happy he found something wrong. Now that they knew what was the problem they would be able to fix it. I was so happy with how this hospital handled me compared to the horrible hospital experience.

Bertha went to medical records and said, "Brian is autistic, it is very important that he get the same people every time he is in here. Can we put it in Brian's file that he gets the same people?"

From what I understood, it's set. And every time since, when I had to go to the hospital I was able to have the same people, if they were working.

The next time we went to see the surgeon he told us, "I know a *female* Urologist who is familiar with autism, would you like for me to make you an appointment with her?"

In unison we both said, "Yes!"

We went straight home and I got a call almost as soon as we walked in the door.

"Mrs. Evans, Brian's appointment is tomorrow at 3:00."

The receptionist told her where it was and what the doctor's name was. She told me what her name was and she said I wrinkled my nose when she told me.

I told Bertha, "I hope she is nothing like the man who messed me up in the first place!"

She said, "She must be related to have the same last name, but I believe she has to be better or the surgeon wouldn't have even bothered setting you up with her?"

I agreed.

When Bertha took me to my appointment the next day with the *female* Urologist, we were hoping for the best. We had been let down so many times and we were running out of options.
The surgeon must have advocated for me because the appointment went very well. We sat in a very crowded little waiting room. I thought we would be waiting for ever. Almost as soon as we sat down we heard.

A very pleasant nurse said, "Brian."

I jumped up and immediately gave her a hug.

She said, "Thank you Brian."

She led us to a room and said, "Mrs. Dr. Scotty will be right with you."

Then I gave her another hug.

She said, "Another hug! Thank you, Brian?"

She had a sweet smile on her face as she left.

Mrs. Dr. Scotty walked in right as she left. She was a small, pleasant acting, smiling and a very happy go lucky doctor. I was grinning from ear to ear. I jumped up again and hugged the doctor. I was so excited I got such a nice doctor.

"Thank you Brian." She responded.

The nurse did a bladder scope on me and said, "Brian! You still have 600 to 900 ml? Did you go as much as you could?"

I said, "Yeah?"

I wondered why she had such a bewildered reaction to the bladder scope.

Mrs. Dr. Scotty did an exam on me and said, "Brian, because you held so much urine, we need to do a Cystoscopy to see what's going on. I don't do surgeries on men so I want you to meet my husband Dr Scotty. He is very sweet, you'll love him."

She left the room and came back in shortly with a man wearing a big friendly smile.

"This is my husband Dr. Scotty." she said proudly.

"Hello Brian! I understand that we need to do a Cystoscopy."

Frantically I pleaded with fear in my eyes, "Can you put me to sleep? It feels like a sword being run through me!"

Dr. Scotty sweetly said, "We don't normally put people to sleep for this procedure but don't you worry because in your case we will!"

I was set up to have a Cystoscopy as soon as Dr. Scotty could fit me in. Dr. Scotty greeted me with so much kindness which is what I needed. He was the nicest doctor I have ever known.

Bertha said, "The best part is he liked you and you just loved him."

When we went to the PreOp department to register for my Cystoscopy, and do pretesting, I was able to look around at all the nurses to see who I liked. I picked who I wanted. Bertha told them I needed all happy go lucky *female* nurses no men. She also said that if they sent me to the inpatient department, the same needed to go for them. She told them I needed knocked out for any and all invasive procedures and I needed to apply Lidocaine one hour before the stick. She also told them that I needed a happy go lucky *female* nurse to rub my head to calm me down and hold my hand while another happy go lucky *female* nurse stuck me with the IV. I was able to choose everybody I wanted. Since they were told exactly what I needed every one of my needs were met.

One of them said, "Why don't we put this in your chart, and then when you go to other departments like inpatient it will be in there and they will know to give you who they need and know what they need to do for you? Would you like that?"

I said, "Yes! I'd like that a lot! Then I can get happy go lucky *female* nurses everywhere I go and they will all know what they need to do for me to!"

When they started the IV, Rosie, Freda, and Anna helped me with my IV. I asked Rosie if she could rub my head to calm me down and hold my hand when I'm stuck with the IV.

She said, "Yes."

So when they were ready, Rosie rubbed my head to calm me down and held my hand while Anna stuck me with the IV and Freda braced my arm down so I wouldn't jerk and also tried to comfort me. It all worked out wonderful. I also told them I wanted the gas, but they still made me do the IV first. When they wheeled me into the surgery room I got to see them all before they gassed me out and hugged them all before they started.

When I went in for the procedure, I noticed all the scary instruments lying on a table next to where I was, and I feared them with my life.

Dr. Scotty reassured me with, "Now don't you worry about the stuff on the table, we are not going to use any of it till you are knocked out okay Brian."

I said, "Okay."

They then put the gas mask on me and said, "You just breathe this gas and relax and go to sleep and you'll never know anything ever happened, because we're all going to do everything while you're asleep and you'll be completely knocked out so you won't know anything."

I fell asleep, and Dr. Scotty began the Cystoscopy procedure. Dr. Scotty was not able to find any blockage. I was left in the hospital for a day with a catheter in me to get the flow readjusted but it did not work. We went to a follow up appointment the next week hoping for some relief.

Dr. Scotty said, "I hate to do this to you because I don't want to hurt you and I want you to know that I would never do anything to hurt you, but we're going to have to do a Urodynamics study to see what's going on with your bladder and unfortunately you'll have to do it awake. After this test you'll never have to do a procedure awake again, but we have to do it this time to see what's going on and it's the only way we can find out for sure what is going on."

Chapter Twenty One

New Experience with a Wonderful Urologist Who Understood My Emotional Needs and Met Them

Dr. Scotty at Dreamer's Hope Regional Hospital saw that I was wide open on my Cystoscopy. Since I was still having trouble retaining too much urine he decided to do an Urodynamics test on me.

Dr. Scotty unfortunately said to me, "Brian, you are wide open but I know you still have a problem holding urine so we need to do an Urodynamics."

I pleaded for mercy again. "Can you knock me out?"

He said, "No, I'm Sorry. I'm not going to do anything to try to hurt you but I really think we need to find out what's wrong."

I was so scared. I would say to Bertha over and over and over again, "I don't want to do it awake!"

She was glad it was scheduled for just a few days later because I was driving her crazy!

There were several nurses in the room. The surgery table was freezing cold when I got on it.

Dr. Scotty said, "Now Brian, hold my hand. I'm right here. I know this is difficult for you but we're going to try to get you through this."

My eyes got even bigger when I saw the catheter that Rosie was going to put in me. Rosie got ready to thread the catheter up my urethra into my bladder.

"I'll go slow and be as gentle as possible, okay Brian? You can do this! I know you can!"

214

Rosie did her best to pump me up to be able to have the courage to do an Urodynamics again. The first Urodynamics, years ago, did not go too well.

Rosie looked at me with her eyes full of sweetness and compassion as she started to put the catheter in.

I screamed loudly, "AHHH!"

I was gasping for air.

"What do you plan to do special after this is over with?" Anna one of the nurses asked me.

Right when I tried to answer her question Rosie pushed a little more.

I screamed, "AHHH!"

"I'm sorry we need to do this." Rosie tried to sympathize with me.

"Do you have any plans this weekend?" Dr. Scotty asked.

Once again right when I tried to answer Rosie pushed the catheter a little further.

My answer was, "AHHH!"

I had a death grip on the edge of the surgery table. My knuckles were white.

"What colors do you like?" Susie another nurse asked trying to distract me as Rosie pushed the catheter again.

I groaned really loudly, "UGH!"

"I'm sorry Brian." Rosie said sweetly then she pushed a little more.

I screamed, "AHHH!" I was in horrendous pain.

"Try not to think about it okay. What do you like to do for fun?" asked yet another nurse, Tina.

My reply was, "AHHH!" yet again.

Finally Rosie smiled reassuringly and said, "You can relax now, we're in!"

The pain subsided till they touched the catheter to squirt water backwards up my urethra into my bladder.

I screamed all the more, "AHHH!"

"Sorry Brian. Now we need you to try to urinate." Dr. Scotty said.

I tried as hard as I could, but nothing would come out. They gave me several minutes to try to go but I just could not urinate. My catheter was connected to a machine with many different tubes connected to it.

"Maybe if we leave you will be able to relax, and be able to urinate. Press this call button after you are able to urinate and we will come back in here okay?"

No matter how hard I tried, I just could not urinate. I really wanted to be able to go, but I was not looking forward to them taking it out. I was scared. Nurses kept coming in my room to see if I was able to urinate.

After over an hour, I was finally able to go just a little. I was desperately wishing somebody would come and check on me.

Anna, one of the PreOp nurses finally walked in the room.

"I finally got to go!" I said proudly.

"I'm glad. Dr. Scotty has other surgeries and we need to get finished so he can do them."

I agreed, "Yeah."

The nurse said, "Now let me try to remove these tubes from you."

I freaked out, I was so scared I panicked and admitted, "It's gonna hurt!"

She tried to encourage me by telling me exactly what she was doing.

She said, "I'm letting the air out then it will just slip out okay?"

I didn't believe her so I frantically watched her pull the catheter out.

I yelled in panic, "AHHH!"

She sweetly apologized to me, "I'm sorry."

After Anna was all done I was shocked and told her, "Taking it out didn't hurt near as bad as putting it in."

She said, "You can get dressed now."

Having done the test he needed to do, his suspicions were right; my bladder was shutting down at only 36-years old! It was a horrible result of being treated for the wrong problem for years. When we talked to Dr. Scotty after the procedure I sure was glad it wasn't too late to do something about it.

Dr. Scotty said, "I'm going to prescribe you a medicine that will force the bladder to work, Bethenecol. You will have to take it for the rest of your life Brian."

I said, "Okay."

We were so happy that we were finally able to find an Urologist who would take me seriously. I still had problems urinating but it wasn't nearly as bad as before. Dr. Scotty eventually had to do an operation to put a pubic catheter in, which I had to wear for two and a half months.

When Dr. Scotty removed the pubic catheter, I was put on the maximum dose of Bethenecol. I still have a little trouble urinating, but it is tolerable.

We were so happy that we were finally able to find an Urologist who would take me seriously. Dr. Scotty found the problem and fixed it as best he could.

Chapter Twenty Two

Trouble Getting Doctors to Believe I Have Hyperthyroidism

Believe it or not I've also had problems with doctors believing me about the heart problem and the thyroid problem as well. Take a wild guess why. You're not 50 years old! They wonder how I could possibly have anything like that wrong.

I came down with Hyperthyroidism in July 1991 and was diagnosed with this disorder when I told Dr. Alan C. Hardwicke of Abilene, Texas about it. At the time I would get these energy spurts that lasted three hours. Then I would start to feel tired and my pulse would rise. My temperature would also rise to a low grade fever. About thirty minutes later I would bottom out.

I told him, "You're going to think this is crazy, but this is what's happening."

He said, "It sounds like Hyperthyroidism."

He verified it on a Radioactive Iodine Uptake Test.

He said, "Just as I thought, your T3 uses up your Iodine in excess. That's when it gives you enormous energy at first. Then when the Iodine is gone you bottom out. Because your T3 sucked it all out of you and there isn't any left to give you energy."

He also found it on a T3 blood test he took by itself. TSH and T4 were normal. T3 would be high one month, normal the next, and high again the next. It was really weird. Every time I told a doctor about this they acted like they thought I was crazy because they couldn't find it on a blood test. Most of them insisted on only testing TSH. That's part of the reason they couldn't find anything. If and when they took a T3 it must have been at the wrong time for it to show high because it was always normal.

]

I went to Dr. Kevin in 2011 and 2012; he said his blood test turned out normal also. When I told him, it won't show up on a blood test he decided to do a thyroid sonogram. It actually showed an enlargement. He also did a Radioactive Iodine Uptake Test and it showed up on the High side of Normal. But because it was still in the normal range, he insisted on Levothyroxine which is for Hypothyroidism, instead of Hyperthyroidism.

I told him that medicine was for Hypo and I had Hyper, but he said, "Your thyroid was normal. I'm just treating the goiter."

Apparently Levothyroxine is for goiter too?

Because of my schooling I know a lot about medical stuff so I said, "Yeah, but the numbers lean toward the high end. The normal range is 5 to 20. Anything below 5 is Hypothyroidism, and anything above 20 is Hyperthyroidism. Don't you think it is Hyperthyroidism? It's a whole lot closer to Hyper than Hypo."

He just said, "I know. Still. I'm just treating the goiter, and as long as the numbers aren't in the high range I'm not worried about it."

Actually, for my condition you are supposed to take Potassium Iodide, Radioactive Iodide, Sodium Iodide, Propylthiuracil, Methamazole or Tapazole according to my Pharmacology book for the Pharmacology class I took in 1990 and 1991. Those are for Hyperthyroidism and the sole purpose of those is to knock down T3. That is what I need them to do, knock down the T3 levels. The only problem is you have to be careful with the dosage or you could get too strong a dose. The medicines you take for this kind of problem are dangerous. They can even damage your liver and cause possible kidney failure. It's a very complicated mess, so I just take supplements when I take something.

I used to take Potassium Iodide supplements. Before that, I took Weight Loss Vitamins with a low dose of Potassium Iodide. Back when I went to Dr. Hardwicke for it, there were no supplements for it, only prescription medications.

In 2013 I took Thyroid Caps. They worked slower but were less dangerous and didn't cause side effects. I tried to restart them in 2015 but they didn't seem to agree with me that time so I just quit retaking them after a couple of pills.

Back in the first decade of this new millennium, my doctors were getting to where they had to raise my Tenormin (Atenelol) because of my weight gain. It got doubled, then tripled, then quadrupled, and even had stuff added to it later. In 2009 I lost weight from 242 pounds to 170 pounds when I did a low carb diet for nine months.

I was able to gradually knock down my blood pressure medicine after that, and eventually got back down to one 50mg per day pill of Tenormin (Atenelol) again.

Then, after the stress of trying to sell our other house in 2010 and 2011, I gained most of the weight back. We had to drive back and forth a 90 mile round trip to our new house. We had to pack up everything at one house and drag it to the new house. Then when we moved into the new house we had to unpack everything and reorganize it all over again. We had to fix up the old and new house in the process just to get the whole thing taken care of. The whole thing was very stressful. I had to eat like crazy again just to handle the pressure of the situation again, just like I did when I worked at my last two jobs. That's how I gained the weight back. I ate myself to death to build stamina to handle the pressure of the situation. I was very tired otherwise. Eating like crazy and shoving caffeinated beverages down my throat on a consistent basis is how I handle it and as a result, the weight came back.

About the spring of 2013, my low dose Tenormin (Atenelol) was starting not to work again.

When I told Dr. Johnny about it, I said "I think I need to double the medicine again because it's not working."

He said, "I think I ought to change your medicine all together." He gave me Amlodopine instead which raised my pulse.

I told him, "The reason I was given Tenormin (Atenelol) in the first place is to treat the symptoms of Hyperthyroidism. When my blood pressure became a problem he kept me on it for that reason too. It was originally given to me for rapid pulse in order to slow my pulse down. I also continued taking it as my blood pressure became a problem. These other doctors just doubled the dose when it no longer helped my blood pressure. I'm tired a lot and I have Hyperthyroidism. I think we ought to just double it like they did. The last time I gained the weight that's what they did. When I lost weight, I didn't need as much and they lowered it again, but now that I've regained most of my weight, I think I need it doubled again."

Dr. Johnny said, "I don't think it's your thyroid. I think it's your medicine. Tenormin (Atenelol) can make you tired."

At first, I was less tired on the new medicine he gave me, but within a week or two I was just as tired as I was when I took the Tenormin (Atenelol). The Amlodopine he gave me dramatically escalated my pulse and made my blood pressure even worse than it was.

Before he switched me, I was having 150/100 with a 95 to 104 pulse regularly. Now that I was taking Amlodopine, I was averaging 174/114 with a 114 pulse. That is dangerous. This guy didn't believe me, and thought I was just anxious, because I came into his office. He thought it was only up because I was nervous.

One day, I went in there, and I said, "Do you know that your nurse got these figures when she took my blood pressure and pulse?"

Dr. Johnny said, "No. I didn't know that. She didn't tell me."

I said, "Well, don't you think that's something I need to worry about?"

He said, "I don't believe it. I think you were just anxious because you were nervous about coming in here. Lay down in this chair for 20 minutes and I will have this nurse come in and take your blood pressure again."

The nurse finally came in there and got the same figures again.

She said, "174/114 Blood Pressure and a 114 pulse, it was the same!"

He finally came in and I said, "She got the same figures again."

He said, "She did!"

He said, "I'm changing your medicine. I'm going to add another component to your Amlodopine, so now you will be taking Amlodopine/Benazaprine and I'm raising the dose."

This only worked better about a week, and then it was worse again. I thought I'd never catch him on the phone. Finally I got through and was put on hold. I thought they forgot about my call and nearly hung up.

The receptionist finally said, "Your doctor wants you to make another appointment to go over it again."

He already messed with it two or three other times before this and I got frustrated and wanted to see somebody else for it. He always would come in the room to talk to me, barely ask me a couple of things each visit, type a note or two on his lap top and tell me he would be back in a minute yet never come back?

A nurse would come in and say, "Well, you're ready to go."

I'd ask, "Ready? This guy hasn't even finished with me yet."

I tried to tell him about my medical problems blew me off like whatever I said didn't matter.

I started writing him letters trying to explain what was wrong with my stomach as far as inflammation, pain, ulcers, etc. I also told him about the childhood heart defects I had in the letters, which he didn't believe. I even told him in the letters how I concluded I had a thyroid problem based on the symptoms I had which matched what Dr. Alan Hardwicke said was Hyperthyroidism, years ago. He got mad.

He had me come to his office and said, "We need to talk. I can't have you constantly writing me letters trying to tell me what's wrong with you. I don't have time for all this. And you're constantly coming in to visit the nurses and trying to tell them what's wrong. You give them papers to give to me to explain things, if you need to tell me something you could just tell me. I also can't ask my nurses to meet all these unusual requests you ask just to get through a needle stick. I have like five other patients I have to deal with and I don't have time to read all your stuff. I don't have time to go over all the details. If you're going to be this high maintenance you need to find another doctor to meet your needs because I can't do it here. I don't have time to go over all this detail trying to figure out what you are trying to tell me what's wrong with you. There is nothing wrong with your thyroid. If there is something wrong with your thyroid I'll tell you there is. So instead of telling me what you think is wrong, you need to listen to me and let me decide what's wrong. I'm the doctor. There's nothing wrong with your thyroid. Just don't keep writing me stuff anymore trying to explain everything or I'm going to have ask you to find somebody else to provide your services for you. See you next week."

I finally got tired of his attitude and his complacency and his unwillingness to work with me on my blood pressure medicine. My pastor suggested I go to Dr. Go Fish and I did. This doctor immediately put me back on the Tenormin (Atenelol) and doubled it as I suggested and it fixed the problem.

Doctor Go Fish said, "Well you know, I'm not really that wild
about that doctor and the way he does things. He could use a little
more wisdom about things. One thing you need to know, doctors
don't like to be told what's wrong. That's the problem. He didn't
like it that you told him what was wrong, and you were right.
He didn't want to admit that because he didn't want to feel like his
own patient figured it out on his own. He wants to be able to feel
like he's the one that figured it all out."

Dr. Go Fish worked out okay for a while, and even had two nice
nurses that happily accommodated me with my blood tests and
comforted and consoled me the way I needed them to with no
problem and no complaints about having to do it whatsoever.

The problem is, every time I tried to tell the doctor I was having a
problem with my stomach or my heart or my ankles or something,
he barely examined me. Sometimes he didn't even exam me at all.
They did actually do an EKG a couple of times and an x-ray on my
foot once because of the clamping problem I was having that was
similar to what my shoulder was doing. He didn't even believe me
about the thyroid thing. He said he didn't want to do a Thyroid
sonogram on me because my TSH was normal. Because of this, I
went behind his back and had the surgeon who did my hernia
surgery, Dr. Wonderful do a thyroid sonogram on me and my
thyroid showed up even more enlarged that time than when Dr.
Kevin did it.

He would say, "Oh I wouldn't worry about it. I think it's just this,
but if you have any more problems let me know, and I'll see you
again in three months."

It got to where I would go in for a follow up and he would say
something like, "So did you go to the lake this weekend? Have
you gone fishing or seen any fish? What are you doing right
now?"

I'd wind up telling him whatever it was. I had no problem with
socializing with him, but that's all he wanted to do.

I would ask, "What about my stomach pain?"

"What about my heart problem or palpitations?"

"What about my ankle problem?" (I would ask about whatever the problem was at that time.)

Dr. Go Fish would just say, "Well at your age I just wouldn't climb any ladders or walk on any roofs but other than that I think you're just fine."

Dr. Go Fish didn't even examine me.

Each time he did the same thing, he never did any doctoring. He even did this if I made a special appointment to see him. It didn't matter whether it was a new appointment or a follow up appointment it was always the same thing.

Dr. Go Fish did this to Bertha too. She had a stomach problem once and he didn't pay a lot of attention.

Then one day Bertha went in and said, "I really need to see Dr. Go Fish again today because it's really bad. I can't wait for next week. I need something done now."

The receptionist said, "Well, Dr. Go Fish can't get you in to day. I'll have to set you up with his partner Dr. Torture. Dr. Torture saw Bertha that day and made her go on an all liquid fast and she barely even had breakfast. I asked them if they could at least let her have lunch before she started the fast. Of course they said she couldn't.

Then because of muscle pain and weakness and numbness problems he made her do this horrible nerve conduction study test and an MRI of the brain and tortured her clear to death. I was mad. Then he wanted her to do a CT the next day. He even made her wait till she was done with the test to eat anything. It had already been two days. Then, they said this guy was out to lunch while we waited for him to get back to find out if she can eat again.

Bertha thought, *"What about my lunch? I'm hungry too. I'm far beyond hungry."*

When Dr. Torture came back he said, "Do the liquid diet until Monday."

She was hysterical and about went ballistic herself. I got very mad at him and the guy that did the nerve conduction study test on her and demanded that she be able to eat something. So we took her over there and the nurse finally talked this guy into letting her eat a soft food diet. He said she had Diverticulitis. They had also done blood tests and x-rays on her in this guy's office before all this other stuff was done as well.

I thought, "This is ridiculous. One doctor at this office doesn't do anything about anything and the other doctor goes too far!"

Bertha got tired of Dr. Go Fish never taking either one of us seriously and just wanting to socialize and shun us off so we decided to find another doctor.

The doctor we went to after this, Dr. Benny did not always agree with what I thought was wrong. If I did believe something in specific was wrong and I wanted him to check it out he was more than happy to check whatever it is to see whether it is a problem or not at first.

Dr. Benny actually did a thyroid blood test on me and wrote down Thyrotoxicosis for the diagnosis and didn't even tell me he did it because he didn't want me to think I figured it out before he did.

When I told him I thought I had Hyperthyroidism he said, "Well, I think it's because you are taking those supplements."

I tried to tell him, "I take the supplements because I have the problem. If I didn't take the supplements it would be worse."

After he talked me into not taking them a while, he retook the blood test and got the same results. I told him it was what I thought it was and I was right the whole time.

Then he said, "Well, actually it's basically normal. Your TSH was a little low but still it was normal. Well, actually you are just a little hyperthyroid, but it's really not that far off. It's pretty much normal."

Believe it or not, there was one thing he actually agreed with me on. He said he thought the Levothyroxine would be the wrong medicine to take because it would just make me all the more hyperthyroid. That, I agree with. That is true. I was hoping someone would figure that one out. At least, he knew better than to give me that stuff if he were to believe I had Hyperthyroidism. I know from my studies that it's true. I told him what you take for Hyperthyroidism is those Iodine drugs like Potassium Iodide, Radioactive Iodide, Sodium Iodide, Methamazole, Tapazole, and Propylthiuracil.

He replied with, "The problem with taking the Iodine drugs is you'll think your fine when you feel better, and then you're dead."

I think this is because there is a danger of liver damage and possible kidney failure with almost all of these drugs. So technically, he's right about that, but what do you do? He said if I kept having problems he'd just send me to an Endocrinologist to see what they could do.

But the problem with that is doctors are so ignorant these days, including the Endocrinologists and they would probably say, "Oh, Hyperthyroidism. That's a thyroid problem. I'm going to give you Levothyroxine."

And when they do, they just gave you the wrong stuff because Levothyroxine raises T3 which is already what the problem is. The Iodine drugs lower T3 but they are dangerous. So, you're basically shot both ways. So, what do you do? Nothing I guess.

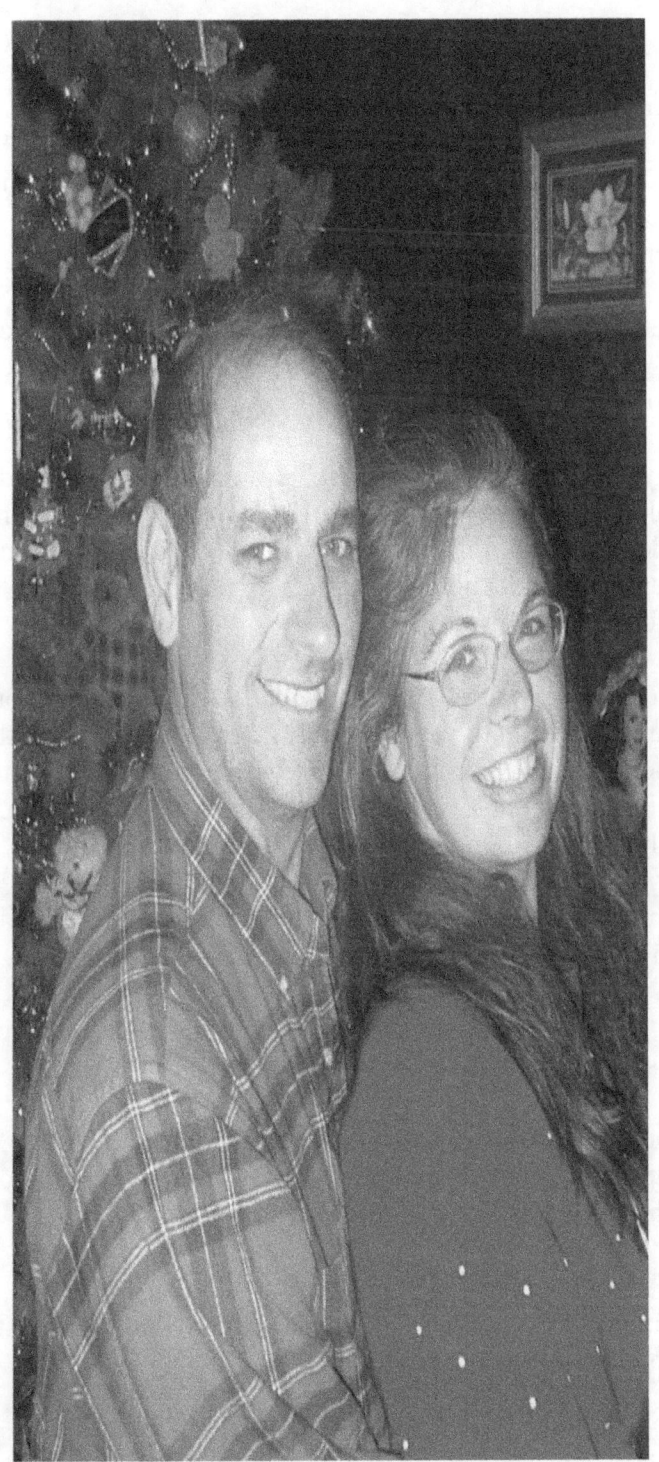

Chapter Twenty Three
Dreamer's Hope Regional Hospital
Wonderful Hospital Experience on October 9 -12, 2012

In October 2012, Bertha and I had to run a lot of errands in town, and we were going to clean the church that day. When we got finished running around I told Bertha I really wanted a nap.

Bertha said, "No, let's go ahead and clean the church and get it out of the way. Then we'll be done and not have to do anything else. I'm tired too. I want to get it over with."

I said, "Okay, I guess we can do it first." I didn't feel well that day because I felt overwhelmed from running too many errands in one day. I decided to vacuum the rugs first. I went to vacuum the rugs in the kitchen when suddenly I had this sharp pain go down the side of my foot behind my ankle.

I thought, "Oh no. I got a bad feeling about this." But I went on anyway. Next, I went in to vacuum the rug in the front door in the sanctuary then I went to vacuum the stage. I started out okay but by the time I got about half way across the stage, all of a sudden, I got this really sharp pain in the left side of the chest that started under my arm, and went from left to center, and went almost all the way from there to the sternum. I had this pain five times in a row. I wasn't sure what to do, and I told Bertha what happened.

I asked her, "Should I stop, or should I keep going?" Bertha said, "I think I'd stop. I wouldn't want to chance it."

We went home for a few minutes to take a nap when all of a sudden it happened again several times in a row and wouldn't go away. Bertha started calling different friends and called my mother.

I called the nurse at the doctor's office and I asked her, "Should I make an appointment to come in?"

Big City Hospitals Don't Like Cowards   Brian Evans

The lady said, "Honey, if you're having chest pain don't worry about making an appointment, go to the Emergency Room now."

I was asking Bertha, "What do I do?"

After talking with two or three other people we decided to take me to the Emergency Room. When I got there I got all happy go lucky *female* nurses in the Emergency Room and they were really nice to me. One lady kept giving me nitroglycerin for the pain until I got it under control.

The ER doctor said, "I'd really rather you not go home until you have a stress test here at the hospital because I think it would be safer if we kept you here."

I said, "Okay."

They sent me to the inpatient ward, and I got all happy go lucky *female* nurses again. All of them were very nice to me. I got lots of hugs, and got to enjoy everybody's company. A little bit later, there was a problem with the IV. Somehow it got loose and the nurses had to reinsert it. These two girls ran in to help me, and tried desperately to reinsert the needle with no luck, and they had to wiggle it around until they could get it to slide back into place the right way.

They had so much trouble that three other happy go lucky *female* nurses came in there and decided to help too. They couldn't figure out why they were having so much trouble. They kept at it for minutes on end, and it may have taken 20 minutes to get it fixed, I'm not sure. I kept screaming and crying and hyperventilating as they did it. They tried to comfort me and console me through the whole thing. I had so much trouble I felt really bad. I was sorry I gave them so much trouble.

I told one of them, "I'm sorry I have such a hard time getting through things like this. I didn't mean to give everyone such a hard time. I tried as hard as I could. It was just hard for me to handle because I have oversensitivity to pain, and I'm not good at handling things like this."

Then one of them said, "You may have trouble getting through needle sticks, and other invasive procedures; but your difficulty with getting through painful situations is a far cry from what we have to put up with from other patients who do better at getting through the painful stuff, but yet gripe and complain about other things continually that are nothing but trivial."

I was so happy they were still okay with me, because I was scared to death I would make them upset for being so much trouble to them, but they were not.

Later, the *female* Radiology tech that came in to give me the stress test had to connect a plastic piece to the IV. Now the problem was the IV was taped up all over the place from where it was reinserted. The girl had to tear some of the tape off and I have hairy arms. She had to keep the needle stable and in place at the same time so it wouldn't fall out. She needed to get to the end so she could stick her end piece from the plastic tube into my IV for whatever she had to do. I screamed and cried horrendously as she pulled and pulled and pulled because it hurt me. Sometimes it jerked on the IV a little bit, which caused me even more pain. She kept having horrible trouble several times over. I was starting to get worried.

She kept asking, "Why can't I get this?"

I pleaded with her, "Please don't be upset with me. I know I'm hard to deal with but this really hurts."

She said, "Now don't you feel bad that you got upset. It's not your fault. I don't want you to think I'm mad, because I'm not mad at all. So don't you worry? I'm completely fine and everything's going to be okay."

232

The whole experience went really well, even with me having so much trouble.

I asked this receptionist at the doctor's office, "Did you have something to do with how nice of people I got and how they treated me?"
She said, "Well, let me put it this way. I told them you were really scared and they needed to do everything they could to comfort and console you to keep you calm and treat you like a little boy, and give you the peppiest acting nurses they possibly could to help you through this because I knew you would have trouble with this."

I said, "Thanks for helping me. I really appreciate it. I had the most wonderful hospital experience this time that I've ever had."

Chapter Twenty Four
Trouble with Cardiologists Believing Me about My Heart
Problems and My Congenital Heart Defects

I told my family doctor in 2005 Dr. Mark about my congenital heart defects but he could never find anything. I decided to go to Dr. Couch out of town and had a Stress Echocardiogram done on me and he couldn't find anything either. I got along great with Dr. Couch's nurses. They were all very nice to me. All of the nurses there were very peppy and sweet and tried to keep me from being scared about whatever test was being done. Luckily no IVs were involved on this test. I think I was afraid there would be and was relieved to find out there was not.

Dr. Ryland did a CT angiogram on me in about 2007 and still found nothing. I loved his APN nurse, whatever her name was, and I asked her if she could comfort me through an IV stick if I went for a procedure.

She said, "I might not be able to, I'll have to see, but you'll probably have to get a surgery nurse to comfort you instead."

What bothered me is when I was sent for this CT Angiogram it was in the Imaging Department connected with Radiology and there were two younger girls that were nurses with chipper, cheerful acting personalities that came after the other patients.

I told Bertha at the time, "I want them to be my nurses. I like them. They'd be perfect."

They acted like they wondered why in the world I liked them so much and what did I want them for?

A "serious trended" female nurse came to get me, which is normally not a good thing. I'm usually bate to that kind of nurse. They're usually mean, but some are just boring. The one that came after me was just a boring nurse.

I asked her to get a chipper acting female nurse to comfort me through the IV stick when she did the IV but she wouldn't get one. She didn't understand and just did the IV stick herself. It's a good thing for her she was a good stick, because if she hadn't been I would have screamed to high heaven and jerked like I don't know what had the needle hurt me as excruciatingly as it normally does.

That was not a good move on her part. I was also upset and disappointed she did not get me someone to comfort me and I did not want her doing the stick on me. I really wanted those two other girls or two other nurses like them, one to do the stick and one to comfort me. That's how I always do it and that's the way I want it. This is what I need. Even if it doesn't hurt I need the comfort of a chipper acting cheerful female nurse when I get stuck. It's very important I get a chipper acting female nurse to rub my head to calm me down and hold my hand through the stick while another chipper acting female nurse does the IV stick, blood test, or shot because it is very hard on me. If you do not, I will not be able to do it. After they were done Dr. Ryland went over the test results with me.

He said, "Your heart is perfect, no valvular defects. No ventricular septal defects. You have the heart of a 16 year old."

Did you know that two Cardiologists and several family doctors threw my Childhood Heart Defect records back in my face because they couldn't believe it because I wasn't 50 years old and I looked fine to them?

Dr. Kevin sent me to Dr. No Way in 2012 when I was having burning in the upper left arm and occasional chest pain. Dr. No Way said there was no way I could possibly have any heart defects unless I was 50 years old, regardless of the fact I told him that some of my childhood doctors had found congenital heart defects on me previously several years earlier. We kept going back and making more follow up appointments with him desperately trying to get him to do something.

His nurse Patty seemed to believe me at first, but because he kept acting like he thought it was all in my head I felt like she was beginning to think it was too. I was trying to get them to do more tests that day and I saw Kimmy that visit and a couple of other times and I kept begging for her to be one of my nurses. I also begged her to help me with an IV if they ordered a test involving an IV.

She said, "You may not even have to have an IV. You don't even know they're going to send you to me for a test yet."

I said, "I know, but I just wanted you to know ahead of time, because I can't handle IVs and if I have to have one I want you to be the one to do the stick."

Kimmy said, "Okay, but I really don't think he's going to send you down here to do a stick. I doubt you'll even have to get one."

She was nice and hugged me, but then she started trying to get out of being my nurse and I didn't understand why. I think she thought, "Why does he have to like me so much anyway?"

On the last appointment I had, they didn't even give me Patty. They gave me some guy nurse I didn't want that was kind of macho like. We told them not to give me any male nurses and they did anyway. I was kind of offended because I thought they probably thought I just came in there to bug Patty and Kimmy, so they threw me off on him so I wouldn't bother them.

Bertha told the doctor when he came back in, "No more male nurses. Brian wants a female nurse. Men tortured him as a child and men scare him. Next time you need to give him a female nurse."

They did another EKG on me and Dr. No Way still insisted nothing was wrong with me.

I tried to show him my childhood heart defect records but he just kept saying, "Oh no. I don't want to see those. I don't believe that. There's no way you could possibly have a heart problem until your 50 years old."

Several other doctors and Cardiologists also laughed in my face in Abilene, Texas as well as Arkansas and Missouri over my childhood heart defect records. All of them threw my records back in my face because they refused to believe that anyone under the age of 50 could possibly have a heart problem no matter what the circumstances.

I'd even had various EKGs and Echocardiograms at all the hospitals I've ever been to and nothing was found there either.

All my family doctors and Cardiologists I ever went to also said, "No valvular defects. No ventricular septal defect."

I would say, "But they found these congenital heart defects when I was 6 years and 9 months old and then again at age 10 and age 12."

These doctors would say, "If it doesn't show up, it's not there. If I don't see it, it's not there."

I was still not convinced and knew there had to be something wrong. I thought they would never find it.

The Childhood records indicated a Ventricular Septal Defect, Pulmonary Flaw, and Possible Aortic Stenosis as well as a Minor IVCD, S1-S2 Juvenile Pattern, Mid Systolic Twang, Systolic Murmur at Left Sternal Border and an Aortic murmur. I didn't believe it, and I knew it was there whether they believed it or not. They just never did the right test to find it.

The next family doctor I went to Dr. Carefree told me he thought all my surgeries I ever had were probably unnecessary. He was referring to the TURP, TURVN, and Sphincterotomy, and maybe even my Ventral Hernia Surgery. He also did not think I had congenital heart defects even though I had childhood records that suggested otherwise. He suggested we do a Heart Catherization test to see if I had blockage because he was more suspicious I might have Myocardial Infarction but he wasn't about to believe I had any heart defects or valvular defects. I wasn't old enough. But I did. The last time stuff was found was at 6 years, and 9 months old, 10 years old, 12 years old five days before my 13th birthday in 1982. Since those dates, no one has ever found anything at all. I never convinced anybody of anything.

Chapter Twenty Five

Tacky Cardiology Clinic

We went to a Cardiology Clinic in Missouri in 2012 to see if they could do some more invasive tests to find my birth defects and any other reasons for the symptoms I've had for a while.

When we went there, we gave them the local Cardiologist's records, which did not find anything and did not believe I had any childhood birth defects or valvular defects. I handed them a copy of the records from my childhood where they thought they found a Ventricular Septal Defect, Pulmonary Flaw, Possible Aortic Stenosis, Minor IVCD, and Juvenile S1-S2 pattern from ages six years, nine months old to 12 years, 11 months, and three weeks old hoping they would look for all these.

When we got there and had the receptionist, Mrs. Careless make copies we noticed that my childhood records were not included.

I said, "Didn't you make a copy of these, too?"

Mrs. Careless crankily said, "We only copied what we thought we needed and that's all."

I told the Cardiologist, Dr. Mystery about it, and showed him the childhood records. He decided to have a Heart Stress test with an IV contrast done to check for it. First the techs in the clinic didn't act like they were going to do the test right.

I told them I needed to be over exerted in order for them to find it. "Don't walk me slow as Christmas like my other Cardiologist did."

They talked like they would do it close to how I wanted it but acted like they might not do it in the exact fashion I had in mind. I got set up before the stress test. I wrote them the letter saying they really needed to do it right if they were going to find it but I also told them I had certain accommodations I needed met.

I told them I needed a happy go lucky *female* nurse to rub my head to calm me down and another happy go lucky *female* nurse to do the stick. I also told them I needed plenty of hugs. These people called me in for a meeting, and had their own Social Worker they drug in there to meet with us, before we went for the test.

I was glad they met with us, so we could explain what I needed to them, until I found out they wanted to steer me their direction, and fix it to where their needs would be met, instead of mine.

They said, "Would you like us to play music?"

I said, "Not really. I just need someone to comfort me through it the way I asked them to."

They said, "What if we talk you through it? Do you need us to do anything to distract you? What can we do?"

I said, "It's okay to talk me through it, but that's not good enough, I need a nurse to rub my head to calm me down and hold my hand while another nurse does the stick. They do that for me at my own hospital all the time."

The head nurse said, "Well, my nurse over here said she would not be uncomfortable doing that?"

I told the lady, "Please, will you just do it for me? I know you don't know me but I really need this?"

The head nurse said, "She just doesn't want to do it for you because it makes her feel weird to have to do it."

I said, "What about that lady over there? I like her. Will you do it for me?"

She said, "She doesn't want to do it for you either."

She said, "We can talk you through it. Is that good enough?"

240

I said, "No."

She said, "This is our team here, and this is who we have. There's this one guy that will also be dealing with you. Is that okay?"

I said, "I'd rather not. I guess as long as the ladies help me, and he just runs the machine."

The lady said, "Well my nurses just feel uncomfortable doing what you need, and I can't ask them to do this for you, because that makes them uncomfortable. We'll give you a hug. We can do that for you. We just don't want to rub your head to calm you down. Is that okay?"

I said, "No, not really."

She said, "Just think about it."

I headed down the hall in the clinic in front of the nurse's desk where I saw the nurse I really wanted to help me with the IV.

I was so excited the time before about just having bought my new house that this lady didn't think I seemed scared to her but I was.

I just wasn't showing as much this time because for once I was distracted about what was going on because I was so excited about getting a new house. I had asked her before, and she wasn't sure she'd be able to get there that early because she normally came in later. I had hugged her the first time I saw her the week before, and wanted a hug goodbye.

She said, "No." and walked away. She rejected me and acted like she didn't understand me.

The Social Services nurse saw this and said, "Here, you can hug me. Let's go outside."

When we got outside the Social Worker said, "I'm so sorry about what just happened. I tried, but I didn't know what to do."

She looked at Bertha and said, "He seems intelligent. Is he Aspergers?"

Bertha said, "No. His intelligence is all learned. People with Aspergers are naturally that way, but Brian was drilled to death by his mother for years just to pass all his regular classes after leaving Special Ed from the 8th grade on, and that's the only reason he's that smart. It's not natural. He wasn't always that smart. People with Aspergers can do things like 10th grade math in the 3rd grade. Brian's not like that. He never was."

The lady said, "He seems so intelligent."

Bertha said, "Well he is but he is just book smart. He doesn't have any street smarts. He is socially and emotionally like a two year old."

The lady said, "Can he do anything? Does he have any special talents?"

Bertha said, "Yeah, he can play a tune on the piano he just heard without even looking but he can only do it with his right hand. And he takes beautiful pictures and just knows where to take all the right shots with the camera. Something in him just knows where to take the picture. It turns out right every time, it's phenomenal."

The lady said, "Have you ever considered savant?"

Bertha said, "Hey, I didn't think of that. He probably is, with all those unusual talents he has, but ask him to do anything else performance wise, and he's stumped. He probably is."

We looked up the savant thing, and sure enough, I qualified for the definition. We decided I must be an Autistic savant, like Rain Man.

We talked about it, and debated whether to go back or not, because I really didn't want to if they were not going to meet my accommodations

I finally said, "No. I've decided I'm not going to do it. I just hope one of these days somebody finds my defects and tells me what all they found but I'm afraid it will never happen."

We called and cancelled the appointment, and the nurse called back.

She said, "We decided we're going to let you do the stress test without the IV. Will you come now?"

Bertha said, "NO! Not unless you meet his accommodations! We already tried a regular stress test before and didn't find anything so you're probably not going to find it on a regular stress test either!"

Then she said, "If we did this other thing over here, will you come?" I forgot what the other thing was.

Bertha asked me and I said, "NO!"

Bertha told her, "No! We're not coming for anything because you were not willing to meet his accommodations, so we're not coming at all now!"

The head nurse called back and she was mad.

"My nurses have their rights! I can't make them do things that make them uncomfortable. They were willing to do the test, and we were willing to work with him, but we just cannot meet all his requests. I can't ask my nurses to do things for him that make them uncomfortable. I've got to think about the comfort of the nurses! It's out of their comfort range to rub his head to calm him down! He should have stuck with it anyway! We were willing to do an easier test since he cannot do this for us, and you're still not going to come!"

Bertha said, "Nope! If you're not going to meet his accommodations, we're not coming period! You need to think about the comfort of your patients above the comfort of your nurses! Apparently you think the comfort of your nurses is more important than the comfort level of your patients! Anyone who does not put the patient's comfort above that of their own nurses doesn't deserve our time and we are not coming because you put the needs of your nurses above the needs of my husband! If we decide to have another test done on him, we'll go somewhere else! We're not coming back to you! You're not seeing him because you refused to meet his needs! I'm not giving you a dime of our money! Bye!"

The next family doctor I went to concerning my heart defects, Dr. Carefree told me he thought all my surgeries I ever had were probably unnecessary. He was referring to the TURP, TURVN, and Sphincterotomy, and maybe even my Ventral Hernia Surgery. He also did not think I had congenital heart defects even though I had childhood records that suggested otherwise. He suggested we do a Heart Catherization test to see if I had blockage because he was more suspicious I might have Myocardial Infarction but he wasn't about to believe I had any heart defects or valvular defects. I didn't know what to tell him after these people in Missouri already refused to accommodate my needs. But, at the time, neither one of us wanted to go with the route of taking a heart cath test, we just wanted to find the congenital heart defects. He would not order any other kind of test besides this one because I wasn't old enough to have heart defects, but I did. The last time stuff was found was at 6 years, and 9 months old, 10 years old, 12 years old five days before my 13th birthday in 1982. Since those dates, no one has ever found anything at all. I couldn't ever convince anybody of anything.

Two years later Dr. Benny, my Family Doctor decided to set me up with Dr. Doubter when I told him about my heart defects and about some of the weird symptoms I was having at the time.

Dr. Doubter decided to do a Myocardial Perfusion Scan and claimed to find nothing wrong as well. I asked my favorite nurse, Jeanine working there who used to work at Dr. Wonderful's office if she could comfort me through the IV stick.

Dr. Wonderful was the nice, sweet lady doctor who had just done my Hernia Surgery and EGD and Colonoscopy two years before. Dr. Wonderful was the one that put her face down to me and said, "You just put your ear on my cheek and I leave my face down here until you fall asleep" when I was scared and wanted a hug from her right before they put me to sleep for my procedure. I really appreciated that. She was very compassionate. Jeanine used to be her nurse but now she worked here and I was glad. I got to see Jeanine there for one of my doctor visits to set up the Myocardial Perfusion Scan test Dr. Doubter wanted done. I asked her if she could comfort me through the IV stick the day I would come for the test. I told her I needed her to rub my head to calm me down and hold my hand while Kimmy did the IV stick. She said she would if she was working but she'd have to fit me in between patients or I would have to do the test really early but she never showed up.

I begged and pleaded with her the day of the test and she said, "I'm sorry. I really didn't know I'd be this busy. There's a student nurse down there. You can ask her."

Kimmy decided to do my IV stick and I was very glad. I always liked her and hoped she would help me. I didn't think she understood me and didn't believe I was as bad as I was about getting through an IV stick as I said I was. She actually acted like she was happy with me this time. I never thought she'd help me because I thought she thought I was just trying to get attention. Now, she would get to see for herself how bad I was with IVs and I was glad because I liked her and I felt like she would comfort me if she saw this problem I claimed to have with IVs was all for real. So, when she started to do the IV stick, I asked the student nurse to rub my head to calm me down and hold my hand during the IV stick and she did.

I really appreciated it but I still felt like I would have done better for Jeanine, but I didn't know if she understood my situation either, like I thought she did. Kimmy, who did my IV even decided to put a wet rag over my head. She had a horrible time getting the IV in and I was incredibly anxious when she did. I screamed in excruciating pain when she stuck the IV in.

I hyperventilated the whole time, panicking. Kimmy asked me to sing "Jesus Loves Me" with her to distract me. I did but still had a horrible time and screamed like crazy very loudly.

She finally got the needle in. I hyperventilated almost the whole time she was sticking the needle in. Then I hyperventilated and panicked even after she was done. I grabbed her and hugged her and held on crying. She said, "Come on buddy, hold on. Just hold on to me okay. You're all worked up. Are you okay? You just hug me and hold on as long you need to. If I didn't know any better I'd think you had a fever because you're warm. Try not to get too worked up there. You're going to throw yourself into a panic attack. You just keep holding on okay. Keep hugging me and keep holding on. You just hug me okay. Try to breathe okay. Breathe, breathe. Oh my, you're about to have a panic attack. Just try to breathe okay. It's alright. Keep holding on to me. Just hold on. I know your having a hard time. Just keep holding on until you can calm down. Get it out but just try to breathe. Okay. Hold on. Hold on. There. I think we're okay now. You had me worried for a minute there. You've been panicking for almost 30 minutes now. I'm glad you're alright. Try to stay calm now. It's going to be alright. We're going to come back for you and do your test in a minute."

When they took me back to do my Stress Echocardiogram before my Myocardial Perfusion Scan, Kimmy came back in and said, "Here. I need you to take your shirt off and put this gown on while we do this EKG."

After the EKG she said, "Now we're about to get on the treadmill. Most guys like to take their shirt off and just go on the thing bare chested but you can leave the gown on if you wish. What would you rather do? Do you want to take the gown off or do you want to leave it on?"

I said, "I guess I'll leave it on."

Kimmy said, "I figured as much. Okay, you can leave it on. I didn't think you'd want to take it off. I just wanted to ask to make sure because most guys do, but I didn't figure you'd want to."

She acted like she knew I was shy.

A few minutes after this they did the Myocardial Perfusion scan and a guy did it, but luckily I already had the IV in me and I think Kimmy stood by me at first until they got it started. I asked if they found anything on it and they said they really didn't see much. I think they noticed a little bit but they didn't see any hole or any valvular defects or anything like that.

They said it was more to test the heart muscle than it was for finding those things anyway. Dr. Doubter finally did an ultrasound and said it was vague but I might actually have an Atrial Septal Defect but I would have to get a Transesophageal Echocardiogram to find out for sure but he didn't want to set it up himself. He said my family doctor; Dr. Benny would have to set it up for me. He was probably afraid Dr. No Way would think he would look stupid to all my ex-cardiologists and all my ex-family doctors if he didn't find anything wrong. I also think Dr. Doubter was afraid if he did find something wrong it would make Dr. No Way look bad because he didn't believe anything could possibly be wrong because I wasn't 50 years old. If I proved Dr. No Way wrong, it could really make him look bad. I think he just threw me off on my family doctor, at that time, Dr. Benny. He wanted to save face with everybody.

I went back to Dr. Benny as he asked me to and asked him if he could set up the Transesophageal echocardiogram. He decided to set me up with Dr. Wacky at Transylvania Regional Medical Center so I made an appointment with them and got in to see them on March 14th to set up the test.

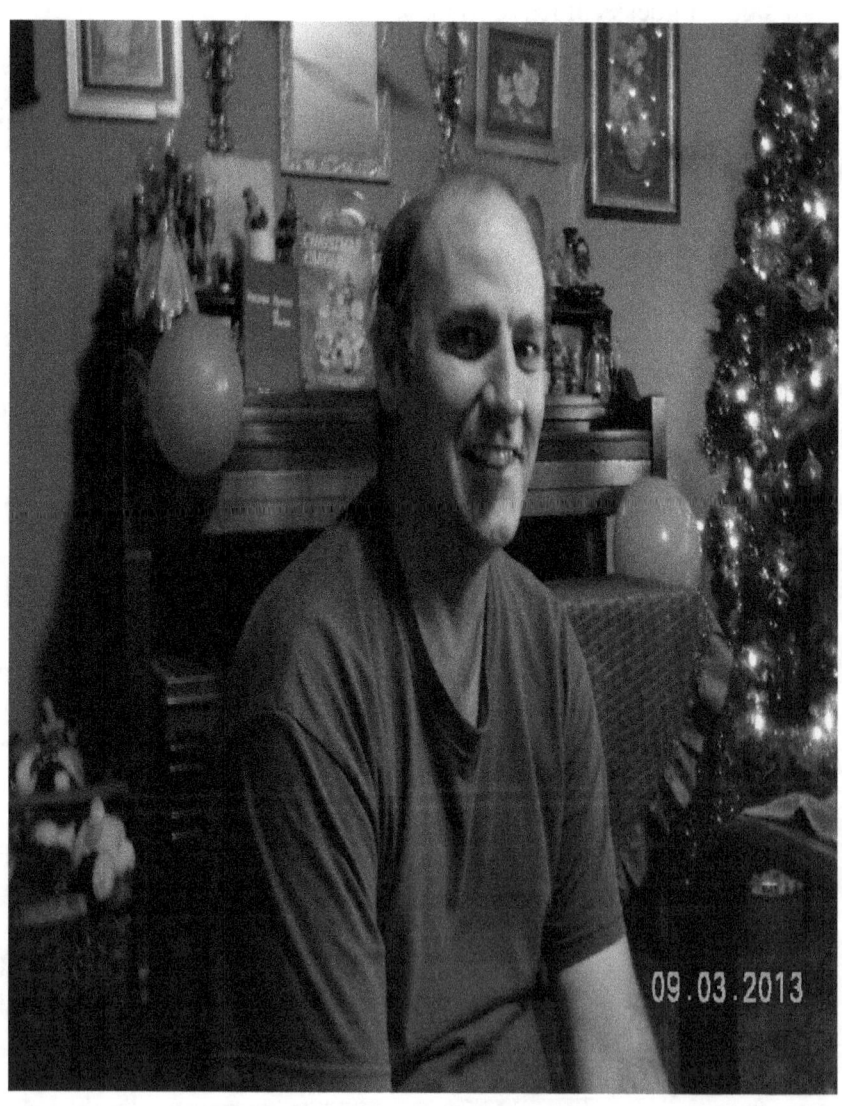

Chapter Twenty Six
Experience at Transylvania Regional Medical Center
Part I: Experience at the Cardiologist's Office

On March 14, 2014 we went to Dr. Wacky's office to check on some bizarre symptoms I was having with clamping in the upper left arm, left chest, and left shoulder blade. This was followed by heavy waves of nerve bands that went down my left arm from my shoulder to my hand and heavy waves of nerve bands rippling down the left side of my chest.

I mainly wanted to get the Transesophageal Echocardiogram that I found out would verify some heart defects that some doctors found on me when I was a child. But because of the symptoms I was having, I was also hoping they would find out what was going on with my arm and chest. Since that was happening I thought if they needed to do a heart cath test to find out what was going on with that problem they could.

Bertha and I had both explained some of my symptoms to the Cardiologist, Dr. Wacky.

She said, "My concern is, we have two problems we are looking at here. One is you want to find your birth defects; we can do the Transesophageal Echocardiogram to find that. The other problem is, if you are still having chest pains after your Myocardial Perfusion scan, I think we need to do a Heart Catherization test to find out what is going on. Sometimes there will be blockage there that does not always show up on a Myocardial Perfusion scan, so I think it would be best to do this test to find out for sure. It is the definitive test. From the things you have told me, I think you may have a blockage in a coronary artery, and your wife doesn't want you to have a heart attack, so I think it would be best if we did this to check it out. Would you be interested in doing a Heart Catherization test?"

I looked at Bertha for reassurance we never would do this test in the past because it sounded very dangerous.

She said, "Yes, with the symptoms you're having I think you should."

Dr. Wacky then said, "Okay we can do a Heart Catherization test as well and we are going to use Coronary Angiography to look for blockage and if we find any we'll need to put a stent in, but only if there is blockage. If it's not too bad, I'm not going to put it in, but if it is really significant or really narrow, then I will."

Bertha had called Dr. Wacky's office ahead of time, and let them know what my needs were. I had a need to hug my nurses. I also needed a happy go lucky *female* nurse to rub the top of my head and hold my hand to calm me down for IV sticks, tube insertions, or catheter insertions. She wanted her to know all this before we even arrived for the appointment.

Bertha told her I was autistic. She wanted to make sure she explained me to her and her workers before I even went there so they would understand. I believe the nurse I talked to at my Family Doctor's office also called Dr. Wacky's office to tell them about my lists of accommodations for both procedures to help be sure they accommodated me. As a matter of fact, I was originally going to Dr. Couch at the same clinic office because of how nice his nurses were to me a few years ago. Since he was unable to see me till August they tried to get me in earlier. They felt I needed a woman doctor, because of my fear of men. So they set me up with Dr. Wacky because she was a lady doctor. They wanted me to have all *female* nurses, and a *female* doctor to avoid making me nervous for this invasive procedure.

Dr. Wacky's office set me up with a nice nurse in the office named Serena, after Bertha called them who was very compassionate and very friendly.

Serena told me what the test entailed and I hugged her and her assistant Natasha. They were both very nice to me and tried to console me about the test especially Serena.

I asked Dr. Wacky for a hug when I saw her at the office and she was fine with my hugging her at her office on Friday, March 14th. Bertha told her how I needed to hug her nurses Serena and Natasha often to stay calm.

She said, "That's fine. I'm not worried about it. That's not a problem."

I asked Serena if she could go to the Cath Lab with me to help me through the procedure and the prep.

Serena said, "I can't be in there because I am not certified in their clinic."

I asked her, "Could you at least go in there to help me, even if it's just to comfort me. Could you as long as you don't do the IV stick, or any of the other stuff yourself?"

She said, "I'm sorry. I would if I could, but they have their own nurses. Don't worry. They've got good ones. You'll be okay."

We gave Serena my lists of accommodations I needed for both the Transesophageal Echocardiogram and the Heart Catherization test I needed all the cath lab nurses to meet. She assured me she would give a copy of the list to every nurse in there.

I will tell you how these lists read and how my definition page of what a happy go lucky nurse is read. The following pages show how these lists read that were given to Dr. Wacky's Office and the Transylvania Regional Hospital Cath Lab:

Big City Hospitals Don't Like Cowards   Brian Evans

Accommodations Needed for Transesophageal Echocardiogram

A very happy go lucky, bubbly, peppy *female* nurse to rub my head to calm me down and hold my hand

A very happy go lucky nurse to do the IV stick

A very Happy Go Lucky, Bubbly, Peppy *Female* Nurse to do the Tube Insertion in my Throat

Please spray a numbing solution in my throat before inserting the tube

Please give me at least enough nitrous oxide to make me numb and tingly so I don't feel the tube going in my mouth and down my throat

Please wait till I am calmed down from the IV stick before inserting the tube down my throat

Remember that the happy go lucky nurse that comforts me through the IV stick also needs to rub my head to calm him down and hold my hand when you put the tube in my throat

If you can, please put me completely to sleep before you even put the tube in my throat because I will be panicked if I am awake

Keep in mind I have a gag reflux, so make sure to watch out for this to happen

Slide the tube in my mouth and down my throat as gently as you can to keep from hurting me as much

Please try not to hurt me when inserting the tube

Please have patience with me over my anxiety and panic attacks over the tube insertion and the IV stick

Big City Hospitals Don't Like Cowards   Brian Evans

All nurses must be very happy go lucky, peppy, *chipper acting
fe*male*s* that deal with me in this department and every department
of the hospital

No Cordial or Mediocre acting *Female* Nurses allowed only Happy
GO LUCKY, Peppy Nurses

No Men at All, No *Male*s

Only the Doctor can be a man, since this doctor is a woman we are
in luck on this one

That works better for me because I am scared of men

All nurses involved must be *female* nurses

I Need this in the Clinic, and the PreOp Department, and in
Inpatient Care, wherever I go, this is what I need.

These happy go lucky *female* nurses will need to comfort me
through the test and talk me through it and try to distract me when
I am in pain.

It will be difficult not to jerk on a test like this one so these nurses
may even have to hold me down to keep me from jerking.

Please, if there is any way you can talk these people into this,
please don't make me do this test awake.

Please ask these nurses to put me completely out with the gas and
the IV.

At least make me numb and tingly enough to handle it, but please
knock me completely out because this kind of test is hard for me to
bear.

Thank you.

The type of happy go lucky *female* nurses I am referring to would be the chipper, peppy acting ones that act like somebody dug up off a Disney movie like Aerial the Mermaid or Anastasia or Mariposa or Barbie's Rapunzel or Frauline Maria on "The Sound of Music" or Eliza Doolittle on "My Fair Lady".

They will all need to do the best they can to comfort me through the test and talk me through it when I'm being stuck with an IV or other instrument and try to keep me distracted when I am in pain.

It helps me when you all act like you're my buddies, and you're going to help me the best way you can, and encourage me through the procedure when I am scared and in pain.

It will be difficult for me not to jerk on a test like this one; so, some of my nurses may have to hold me down to keep me from jerking.

You may have to have one of the nurse's hold my arm down for the IV stick to keep me from jerking.

Please ask these nurses to put me completely out with the gas and the IV.

At least make me as numb and tingly as you possibly can to keep me from feeling anything to make it easier for me.

The best kinds of nurses for me are the ones that act like someone a person dug up off of a Disney movie or something.

If you see how *bubbly acting* the Disney movie characters Anastasia, or Ariel, the Little Mermaid, or Barbie's Rapunzel, or Frauline Maria from the "Sound of Music" or Eliza Doolittle on "My Fair Lady" act and notice the same personality tendencies in a real live person that's a nurse, this is the personality types I relate to the most.

Some people may think there is no such thing as a person that acts like this, but if you really think about it, there are some people that when you see the way they act might make someone want to say, "You know, you act just like Frauline Maria" or "You act just like that character, Aerial on the Little Mermaid" or "You sure act a lot like that girl named Anastasia on that movie. Have you ever seen that?"

Ever heard people make these kinds of comments about people they've run into.

They may not be Anastasia or Eliza Doolittle or Frauline Maria or Ariel or Barbie's Rapunzel, but when you see the way they act in public you might think, "Boy, they may not be that person, but they sure do act like it. If I didn't know any better, I'd think it was them." Even though, they're not them, they just act like them.

<u>Accommodations needed for Heart Catherization for Stent Placement or Surgery</u>

Please do not make me do this surgery awake.

Catheters hurt me worse than IV's.

Catheters feel like a sword is being run through me.

Dr. Scotty puts me completely to sleep when using urinary catheters because he knows it will be too excruciating for me to handle.

Just think how much more excruciating it would be if I had to have a catheter threaded all the way from my groin to my heart awake.

That goes for the alternative in the arm too.

That's what a guy at church told me they did to him.

I thought, "There's no way I can handle this test awake."

This is the following list of things I need for this type or test or surgery:

I need a very happy go lucky *female* nurse to rub my head to calm me down and hold my hand through the IV Stick and the Catheter Insertion.

A very happy go lucky *female* nurse needs to do the IV stick.

A very happy go lucky *female* nurse needs to insert the catheter.

Several other happy go lucky *female* nurses to assist with the procedure.

If they refuse to knock me out, at least give me enough Nitrous Oxide to make me numb and tingly to help me not feel it and/or put numbing stuff in my IV.

A patient at a clinic suggested I might have them put Novocain on the site of the catheter puncture.

The following will be necessary if they refuse to knock me out:

In addition to the above list, the following will also need to be done.

One Happy Go Lucky *Female* Nurse needs to hold down the right arm.

One Happy Go Lucky *Female* Nurse needs to hold down the left arm.

One Happy Go Lucky *Female* Nurse needs to hold down the right leg.

One Happy Go Lucky *Female* Nurse needs to hold down the left leg.

One Happy Go Lucky *Female* Nurse needs to hold down both feet.

If this nurse doesn't think she can hold both feet down at once, you will need to have an additional happy go lucky *female* nurse to grab the other foot to hold it down.

This is to keep me from jerking.

I guarantee if I am awake that this will be a problem because the pain will be so excruciating to me that they will have no other choice.

It will be very difficult for me not to jerk.

It is very important I get all happy go lucky *female* nurses for this.

If I get a cordial or mediocre nurse when I'm already nervous about the IV and the catheter, I will be twice as likely to jerk, as I would if the people I wanted did it.

I may still jerk, but, they would be less liable to hurt me if they got all the happy go lucky type nurses I like.

If they don't give me the type of nurses I like, they are asking for an absolute disaster, because I will probably be so frantic, and jerk around so bad, that they could unintentionally hurt me.

Even if I do get the kind of nurses I want for this procedure, I will be screaming in excruciating pain through the entire procedure, and not be able to tell them what hurts less that something else.

It will all hurt equally the same throughout my body, and be excruciating everywhere the catheter moves in my body.

So, please, I beg you; tell these people to knock me out completely for this procedure before inserting a catheter.

The pain is too excruciating for me to bear.

Thank you.

Remember, they need to get very peppy, happy go lucky *female* nurses that act like someone somebody got off a Disney movie.

These are the kind of nurses that can help me through an invasive procedure like this.

No one else will work, especially for a test like this.

Remember, no men.

All nurses must be very happy go lucky, peppy *female* nurses only.

This goes for the clinic, and the PreOp department, and the hospital, and the hospital inpatient care.

I need this kind of nurses at all times, everywhere I go, no matter what is being done, or where I am sent to, or wind up at.

Big City Hospitals Don't Like Cowards   Brian Evans

This is what I need.

Please see to it that this is what I get.

Thanks.

MY DEFINITION OF A HAPPY GO LUCKY NURSE

PEPPY
HYPER
CHIPPER
COMPASSIONATE
FUNLOVING
SWEET
MOTHERLY
BOUNCY PERSONALITY (PERKY ACTING, UPBEAT,
VIBRANT)
KEYED UP, IN A GOOD WAY (PUMPED UP PERSONALITY
LIKE FRAULINE MARIA)
COMFORTING
ENCOURAGING
DETERMINED TO HELP YOU THROUGH AN INVASIVE
TEST THAT TERRIFIES YOU WITH A CHIPPER,
ENCOURAGING, APPROACH (TALKS YOU THROUGH IT
AND TRIES TO DISTRACT YOU FROM YOUR FEAR BY
MAKING YOU TALK ABOUT THINGS THAT MAKE YOU
HAPPY AND DO WHAT YOU NEED THEM TO DO AND
COMFORT YOU AT THE SAME TIME, IN MY INSTANCE
RUB MY HEAD TO CALM ME DOWN AND HOLD MY
HAND THROUGH AN IV STICK, TUBE INSERTION, OR
CATHERIZATION PROCEDURE

HAPPY GO LUCKY NURSE VERSES MEDIOCRE/CORDIAL
NURSES

A CORDIAL NURSE (Or Mediocre Nurse) just walks in the room
casually, usually in slow motion and matter of factly says, "Hi.
I'm Jane. I'm here to take your blood. Come with me, please. We
need to do a blood test." This person may be nice and even smile,
but they are not much help.

A HAPPY GO LUCKY NURSE USUALLY WALKS IN
PUMPED UP WITH A GO GETTER PERSONALITY THAT
PRACTICALLY SHOOTS OUT THE DOOR TO GET YOU
AND ACTS PEPPY AND FRIENDLY AND SAYS,

"Hi, I'm Jane. Come in with me and let's take your blood!" And
then, when you act scared, they say, "It's okay. We're going to be
just fine! Come on buddy! You just come with me and we're
going to get you through this! You just wait and see! You're
going to be just fine!"

When I start screaming and hyperventilating through a blood test
or IV, whichever one I'm having done, they usually say something
like, "Breathe! Breathe! Take a deep breath! Try to relax okay!
Stay with me buddy! Try to hold on! We're going to get you
through this! You just bare with me and we'll be done in a minute!
I'm sorry this hurts but I'm going to be as gentle as I can, okay.
It's going to be okay, buddy! You're going to be okay!
Everything is going to be just fine!"

Then when they're done they say, "See, we made it just fine.
You're going to be okay. Now let's set you up and you let me
know if your dizzy or not and then I'll help you up!" That, or,
'Well, we're ready to go to surgery now. We're getting ready to
put you to sleep. So you just rest and have a nice nap while we do
our thing and you'll never know anything ever happened. There
you go. Goodnight!"

Big City Hospitals Don't Like Cowards   Brian Evans

This is a letter we give to the doctor's that deal with me that Bertha has written to advocate for me.

Dear Physician,

I wanted to tell you a little about my sweet, dear, autistic, husband Brian Evans. He is the opposite of most people who have autism. Brian likes to hug…a hug to Brian is not a wrap his arms around you hug; he hugs by pressing his ear to the other person's cheek.

Brian can talk but it is very hard for him to get what is in his head out his mouth. It is much easier for him to write it. So, expect a letter each time he has something to tell you about.

Brian also has an anxiety disorder. He always worries about everything and details are very important to him so explain in detail any diagnoses, treatment plan, etc.

The most important thing you need to know about Brian is he has a MAJOR needle phobia! He needs 3 people to give him a shot or take blood. They need to be happy go lucky. Brian needs to have one hold his hand one to gently caress the top of his head (just like you would comfort a child) and one to give the shot/take blood. Brian is a sweet little boy stuck in a man's body.

Men scare Brian so if you have a *male* nurse please do not use him with my husband only sweet happy fe*male* nurses please. Brian was tortured by men as a child in a Military Hospital. Thanks.

In Christian Love,

Bertha Marie Evans

Big City Hospitals Don't Like Cowards   Brian Evans

This is what she gives to the nurses…

My sweet dear autistic husband Brian Evans needs hugs to reassure him that everything is alright. Brian is like a sweet little two-year-old stuck in a man's body. It is very important that he is treated just like a child, be kind, smile and give him lots of hugs. Thank you. May my Heavenly Daddy, God, Bless you?

                    In Christian Love,

                    Bertha Marie Evans

Chapter Twenty Seven
Experience at Transylvania Regional Medical Center
Part II: Meeting the Creepy Three at the Heart Cath Lab

On March 18, 2014 we were taking a trip to Abilene, Texas to see my mother and stopped in the Cath Lab to talk to them where they were at in Arkansas on my way down. We reluctantly showed "these three creepy acting *female* nurses" with "serious trended personalities" my lists of accommodations. We made sure to give them a copy of these lists of accommodations just in case they didn't get one. They were all around 40 years of age or older and had dark brown hair and a dark, copper tone-like complexion to their faces. They were all three slim. They all three had this creepy glare in their eyes when they looked at me, like they thought I was their next victim. They looked at me like a lion looks at their prey. They acted like they could not wait for me to go in there for my procedure so they could torture me to death. I didn't understand why they were looking at me like that. I was scared of them. We went in there to see them trying to figure out where the Cath Lab was.

When we went there they said, "The cath lab is not in here."

Then we went to the registration office, then back where they were, and we asked these ladies, "Where is the cath lab at?"

They said, "This isn't actually the cath lab. The cath lab is upstairs."

Bertha asked, "Are we even in the right place? How do we get there?"

I asked, "Is there a way to go upstairs to get to it to find it?"

They creepily said, "No. No one is allowed upstairs. You have to get up there from down here!"

Scared to death, I asked, "Well, where do we go, then?"
They told me in a creepy tone of voice, "You'll be coming to us!"

I was about to shiver with fear and thought, "You! Oh, please no!"

Bertha reluctantly gave the meanest looking one my lists of accommodations and my explanation of what a happy go lucky nurse was, and that lady finally threw her hands in the air.

She plainly said, "I won't be here!"

That lady looked in a log to see who would be working on April 1st, and said, "Your nurses will be Lacy and Katie."

I asked, "Do you have any pictures?"

They said, "They'll be here tomorrow if you want to talk to them."

I said, "We would, but we're on our way to Abilene to see my mother for two weeks before we come back for the procedure. Do you have any pictures?"

She said, "No. One's blonde. The other has brown hair. One's 40 and the other one is in her mid 20's. You'll like them. They're sweet."

I thought, *"Good! I sure don't want you! You're creeping me out!"*

These three ladies never smiled and acted almost like gangsters acting mysteriously as if they were trying to come up with a plot for how they wanted to manhandle me the day I would go in for their test. They looked like lions that looked on their prey like when they are about to be their lunch with their serious look and strange glare in their eyes, and kept sending us on goose chases till they finally let out the punch line, "You'll be coming to us!" in a creepy tone of voice. It was almost like, "Let's not pounce on him now. Let's wait till the day we come and then will pounce! Then we'll have him" or "Welcome to my dungeon! I'm glad you came! Ladies let's get him!" or "Oh there's no door over there. You can't get out that way either. Oh there's no window either.

That door's locked. You can't get out! Sorry! Going somewhere! Grab him, now!" I can't prove it but it sure seemed like it. It was really weird. And the nurse I did get with her bunch acted guilty like they would have done everything I feared they would have done and my fears were not in vain. It sounds fishy doesn't it? Makes you think don't it?

Chapter Twenty Eight
Experience at Transylvania Regional Medical Center
Part II B: The Creepy Three, What if I Would Have Got Them?

Does that whole situation seem creepy to you? It did to me.

Here's what I thought would happen if I got these three ladies instead of the nice people on the day of my procedure:

Because these ladies looked at me so creepily I was scared to death of them. I was afraid that they would drag me to the bed, force me down, stick me as hard as they could with the IV, and gripe about it when I screamed if I got them instead of the nurses they told me about in their schedule log. I had nightmares about these three ladies for the next two weeks. I accidentally remembered them saying these two girls they told me about in the schedule log would come from upstairs to get me.

Then I thought, *"Wait a minute! Why are they coming from upstairs to get me instead of downstairs? Are these two girls going to come for me right away and help me with my IV stick, or are they going to come down after these other three ladies are done with me? That one lady nurse said they would not be here that day but she didn't say these other two creepy ladies I saw on March 18th wouldn't be working on April 1st. They never really said who would get me first, them or the other two girls they told me about."*

I thought, *"What if they're just pretending like Lacy and Katie are going to come for me and tell me to go change into a hospital gown first? Are they going to trick me into thinking these two girls are coming for me and then say, 'You won't be getting them? You're going to get us!' after I've already changed into my hospital gown?"*

I thought I could just see these creepy acting ladies say, *"Go change into your hospital gown and Katie and Lacy will be here to get you in a minute."*

Big City Hospitals Don't Like Cowards   Brian Evans

I thought if I asked, *"Are Lacy and Katie coming now?" after I've already changed into my hospital gown they would say, "No, they're not coming! You're getting us!"*

I was afraid they would do this in order to trick me so they can have me right where they want me as fair game so they can torture me.

I feared they might actually do this to me because a cranky lady actually did pull this kind of trick on me a few years earlier for a Intravenous Pyelogram. When the nice friendly young girl that worked with her told me to change into a hospital gown for her said, "Let me know when your ready and I'll be in to help you in a minute." I changed into my hospital gown just as she asked me to and came back out to let her know I was ready. When I looked out the door she was gone. When I asked the cranky lady that worked with her "Where did that sweet young girl go that was here a minute ago that was supposed to help me?" That lady back then said, "She went to lunch! We're going to have to get somebody else!" and then she got a male IV tech to ram the IV in me as hard as he could while she yelled and screamed at me and then said, "Take it out! I can't take it anymore!"

I thought, the way these ladies act, they act just like her. I don't trust them not to do the same thing as she did. She tricked me back then and tried to torture me when she made the nice person go away and got me to herself. How do I know these creepy acting ladies won't do the same thing? They act just like her, and others I've gotten in the past that are just as mean as or meaner than she was. I would have shivered in fright if one of them would have suddenly grabbed me telling me as they drug me into the room, "Come on! Get in here!"

I thought one of them would grab an IV while the other one held down my arm and crankily say, *"Do you have the IV?"*

And the other one would say, *"Yes!"*

268

Then I thought the person that grabbed me would say to the other nurse, *"Stick him!"*

I thought while I screamed at the top of my lungs in excruciating pain the one holding me down would say, *"You want to give us a problem! You want to give us a problem! If you don't cooperate with us and you keep giving us problems we'll make your life miserable and you'll wish you never met us!"*

At this time I would be screaming in excruciating pain.

After rehearsing this nightmare of what I thought these ladies might do to me, I thought, *"Wait a minute! I know! I'll refuse to change into my hospital gown until Lacy and Katie come for me. Then they'll have to let Lacy and Katie insert the IV instead of doing it themselves, then I'll be safe!"*

After that I thought, *"On second thought, that's probably not going to work. These three ladies seem pretty mean. I don't think they're going to take 'No' for an answer. Somehow, I get this feeling if I refused to change into my hospital gown for these three ladies I might get forcibly stripped! I don't think they are going to let me by that easily. They don't act like they're going to be nice enough to say, "Fine, if you don't want us we'll let you wait for these nurses you are more comfortable with than us."*

You're probably thinking, "If they scare you that much, why don't you just ask them to give you someone else?"

Do you really think these three "creepy acting", "serious trended" female nurses would have taken "No." for an answer?

No! These ladies are evil and they act like if I even dared say, "No" to them they would take me down so fast I'd wonder what just happened. I don't think they're going to just let me by and just give me whoever I want. These three ladies are cranky and they're not going to take "No" for an answer! They're going to make me cooperate with them if they have to strip me down to make me cooperate with them! I know!

I've ran into their type several years ago at the military hospital I went to when I was a kid and that's exactly what they did when I would refuse to cooperate with them! I know they would do this to me. It's written all over their face!

And, you're probably thinking, "I thought you said it was all these "male" doctors, nurses, and techs that would treat you this way?"

It was, but there were a few exceptional circumstances where I actually did get a female nurse and when I did they were nearly always the "serious trended" female nurses and they were mean, and they had the attitude back then, "You'd better do what I say or else because if you don't I will personally strip you down myself and make you do everything I ask. So you better change into your hospital gown yourself if you don't want us to do anything to you, because if you don't, we will do it for you!"

They were very gruff and they were very mean, just like the men were. I got the men 90% of the time, but I got these "serious trended" female nurses the other 10% of the time, and that's the way they handled things themselves.

This is the scene that flashed through my mind of what would happen if I refused to cooperate with these ladies and change into my hospital gown for them. I never caught their names when I met them. So, I wouldn't be able to tell you for sure who they were if you asked. But, I am using fictitional names here anyway so let me give them names to help explain what I think they would do.

I'm going to call the one that creepily said, "You'll be coming to us!" Veronica.

And I'll call the other two Janet and Magness.

I started envisioning this scene in my mind about the creepy three I just saw:

My nightmare went something like this:

Janet says, "Go change in to your hospital gown and Lacy and Katie will be here to get you in a minute."

I change into my hospital gown and ask, "Are Lacy and Katie coming now?"

Janet says, "No! They're not coming! You're going to get us!"

I wind up shivering in fright when I see them. Then one of them says, "Come on! Get in here!"

Janet says to Magness, "Do you have the IV?"

Magness says, "Yes!"

Janet says, "Stick him!"

I start screaming at the top of my lungs!

Janet says, "You want to give us problems? Do you want to be a problem? If you give us problems, we'll make your life miserable!"

Janet says to Magness, "Stick him again! We'll teach him to give us a problem!"

In my nightmare I would be like, "Ahhhhh!"

Janet says, "You want to be a problem!? You want to be a problem!? Huh! Huh! We'll make you wish you'd never come in here!"

After rehearsing this nightmare in my mind I thought, "Wait a minute! I know what I'll do if I get these three creepy ladies! I'll refuse to change into my hospital gown! Then, I'll be safe!"

I kept thinking this through my mind for days, "Just refuse to change into my hospital gown if I get Janet, Magness, and Veronica, and tell them I'm not going to change into my gown until they get Lacy and Katie to come for me, and then I'll change, and they'll sure be the ones to do the IV stick".

After I rehearsed this in my mind a few days, thinking I had a solution to the problem, if I happened to get these three ladies instead of Lacy and Katie, I thought, "No way! They wouldn't, would they?"

Another scene flashed through my mind of what they might do to me if I refused to change into my hospital gown until they got Lacy and Katie down there.

Janet says, "Go change into your hospital gown and Lacy and Katie will be here to get you in a minute."

I say, "No, not until Lacy and Katie come for me! I'm not falling for it!"

Then Janet says, "What do you think you are doing?" when she sees me standing in the hall waiting for Lacy and Katie to come for me.

I say, "I'm waiting for Lacy and Katie."

Janet comes to me and says, "Are you going to be a problem? You want to be a problem? Are you going to change into your hospital gown or are we going to do it for you?"

I say, "I want Lacy and Katie! I'm not doing it till they come!"

Janet grabs my wrists hard, drags me to the room, spins me around the door, and then puts my arms behind my back. She then puts my wrists together and grabs me with a death grip around both arms on both wrists in one grip.

Magness is at the opposite end of the bed waiting for me that I wasn't expecting to see.

Janet says to Magness "Do you have the gown ready?"

Magness says, "Yes."

Janet says, "Take his clothes off and put the hospital gown on him!"

Magness yanks my clothes off and shoves the gown on me. Janet and Magness together drag me to the side of the bed.

Janet has a hold of my arms, says, "I've got his arms! You grab his legs and push him on to the bed! Now turn him around, so, he'll lie down on the bed! Now pin him down, hard!"

Janet says to Magness, "Do you have the IV?!"

Magness says, "Yes!"

Janet says, "You don't cooperate with us, this is what you get! If you don't want stripped you'll do what we ask! If you don't do what we ask you will get stripped! This is what happens when you don't do what we ask! If you don't cooperate with us we will make your life miserable! So, if you don't want stripped and you don't want us to be this forceful with you you'd better do what we say or else!"

Janet says to Magness, "Do you have the IV?!"

Magness says, "Yes!"

Janet says, "Stick him! Now!

I scream, "Ahhhh!"

Janet says, "Do you want to be a problem? Do you want to be a problem?! You give me any more trouble and I'll make her stick you again!"

Janet looks over to Magness and says, "Stick him again! We'll show this coward how to give us trouble! Get him hard! Come on! Jab him! Make his life miserable! I'll show him how to give us trouble! Get him good!"

Keep in mind, this particular scenario with Janet, Magness, and Veronica never happened.

This *nightmare scenario* I just told you about taking place is only what I *feared* would happen if I got them after Veronica so creepily said, "You'll be coming to us!" two weeks earlier and looked at me like a lion looks at its prey.

I've never been forcibly stripped by a nurse as an adult. However, I never refused to change into a hospital gown for them either, even if they were "serious trended" female nurses.

I feared if I ever did refuse to change into a hospital gown for a "serious trended" female nurse again as an adult I would get forcibly stripped again by a "serious trended" female nurse for the first time in my adulthood because that's what happened when I was a kid.

I was going to begin to refuse to change into a hospital gown for "serious trended" female nurses for the first time in order to force them to have to give me a "Chipper acting" female nurse instead of them.

That's why I was afraid I would was afraid I would begin to be forcibly stripped by "serious trended female nurses" again as an adult, is because I was going to refuse to cooperate with them ever again and insist I get a "chipper acting female nurse" instead.

That's when I figured I was in trouble, because I figured they would not take no for an answer if I was required to change into a gown for them because I figured once I made the wrong move, they'd rip my clothes right off of me to force me to cooperate with them, just like those nurses like them did to me when I was a kid. I figured that was a dangerous move, but I was going to take a chance just to see if I could get out of getting them and get someone I really wanted that I was more comfortable with.

I figured for the first time ever, that the forcible stripping thing that happened when I was a kid would begin to happen again. I figured it would only make them mad if I refused, and they would refuse to give me a different nurse I really wanted and take me by force and say, "You either take your clothes off and change into your hospital gown or we will do it for you! If you refuse to do what we say we will take you by force! You will do what we say! And, we will get the job done one way or the other! So you might as well do what we say! Are you going to change into your hospital gown or are we going to do it for you? Alright buddy, you asked for it!" One serious trended female nurse says to another serious trended female nurse, "Take his clothes off and put the gown on him!"

That's what happened when I refused to change into my hospital gown for a "serious trended" female nurse when I was a kid, and that's what I figured would happen again as an adult if I ever refused to change into my hospital gown for a "serious trended" female nurse again.'

Now you now why I feared this would happen.

The "creepy three" in this story never smiled and were all three "serious trended female nurses". They were also very serious, unenthusiastic, never got excited about anything and acted very mysterious and mischievous and very scary.

The reason I feared this would happen is because of how mysteriously these three ladies acted and then creepily said, "You'll be coming to us!" before they found out a different batch of girls was working the day of my procedure.

My actual procedure day was two weeks later.

When I went for the real procedure I told Melba what happened and said I feared these ladies would do all this to me. Melba inferred she thought everything I feared Janet, Magness, and Veronica would have done to me would have actually taken place had I got them instead of her and Katie and Lacy that day.

Melba acted guilty when I said, "I don't think those three would have understood me!"

She said, "No! They wouldn't have!"

She acted like she knew they would do something like this to me and that my fears were not in vain.

So this fictional story of what these three creepy acting ladies might have done might actually have become a reality, if I had got them instead of Lacy and Katie and Melba.

I told my wife, Bertha about my fears of what these three creepy acting nurses we saw would have done

I asked her, "Do you think it's just me or do you think they would have actually done all this stuff?"

She said, "If I had not seen the way they looked at you for my self, I would have thought it was just your imagination, but they scared me too."

I asked, "So, do you think they would have actually done all this if they would have been the ones?"

She said, "Yes, I do."

I asked, "Do you think if I would have actually refused to change into my hospital gown until Lacy and Katie came to get me, they would have forcibly stripped me and put the gown on me themselves? Do you think they would have done this and then forced me to do everything they wanted me to do?"

Bertha said, "Yes, I do. I think they would have if you would have refused."

I said, "That's what I thought. I was afraid they were actually that mean. They looked like they were. Luckily, I didn't get them."

After this, I also remembered how those other three "serious trended" female nurses treated me at that hospital I went to 10 years before this. I remembered how Paulina at the other hospital acted just like Scarlet at the institution and I was afraid she might forcibly strip me too if I refused to cooperate with her. That's what Scarlet would have done. I know that from experience. And that's the way those mean ladies acted at the military hospital I went to when I was a kid too. That's what made me think these three ladies would do this because they acted just like them. I wasn't to sure Tracy wouldn't have done this to me either. She was pretty controlling too. I don't think either one of them would have taken no for an answer if I would have refused to change into a gown for them if I would have got them first instead of PreOp. I wasn't planning to go back to see them either. I was glad I wasn't going back to them, and I was glad I didn't wind up getting these three at this hospital either. However, the ones I did get that started out nicer wound up just as evil in the end, so it really didn't help matters any to get who I got.

Chapter Twenty Nine
Transylvania Regional Medical Center Part III:
The Phone Call with the Head Nurse of the Cath Lab

On March 19th, Bertha called Angie, the head Cath Lab nurse of Transylvania Regional Medical Center's Heart Cath Lab to tell her about my fears I had over the upcoming procedure and what accommodations I needed met. She told Bertha on the phone that she had gotten my lists of accommodations for both of the tests they were doing and that every nurse got a copy because Serena had given a copy to every nurse.

She said, "We got your list of accommodations, and all your needs will be met! So you don't have a thing to worry about!" in a positive, excitable tone of voice.

The only problem is, we also asked her to have the nurses that would be working with me on April 1st to call me to calm my fears, because I was worried about whom I would get.

She told Bertha, "I'll have a nurse call him before he goes in for his procedure."

Nobody ever called me though. We left a message the following Monday on her phone telling her how I was worried about getting those first three ladies we saw on March 18th. We wanted to be reassured whoever I got would not be them, and that they would be *chipper acting*, cheerful acting *female* nurses who would give me lots of hugs and meet all my emotional needs that were on my accommodations list. We asked if I was actually going to get Katie and Lacy who were mentioned to us that were supposed to be in the log that day, because if I was reassured I would get them I would feel a whole lot better. I was assuming they would probably be sweet from what I was told. Angie never returned the message we left that day and Katie and Lacy never called us to give me reassurance before my procedure nor did any other nurse.

Instead I almost immediately got a call from a lady wanting to register me for the procedure, not the nurse that would be working with me, just a business office person. I continually wished they would call.

I was relieved when it was actually the morning of April 1st, just so I could see if the nurses I got would be the nice ones or not. The whole thing was driving me crazy and I was driving Bertha crazy.

Chapter Thirty
Transylvania Regional Medical Center
Part IV: The Day of the Procedure

On April 1, 2014, we went to the Transylvania Regional Hospital cath lab prep room at 5:30 am, thirty minutes before my arrival time of 6:00 am so Bertha could talk to the very ones that were going to work with me. She did this to be absolutely sure they got the lists of accommodations and knew what to do for me to help me through my procedures and my IV stick.

Things started out okay with the batch of girls I did get but it didn't take long for things to get ugly.

Cora took me back to my patient room and asked me to change into my hospital gown. Cora was a sweet, chipper nurse.

She said, "Everything has to come off but if you want to you can wear your socks. If you don't want to wear your socks, that's fine too. Either way is okay. Just decide what you want to do and let me know if you left your socks on or not."

At that point I decided to leave my socks on.

After going over the contents of what I had they had to keep in a bag, she proceeded to shave me for the procedure.

Cora shaved the site where they wanted to stick the heart cath at before Melba, Lacy and Katy took over to help me with the IV stick. Cora was very nice to me, and I almost wished I would have asked her to comfort me through my IV stick, instead of Katie. I think I actually told Cora I'd like her to do that for me, but wanted to check to see who they had first, to see who I would be comfortable with. Cora acted like she'd be fine either way.

Then Melba comes on the scene and I asked, "Who's going to help comfort me through the IV stick?"

She said, "We'll find somebody."

I didn't know who anybody was yet so I looked at Katie, Lacy, and Cora all three and said, "I like that one and that one, and I guess that one too, referring to Lacey."

Melba said, "I think I'm going to go with Katie is that okay?"

I was kind of undecided between Katie and Cora, because I liked them the very best and I said, "I like them both. I guess either one would be okay or that one over there if you want them."

Melba said, "I'm just going to go with Katie. That's what we had in mind. Is that okay?"

I said, "Yes."

After Melba picked out the nurse that would help comfort me through the IV stick, I told her about the creepy three ladies I saw on March 18th, and said, "I'm glad you understand me. I don't think those other three ladies would have."

When I said that, Melba suddenly turned her head, and tilted her chin down. She went from having a jolly look on her face to having a strangely serious look on her face. She looked guilty, like she knew who I was talking about. Either she knew what they were going to do to me, or knew they really would have done something horrible to me, but didn't know what. She acted like she knew something she wasn't telling me.

Melba said, "No. They wouldn't have."

I told Melba these three ladies were looking at me like a lion looks at their prey. I told her how these three ladies I saw two weeks earlier gave me this feeling they were just dying to manhandle me.

When I described the things I feared these ladies would do to me she said, "I'm sorry you had to see that."
After I kept at her trying to tell her every last thing I was afraid these three ladies would do to me, she acted guilty again.

She then said, "Well, it's a good thing you got me and Lacy and Katie anyway."

Melba acted like these three women would have actually done everything I told her I feared they would do, but just didn't come directly out and say it. She sure acted like she was letting me know my fears were not in vain, though.

Before Katie came in the room I kept having to go to the bathroom that was around the corner from the nurses' station. I was having to walk in front of the nurses' station and go around the back end of it feeling embarrassed and Katie was sitting right there the whole time grinning at me. I kept feeling really self conscious and kept casually walking to the bathroom in an animated fashion almost tiptoeing when I walked to it.

Katie finally came in my patient room to see about me. Bertha showed her how I needed her to rub my head to calm me down and hold my hand.

Melba said it was time to put the IV in. She actually let Lacy do the stick, while Katie comforted me; Katie actually did exactly what I needed her to do. Melba was a "serious trended nurse".

Lacy was the older one around 40 that I was told about by the creepy three women two weeks earlier, she was semi-chipper. Katie was the one in her mid 20's that was blonde. She was a little more chipper but not in the same way as nurses in the past I had. Something seemed different about her, like she was a slightly more sophisticated nurse than what I was used to and later I would find out she was a little bit reserved. She seemed a little tacky.

The girl named Cora at the beginning was the most chipper of all, and the sweetest one of the bunch, but they used Katie and Lacy instead for the IV sticker and IV comforter.

Melba recommended Lacy use a certain vein in my left hand to stick the IV in, but Lacy picked a different vein for some reason.

I hyperventilated and grimaced when Lacy stuck me, and she said, "Well we weren't able to get it in. Your veins are narrowing out because of your anxiety. We will give you a little break then try again, only this time we're going to use the middle arm by your elbow."

I was so scared to have to do it all over again. Katie stood by the head of the bed, and rubbed my head to calm me down and held my hand like I asked her to this time too.

Unfortunately they were not able to get it in this time either. Come to find out they actually did get the needle in, and even drew blood for their blood test, so I thought they were good to go. At first, it looked like Lacy had the needle in. Bertha said she thought they took it out, because they must not have gotten it in a vein.

Bertha thought about that later and thought what I thought.

She asked me, "If they weren't able to get the IV needle in the vein how were they able to draw blood before they took it out? That just doesn't make sense."

I told Melba, "I'm really sorry. I really am trying. The pain hurts worse in the left arm than it does in the right, and I've never had an IV done in the left arm because of that. I've always had it done in the right arm."

Melba said, "I know, but because they have to put the other IV in for your Heart Cath in your right arm they have to put this one in your left arm. I know that sounds strange, but that's the side they use to do it. I'm really sorry. It's not your fault. You're just anxious, and your veins just keep narrowing out because of your anxiety. It's not your fault."

Melba said, "I'm going to talk to Dr. Wacky to see what she wants to do."

When Melba told me she was going to talk to Dr. Wacky about it, I thought, *"Oh no. I wish she wouldn't tell her about it, and would just try to figure something else out. I'm afraid Dr. Wacky might be upset with me for this."*

At one point while she was in there that time I was trying to decide whether to take my socks off or not.

Melba was checking my pulse in my ankles when I thought of this and I said, "I really want Dr. Wacky to look at the swelling and edema around my ankles. I want her to see whether she thinks it's anything to worry about or not."

I took my socks off and showed Melba the swelling and edema. I said, "Do you see that? Do you see how they are swelled? Do you see the edema? I wanted Dr. Wacky to be able to see this."

Melba said, "Are you going to take them off? Do you want to take them off?"

My being shy I was like, "I think I might. I'm not sure. I didn't know what to do. Did you notice it? Do you think she would look at it?"

Melba said, "Well, she probably would look at it if you asked her too. I don't know if she would or not but you could ask her to look."

I told Melba, "I guess I'll take them off then."

Melba asked, "You want them off or on? Do you want me to take these? Are you sure? Do I take these or not? You want me to put them with your other clothes?"

I said, "Okay yeah go ahead."

Melba said, "I'll put them right here in your drawer. You can get them back when you come back from your procedure."

They had this very hot wool blanket over me anyway and I was about to burn up and it was making my feet hot anyway so it actually felt better to have them off anyway. The only problem is now I felt like I was going to get embarrassed if anybody saw them. I was really self conscious but most of the time I was in there they had that hot wool blanket covering my feet where no one could see anyway. After this, Melba went to talk to Dr. Wacky like she said she was going to do earlier.

Melba came back and said, "You actually threw Dr. Wacky off a patient, but that's okay. We'll get this figured out somehow."

Melba said, "We're going to need to have a little pep talk, then we're going to give you another break. At 8:00am we're going to have the pick team come in. There will be several ladies coming in here to help you. There should be about seven of them. They're really nice. I think you'll like them, and I think you'll do really well with them."

I was relieved after she told me this, because I thought if a team of friendly ladies came in to all help me out, they would surely be able to get the IV in the next time. I thought they'd especially be able to get the IV in if one of them held my arm down so their IV person could do the stick.

Then Melba asked me, "Do you have any more Lidocaine?"

I said, "Not on me. Bertha left it in the car. I knew I should have brought it with me. I always keep it on me even after I put it on just in case."

Melba told me, "You need to go get your Lidocaine because we're getting ready to stick you in the upper left arm and this is going to hurt."

Bertha said, "Don't worry. I'll go get it. I'll be back in a minute."

Bertha came back with the left over Lidocaine bottle and spread the Lidocaine cream on my upper left arm as thick as she could as fast as she could.

Melba said, "It's only going to be 30 minutes, so you'd better put it on thick because this is really going to hurt. They're going to be coming in at 8:00 am so you guys need to try to hurry."

I waited till 8:10; well after I expected to see a pick team of friendly lady nurses come in which never came.

Instead, this grumpy lady, the so called pick team lady, walked in with her ultrasound machine. Come to find out, there was no pick team. There was just this ugly acting lady that came in with Melba and Katie to do the 3rd stick. They claimed she was the pick team lady nurse.

I asked Katie if she could come over to rub my head to calm me down, and hold my hand again to help comfort me through the 3rd IV stick.

She said, "No. I'm going to stay right here. I can't get over there. The machine is in the way."

Katie stood at the foot of the bed, and put her hands on the bed railing. Then she looked forward at me and smiled. I was really disappointed. I also felt funny I was no longer wearing socks and she was standing right next to my feet. I was glad they were covered by the blanket and hoped she wouldn't notice I was barefooted under my blanket. I feared I'd feel really embarrassed if she saw. What upset me the most was the fact she didn't go to the head of the bed to rub my head to calm me down and hold my hand during the IV stick. I wondered why she didn't just go around the machine. I was beyond frightened, I was scared to death I wouldn't be able to handle the next IV stick without her help. It was really stressing me out. I desperately needed Katie's help really bad, especially with this ugly acting woman in there.

Bertha thought Katie should have went around it, or crawled over there some way. When Katie didn't do this for me, she crawled over there herself to do it.

The grumpy pick team lady that came in the room sat beside me to look for a vein in my upper left arm and gave me dirty looks. She acted mad at me for no reason; this made me a nervous wreck.

Katie tried to keep me distracted, "Look at the ultrasound machine, and look at your veins. Isn't that neat? They're trying to find a vein so they can get the IV in."

I had no interest in looking at my blood veins just saying the word blood or needle freaks me out. I don't have to see them.

Melba was also trying to distract me by yelling, "Look at me! Look at me!!"

I would frantically look at the pick team lady. She wasn't the best looking person you ever saw, probably average looking. She wasn't very nice at all either. She was an old grump, in her mid 50's, with a big grey hair perm.

Melba kept saying, "No! Don't look over there! Look over here! Look at me!! Look at me!!!"

She was very rough with the needle, and practically swung at my arm with it. She stabbed me really hard with the IV at a straight shot in the upper left arm. I jumped, and pulled my arm away screaming my head off. Melba was very angry.

Melba yelled at me and said, "That's not allowed!"

I sulked and said, "I'm sorry. I can't help it. It hurts."

Melba said, "I know. I just had to distract you. What if she had got stuck? You can't do that! That's why I had to get your attention."

I was petrified, crying and shaking, and trembling in fear.

I told Melba, "I told Serena, the nurse at Dr. Wacky's office on March 14th I would probably scream when they did the IV and the procedures and she said, 'Scream all you want. We'll just deal with it.'"

I also told Melba, "The nurses at my local hospital I normally go to deal with this all the time. When I scream there, they just tell me I sound like a woman in labor."

Melba looked at me like she was not willing to accept my excuse for my screaming regardless of what I told her.

The pick team lady stuck me with the IV a second time. This time she did it at more of an angle. I still barely got through it. I had to grit my teeth to get through it without screaming. I was terrified. Bertha said that Katie actually went and held my arm down during my 4th IV stick. That's probably the only reason they got it in. Katie did not comfort me that time, either.

I think Katie thought, *"I'd better hold his arm down this time, or this will happen again."*

Considering how much trouble I already had with the first two IV stick attempts that Lacy did on me, you would think that Katie would be worried I might jerk my arm when she saw this grumpy PIC Team lady come in the room. She should have known it was going to scare me by how mean that lady acted.

My lists I gave them said that they could hold my arm down to keep me from jerking if they thought it was necessary. They were sure going to have trouble with me jerking with a woman like that lady coming in the room. That lady swung the IV at me like it was a shot, like I said, and Katie just stood there and did nothing. Since Katie did not hold my arm down for the 3rd IV stick, I failed to get through. Then I got blamed for it when it happened. They should have known if someone came in that made me nervous, and got rough with the needle, this would happen.

I already warned them this would happen if someone made me nervous on the lists I gave them. I told them not to send a lady that acted like the pick team lady did in there.

I already told them people like her made me nervous and not to give them to me for a nurse. They should have known better than that and sent another sweet acting, chipper nurse in there to help me instead. That or give me the seven other pick team ladies they lied about giving me that never showed up. They knew that would scare me. As a result, I got blamed by Melba when I jerked my arm on them. I felt like the ugly acting pick team lady nurse jabbed me hard on purpose the first time she stuck me. It was technically my third IV stick, but it was only her first attempt. The lady stuck the IV in my upper left arm like it was a shot the first time she did it. Katie did not comfort me through either of the last two sticks I had done. I did even worse with getting through the IV stick when the second lady stuck me that they called the pick team lady nurse. There was no way I was going to do well for her, either. She was much meaner and rougher with it, and Katie refused to comfort me this time. All this did was make matters even worse. It didn't make anything better to send that ugly acting pick team lady in there. All it did was make me react even worse than I did to being stuck with an IV and made me really flip out on them.

I started hugging Melba, and holding on to her, crying and saying, "I don't want to make you mad at me! You act like I made you mad!"

Melba said, "Are you okay? I'm not mad. I just had to distract you. That lady was above me, and what if she would have got stuck? I had to get your attention. That's all. I'm not mad. Everything's okay."

The second time this pick team lady nurse stuck me with the IV needle she got the needle in but I gritted my teeth not to scream. This was her second attempt, but technically my 4th stick.

Melba then said, "You did well. If you had not done well that time, there's a man standing out there outside the door that would have come in here next."

The head Cath Lab nurse, Angie was also supposed to have gotten a list of my accommodations that stated if I got a nurse that made me nervous I would be more likely to jerk from a needle stick if they did it instead of a nice acting person.

I got someone ugly for the 3rd and 4th IV sticks, and that's exactly what happened. Bertha said I just grimaced when Lacy did the first two IV sticks on me.

When this old grumpy acting pick team lady nurse got a hold of me, that's when I jerked, and screamed at the top of my lungs. I had stated on the lists of accommodations that it would not be my fault if I jerked on them. It is something I cannot help due to my severe oversensitivity to pain when getting IV sticks, catheters, and tubes put in. They should have known this would happen, after I pointed it out, long before I did it.

Plus their head cath lab nurse, Angie called Bertha on March 19th said, "I read the list and every nurse got a copy of it, and all his needs will be met! You don't have anything to worry about!"

Now not only does Katie not comfort me through a procedure, but she backs away somewhat the last time I hugged her. I didn't understand why she was doing this to me all of a sudden, because I needed her comfort.

A few minutes later Melba walked in to take me to the procedure room upstairs.

I said, "I need to be able to hug all my nurses in the procedure room upstairs also before and after the procedure."

Melba said, "I don't think you're going to be able to hug very many nurses up there! Most people up there like their space! The nurses have their rights! They don't have to hug you!"

290

Melba also said, "Katie said she doesn't like your ear on her cheek, so she doesn't want to hug you either!"

They'd already promised before that I could hug all my nurses, but now the story was being changed.

During the first two IV sticks, Melba, and Katie, and Lacy were all three nice to me, and met every accommodation I asked them to meet.

That all changed, after they informed Dr. Wacky I wasn't able to make it through the first two IV sticks.

When Melba said she was going to ask Dr. Wacky what she wanted to do about it, I thought, *"Oh no. I wish they wouldn't tell her about it, and would try to figure something else out themselves. I'm afraid Dr. Wacky might be upset with me for this."*

Now that Dr. Wacky was probably mad about my putting her behind, and they had an ugly woman helping with the IV instead of Lacy, Melba turned on me, and so had Katie.

I suspected Dr. Wacky may have told them to be mean to me by torturing me to punish me for not getting through the first two IV sticks. Melba apparently lied about the so called pick team of seven ladies that would be nice to me and help me through the procedure to make it even easier for me to get through it.

She told me she thought I'd do well if they came in there and they never did. There was only one pick team lady, and she was downright evil.

I kept rubbing my left arm because it was really hurting me and Bertha kept telling me, "That's not where the IV is. It's in your lower upper arm."

About an hour and a half later, at 10:00 am right before they took me back for my procedure I felt the place hurting me again.

I pulled my hospital gown sleeve up to rub on my arm and was shocked at what I saw.

I said, "Look at this! She left the tourniquet on!"

Bertha got Melba and asked, "Is that supposed to be there?"

Melba said, "No, its not."

She took it off my arm and got me a warm wash rag to put on it. There was a big red whelp around my upper left arm left for the next few days. Apparently this ugly acting pick team lady nurse left the tourniquet on my arm. She was long since gone by the time I figured out she did. Angie, the head nurse of the cath lab had already called Bertha two weeks before the procedure to assure her all my needs would be met. Now they were not being met at all.

Melba said, "Would you like to see your doctor before you go to the procedure?"

I said, "Yes."

Dr. Wacky went in there and I asked her if I could have a hug, and she lied and said, "I'm sick. I'm not contagious."

I was shocked because Dr. Wacky was fine with my hugging her at her office on March 14th.

On Friday, March 14th at Dr. Wacky's office Bertha told her about my hugging her nurses and how I had a need to hug, and she said, "That's fine. I'm not worried about it. That's not a problem."

Now, on April 1st she was acting totally the opposite about it.

After Bertha told her I really needed to be able to hug her she finally came over and hugged me. Because I saw how cross Dr. Wacky was acting toward me and I get easily embarrassed about my feet and I'm shy about people seeing them I wasn't about to show her my feet now.

 I went to all that trouble to take my socks off earlier, fearing embarrassment, just so she would look at my swelled ankles with the edema around them to see if she thought I had anything to worry about. That way if I did she could attempt to take care of that problem as well.

But since she was going acting mean I didn't want to show her now because I feel intimidated and embarrassed.

I asked her all the questions I had regarding my procedure before I went back.

Then she said, "I guess we can do your procedure now, if you cooperate with me."

Bertha had a shocked look on her face and Dr. Wacky said, "Or, we'll deal with it."

I was kind of offended and scared out of my mind so I started thinking thoughts like, *"What is she going to do, jab the tar out of me with the catheter, and get mad if I scream like Melba did over the IV, and allow the nurses to refuse to comfort me through the procedure as I asked?"*

I felt like Dr. Wacky was accusing me of not behaving myself by causing these nurses to have trouble getting the IV in me. I was afraid that she was only going to put me partially to sleep.

I was afraid she was going to scold me if I gave her trouble during the heart catherization procedure. I hoped she would put me completely out, but had my doubts the whole time that she would. She acted like I was going to be subconscious, like I would be partially aware of what was going on.

I was afraid that Dr. Wacky and her procedure room nurses would refuse to comfort me, because she thought I was supposed to take it like the average patient would. Bertha reminded her that I had an over sensitivity to pain.

Dr. Wacky said, "Oh I think it's mainly just his nerves. I've noticed that since you've been here. We just need to get the nerves down."

I thought, *"She apparently doesn't comprehend I feel pain ten times louder than everyone else does."*

I told Dr. Wacky, "I'm worried I'll have spasms in the right arm and in the heart after the procedure, and will need a week supply of pain medication to tame it down."

I pleaded with her, "I've had urinary catheters put in me before, and I had shooting pains from them, and I'm afraid the heart catheter might cause me to have shooting pains in the arm, and in the heart. That really has me worried."

I told her, "I also had shooting pains after a hernia surgery I had two years ago."

Melba said, "You won't have to worry about that. We give nitroglycerin before we even start the procedure and it blows up your veins."

Then I asked Dr. Wacky, "Could you still give me a week's supply of Hydrocodone? I'm really worried I'll be in pain afterwards and may still need it to tame things down even after the procedure?"

Dr. Wacky said, "I don't ever give Hydrocodone for a procedure like this one because this procedure is routine."

Bertha gasped, "Routine! It may be routine for you, but it's not routine for us. We've never had this kind of procedure before."

Big City Hospitals Don't Like Cowards   Brian Evans

I thought I was in trouble. Luckily, I didn't have spasms till April 4th. The pain was kind of overbearing that evening and it finally quit spazzing out about an hour after I took two Tylenol, which is unusual. Luckily, I didn't have any arm and chest spasms until the evening of April 4th.

After I talked to Dr. Wacky about the procedure and the medicine, this blonde girl, Marigold came in the room to wheel me to the procedure.

Melba introduced me to Marigold.

When she came to the side of the bed, I nicely asked her, "Can I have a hug?"

Marigold yelled at me and said, "You just lay back down there!" in a very mean condescending tone of voice.

She acted like she was going to let me have it if I didn't watch it because she was probably going to hurt me someway if I reached out to her for comfort. Marigold whipped around the bed, and grabbed the back of it like she wanted to move the bed furiously out of the room as quick as she could, and practically shove it out the door with me in it. I was scared to death.

I panicked and thought, *"What are you going to do to me?"*

I held on to the bed railings with my hands tight.

Bertha said I was white knuckled, holding the rails tight with my eyes darting back and forth in panic. I hugged her several times before I left. She was also worried they would do something terrible to me.

She thought because I was so scared I would have a heart attack before they even started the procedure.

When Marigold started out the door with the bed I was in Bertha asked Melba, "Can't she even smile?!"

Melba said, "She is smiling!" and the blonde girl got a big smirk on her face and Melba stomped out of the room down the hall behind her.

Marigold pushed my bed furiously down the hall, and into the elevator. We got off the elevator and she hurried down another hall upstairs. Then she turned the corner down a back hallway and into a room. She placed my bed on wheels next to an examination table.

The first person I saw come into the room was Fanny.

She walked toward me and I pleaded with her, "Can I have a hug?"

The girl just looked at me angrily and didn't say a word but she stormed off to her machine clear across the room from me.

I asked the second girl I saw, Jessica, "Can I have a hug?"

She just looked at me like she was mad, didn't even bother responding to my question and practically stormed across the room to her machine just like the first person.

I frantically asked everyone in the procedure room, "Didn't you get a list of my accommodations?"

Jessica stormed across the room and yelled, "Yes!"

She yelled her answer to me like she was mad as a hornet at me. She may have admitted they got the list of accommodations in anger but neither she nor any of the rest of the girls in the room was meeting them. All of the young *female* nurses in there appeared to be in their mid 20's. That's what really shocked me. They even looked like girls that normally would have been nice and friendly and compassionate, but they were not. They were completely uncompassionate. In the past the youngest nurses I ever had were always the friendliest, but not at this hospital.

The third girl Cora, who was nice to me earlier in the prep room finally came up to the head of the bed and in a very sweet tone of voice said, "Hello!"

I asked, "Can I have a hug?"

She said, "Sure."

A fourth girl, Sandy went to the other side of my bed at the head of the bed and I asked, "Can I have a hug?"

She said, "Yes." and gave me a hug.

This made me feel better for a moment but I still felt rejected by everybody else. Then I accidentally overheard one of the first two girls call the fourth girl Sandy when they asked her a question. So I figured out who she was. Just about the time I thought things were about to turn around, things immediately got grim again.

A fifth girl, Sally walked in the door and I asked her, "Can I have a hug?"

She said, "No!"

I felt rejected again and felt like I could not bear my situation. Sally had come over to the side of my bed just past were Cora was standing.

She backed away when I asked her for a hug. She came back at me again with a plastic tube that had a plastic piece on the end of it, and she said, "Are you ready?"

I said, "Yes!"

I looked at the foot of the bed, and saw this other girl standing there.

She said, "I'm going to put this on him."

She lifted the bed cover just above my foot. She put what looked like a blood pressure cuff on my leg just above the ankle.

I didn't know one of them was going to uncover my foot to put a blood pressure cuff around my ankle and I felt a little strange because she saw me in my bare feet because I didn't have any socks on.

Then I looked back the other way where I originally saw Cora and Sally and no one was standing there anywhere.

I thought, *"Everyone's abandoned me!"*

I thought, *"They must have left me here to lay here and suffer!"*

Then I thought, *"They probably want the doctor to torture me and refuse to comfort me!"*

I thought, *"Everybody must be going to watch from a distance and gawk at me, and laugh at me, while the doctor tortures me with no one standing there to help me, and have a hay day enjoying the show!"*

I thought, *"Where did everybody go?"*

Then I thought, *"What if Cora saw I wasn't wearing socks when that other girl uncovered my foot to put that blood pressure cuff on above my ankle? I left my socks on after she asked me to change into my hospital gown earlier. She probably wonders why I took my socks off later and wonders why in the world I'm barefooted all of a sudden. She's probably thinking, 'Why did he take his socks off after leaving them on earlier? Is there something weird going on here?' I hope that wasn't the reason she suddenly disappeared. I hope she didn't leave because of that and think something weird was going on. I don't know for sure if she thought that or not, but I hope that's not why she suddenly disappeared all of a sudden.*

I figure she must think there's something fishy going on since I took my socks off after all after leaving them on earlier when she saw me the first time. I hope I didn't run her off. I didn't mean to give her the wrong idea. I don't know where she went."

Then I thought, *"Maybe the doctor just sent them away and told them to go somewhere else so she could have a hay day torturing me and they wouldn't be there to help me or comfort me if she did. I'd be fair game to her then and they wouldn't be able to do a thing about it because they wouldn't be there to comfort me and console me in my distress."*

I thought, *"They must have ran off so the doctor and her other girl nurses could torture me without comforting me."*

I paused a minute, looking the direction where Cora and Sally were originally standing wondering, *"Why don't I see anybody?"*

I looked in front of me, then toward the wall, then in front of me and toward the wall again and couldn't see anybody.

I was scared and thought, *"Everybody left me! Why did everybody leave? Please, somebody help me! Don't leave me here alone!"*

After I looked and looked a minute or two, and still didn't see Cora and Sally I was still wondering why I didn't see anybody, and suddenly I was out cold. I didn't know anything else.

When they were done they took me back to the prep room where I woke up again.

I asked Melba, "Could you please have someone comfort me when you take the IV out?

Melba said, "No! I'm not going to get anybody. I'm just going to pull it out!"

Melba just pulled the IV out, and it really hurt me. She just let me suffer without any help or any compassion from anyone. It really hurt me and I was afraid.

When Melba said, "You can get dressed now." After Bertha came back in the room, I flung the bottom of my sheet to cover my feet and frantically said to Bertha, "Hand me my socks out of the drawer, quick!"

I grabbed my socks and pulled them under my sheet with most of the sheet raised up and quickly put my socks back on as fast as I could.

Melba looked at me like she was thinking, "What on earth are you doing?"

Bertha said, "You're showing them parts of your body most people don't want people to see when you raise the sheet up like that."

I said, "I'm putting my socks back on under the sheet. I don't want anybody to see my feet."

Bertha said, "Well, while you're trying to hide your feet from these people trying to put your socks back on, your showing everybody something else because you have your sheet raised up and when you jerk around under there trying to put your socks back on so they don't see you, they're seeing something else instead."

She said, "They probably don't know what was going on. They don't know you're embarrassed about your feet. They never would have guessed that's the reason you got all anxious and rushed to put your socks back on under the sheet. Try to hurry and put your socks back on and put the sheet back down. They're standing over here shocked acting like they don't know what to think."

I didn't want to anybody to see my feet, so I did that to hide them. For some reason probably because they gave me a pill for anxiety earlier my self-consciousness was not hitting me as hard at the moment that girl uncovered my foot in the procedure room but it was really getting to me now and I was severely embarrassed. Bertha thinks it was because I was under a tremendous amount of anesthesia too. It bothered me now, something fierce.

While I was in the procedure room, Bertha thought sure Melba was going to overdose me to get back at her for asking for my needs to be met. Bertha was pacing back and forth, and crying in front of the hospital the whole time I was in there. I never cared for Melba to begin with and she just made me nervous the whole time. I wished she would have just let Lacy and Katie at it to begin with and stayed out of it. If she would have stayed out of the equation the whole thing might have never happened.

Angie the same lady that assured her my needs would be met on March 19th, walked up behind Bertha while she was crying.

She hatefully snaps at her, "Mrs. Evans! What seems to be the problem, here?"

Bertha said, "The problem is, I was assured that every one of my husband's needs would be met!"

She said, "The procedure is going well! His needs are being met! We can't meet all his requests, but all of his needs are being met!"

The patient advocate even came along, and took the side of the head Cath Lab nurse, Angie, instead of Bertha. They were more of a patient condemner than a patient advocate. A security guard came along, and also gave Bertha problems.

Cherry, a friend of ours from church was to come help me. She knew I was nervous about the test from when I called her earlier in the week about it. She didn't get there in time though; they had already taken me upstairs. When I woke up the nurses would not let Cherry even come see me afterwards.

The head Cath lab nurse, Angie came to the waiting room to talk to Bertha. Cherry was sitting next to her trying to calm her down.

She asked Cherry, "Are you a nurse?!"

Cherry said, "I don't think that's any of your business."

Angie, the head nurse of the Cath Lab department, and the security guard, and the patient advocate, all three continually hounded Bertha and Cherry the whole time I was in the procedure room, and wouldn't leave them alone.

They acted like they thought it was horrible that Bertha would ask them to stoop to such a level where they would have to try to comfort me, because they thought the rights of the nurses were far above the genuine needs that I had they needed to meet.

Angie kept saying, "The nurses have their rights! I'm not going to make my nurses hug him! His needs are being met but I can't meet his requests and I can't make my nurses hug him!"

Angie made Bertha feel like she thought my requests were inappropriate, and that everything Bertha was asking them to do for me was inappropriate. Melba told Bertha it was not in their job description to meet my requests.

When I finally got out of there, I saw Cherry and I excitedly shouted "Cherry!"

I was glad to get out of there. We decided we were never going back. Let me tell you something. I know something about the nursing world they don't know I know. Two ladies begged me to take Medical Assisting several years ago when I was taking a Pharmacology class in order to get hired as a Pharmacy clerk by a Pharmacy in town, and wishing their college campus had a major in Business that they did not have.

These two ladies noticed I was good at what I did, and said that if I majored in Medical Assisting they would help me with my fear of needles in the two classes that required shots and blood tests. It just so happens, I was not interested in a clinical degree, but a clerical degree, and you could be whichever Medical Assistant you wanted to be, but still had to take two classes involving needles I really didn't want to take, because I just wanted to do paperwork in an office. At that time I took a Medical Administrative Assisting class.

The Director of the entire Medical Assisting Program got up in front of the class one day, and said, "I want to tell you something. In the nursing world it's not about your rights. The patient comes first. The patients have a set of rights that you have to meet, and you are required to meet them. That means that if someone comes in to your doctor's office or hospital with a fear of needles, and they tell you that there are certain things they need for you to do to get them through a needle stick, or there's a certain type of person they need to help them through a needle stick, then you are required to do whatever it is they need to get them through it."

That's right; my teacher said it, the director of the department. As a matter of fact, it's in their medical school books too. They have a nurse's creed, and an oath they have to promise to. They are required to comfort and console the patient through any painful experience they may have because of needle sticks or invasive procedures. Nurses are required to do whatever it takes to get that person through it and meet their requests exactly the way they want you to. That means if men scare them, and they feel more comfortable with a *female* nurse, you have to give them that.

If one *female* nurse acts too serious and makes them nervous, and another one is bubbly with a motherly personality, you have to give them that, too, if they ask you to. And it doesn't mean if you decide you want to play music for them, or just talk them through it as an alternative compromise, because it is what you want to do for them, in order to get out of having to touch them.

It doesn't mean, if they ask you to rub their head to calm them down and hold their hand that you can do what you want to do to help them instead of what they are asking you to do, which is what works for them. You have to rub their head to calm them down and hold their hand if that's what they want and that's what works for them. You can't withhold this from them just because you don't want to have to do something like that, because you don't want to have to stoop to that low a level to have to play the role of someone's mother to get them through something. If that's what they need, and they ask you to do that for them, that's what you are required to do according to the nursing profession's own rule book.

One Cardiology clinic facility in Missouri told Bertha years ago they didn't think their nurses would be comfortable doing that.

They are the ones that said, "Well, we don't feel comfortable doing that for you, can we play a tape of music for you instead or talk you through it?"

The answer was, "No, I want them to do what nurses have always done for me, because that is what works for me, to rub my head to calm me down and hold my hand."

Well guess what! You as nurses have to not only because I need it but, because your own school books tell you if that is what I need, then that is what you have to do or at least find someone who will.

At Dreamer's Hope Regional Medical Center in Arkansas, all the nurses everywhere in every department are way nicer to me there than they were at Transylvania Regional Hospital in the Cath Lab I went to. Dreamer's Hope Regional Medical Center never gave me any problems. I've probably been to Dreamer's Hope Hospital a dozen times in the past ten years, and the nurses at their hospital have done exactly what we asked them to do for me every time with no complaint where we normally go.

Unfortunately, Dreamer's Hope Hospital didn't have a cath lab when I needed this procedure done, so we had to go to a bigger city hospital just to get a Heart Catherization or Transesophageal Echocardiogram done on me. That's why we went to Transylvania Regional Hospital's cath lab in the first place, because they do all that. If my own local hospital at Dreamer's Hope Regional would have had this, I guarantee you I would have never went to this cath lab at Transylvania Regional's Hospital. I would have just waited till I had an emergency, and gone to the emergency room for it at my own hospital if they would have had something like this, and the people there would have been way nicer than this to me.

No one ever treated me with the cruelty at Dreamer's Hope Regional that Transylvania Regional Hospital treated me with. That was terrible, and the whole thing is ridiculous.

A month after this, my family doctor informed me she wanted to do a retest in one year. I was told I'd have to go back the next March or April. We even tried to get a different Cardiologist at a different hospital to help me, but their hospital didn't trust their own nurses. They feared their nurses would do me the same way as Transylvania Regional did, and tried to discourage my even going to them. Now, I feel stuck with having to go back to Transylvania Regional Hospital, and hoping these people will be nice this time. I'm just not ever going back to them.

When you look at my story about the nightmare I had about what these nurses might do to me you might think, *"Oh, Brian. It's just your imagination. Nobody's ever going to do something like that to you."* But for one thing, think about what really did happen with the ones I did get that were supposed to be nicer.

Keep in mind that I told Melba all about it and she kept acting guilty, and openly admitted these three lady nurses I saw two weeks earlier would not have understood me.

They definitely would not have been nice about anything even according to her and she made it quite obvious that my fears were not in vain.

The trick I feared they would play on me by pretending I would get a nicer nurse when they asked me to change into my hospital gown and then snap at me and say, "You're getting us!" was actually played on me by a hospital in Texas in 1994. In that setting the nice person went in, and had me change into my gown and then disappeared.

The evil *serious trended* fe*male* nurse took over when they were gone and had her tall, husky, *male* nurse torture me with an IV while she griped at me for screaming in pain and had a hay day with it. There have been several instances in my life time where the more serious acting, mediocre, straight faced nurses were grumpy, acted domineering and dictatorial toward me and considered me to be their property. I was someone they could run over at will without my being able to do a thing about it.

This "serious trended female nurse" had the idea that because they were the nurse and I was not, they were in control. So they felt like they had power over me and I couldn't do a thing to stop them. That's the way these three creepy acting serious trended fe*male* nurses acted.

They crossed me as being nurses that would say, "You do what I say or else!"

They probably would control my every move if I refused to cooperate with them. I have been threatened in several instances in my lifetime by these type of nurses who told me back then if I did not do what they asked, they would strip me down against my will to force me to cooperate with them whether I liked it or not. They would let me know they would make my life miserable if I did not cooperate with them.

They all claimed they were not about to put up with my cowardly squeamishness, or tendencies. They were that mean.

They acted like, "You think you're scared now, you're really going to be scared when we get done with you!"

Brian Evans# Big City Hospitals Don't Like Cowards

They were horrible. Besides this, there is a paragraph in Transylvania Regional Medical Center's booklet that says something about restraints that would go right with my theory of what these creepy three ladies would have done.

It says, "As a patient, you have the right to be free from restraints or seclusion unless medically required to keep you or others safe. You have the right to safe use of restraints or seclusion by trained staff when needed. You have the right to be free from any type of restraint or seclusion put in place as a means of intimidation, punishment, or convenience."

Sounds fishy, doesn't it. It makes it sound like they must have a problem with things like this at their hospital, or it would not be in there. My own local, friendly acting hospital I normally went to didn't even have a rule booklet about them at this time.

They act nice to everybody to begin with in most of their departments so why would this other hospital have a booklet with something like this in it if it is not a problem? If it is a problem, they need to make this kind of statement, but if it was not a problem it probably wouldn't even be in there in the first place, because no one would ever have to worry about it.

This makes it sound like the creepy three really would have done everything I feared they would do, especially since Melba acted guilty, like she knew they were going to if I got them, when I told her about it.

So in my opinion if I would have got the creepy three, I believe they would have done everything I stated in the story I feared they would do to me, and Bertha agrees with me. If I were to be thrown into their ball court the next time I went in for my retake procedure, we could have a horrible situation on our hands, and everything fictitious about what they would have done would suddenly become a horrible reality. There wouldn't be anything fictitious about it anymore, because if I got them, it really would happen and there wouldn't be any maybes about it anymore.

Big City Hospitals Don't Like Cowards

Everything I feared would come true and it wouldn't be a fiction anymore. If I got them, what was fictional would become real, and I would be in serious trouble.

I could tell by the way they acted they were really that way. Melba acted like she thought so too and so did Bertha. I hope if I ever did go back, I wouldn't get them the next time. Even if I did get who I got the last time, they could be nicer than last time but they probably actually wouldn't.

Chances are if I ever got them again, they would try to get revenge for my trying to get them in trouble for what they did and do even worse things to me than they did the last time. I don't trust anybody there anymore. I'm afraid of those people.

I'm scared to death of those people. I'm afraid of what they might do. There's no telling what they might try if they thought they had the power to get by with it. That's exactly what I'm afraid of. The power to get by with it is what already caused this to happen.

If these nurses at this hospital feel they have all the more power to do something horrible to me next time, they may feel like there's nothing left to stop them from doing anything they wish to do to me because the figure no one will ever do anything about it.

I also found out these people did this to a man with a cane, when I was looking for a different doctor's office and didn't get in because they were connected with this hospital.

I also found out one of my church friends, a *female* senior citizen went to these people, told them that she had trouble with IV sticks because she had bad veins and these people promised her they would be nice to her. When they failed after several tries, they got angry with her and decided they were going to get rough and tried to torture her as well.

One of their own ex-employees from the business office left a review about them saying nurses were keeping charts back from patients so stuff would not come back on them.

I think something is going on, and they don't want people above them to find out what their doing. I think they're treating people with cruelty and documenting some of the things they do to them. If they got caught they'd get found out and get in trouble. Someone needs to make sure they are not treating their patients with cruelty behind everyone else's back. If they don't, they will feel like they are getting by with this and continue to torture future vulnerable, gullible victims that can't defend themselves.

We reported the incident. We are hoping if they get in trouble for this they'll think they'd better be nice or they might lose their job.

Chapter Thirty One
Wannabe General Hospital

Now that I've told you all the different terrible experiences I went through with different hospitals, I want to tell you about a plea I had with a Cardiologist at a different hospital in Missouri I contacted telling her all my needs. I let her know I saw her website, and 3/4ths of her nurses looked really friendly. I told her I picked the ones I liked. I had made a list of who I wanted for them and myself. They had pictures of people in about four different departments. A couple of the pictures must have had 15 or 20 people in each picture and the other two pictures had four or five nurses a piece in them. Out of about 50 possible nurses, I actually picked 36 people I liked the looks of and told her they were the ones I wanted.

I told this Cardiologist, Dr. Jenny, one of the ladies in the picture with only four or five people in it that there was one person in that specific picture I liked I thought would be more motherly acting than the others. I liked them all, but this one just sort of stuck out at me like she would have that extreme peppiness the others have, but also have a calmness about her that made me feel calm, similar to that of someone I picked out at my own hospital that I go to for procedures that helps me with my IVs there. This lady is probably even more upbeat than she is. There was just something about her that gave me the feeling she had some of the same personality qualities as the one that helps me now as the one that already helps me at my own hospital. The one that usually helps me now is upbeat alright, but she has this unusual calmness about her also that makes me feel calm. That's what feeling I got about the woman I saw in the picture.

Dr. Jenny is a fictional name for a real person by the way and so is the name I am going to give you of her nurse I liked. I'm going to call her, Myra Sylvester, also a fictional name for a real person.

I actually wrote Dr. Jenny a letter explaining how I had special needs and how certain nurses that were not my type had treated me with cruelty and lack of compassion.

310

I told her the ones I did like that were more *bubbly acting* were more understanding and eager to help me with my fear of needles and comfort me and console me in the way I asked them to and they way I needed them to:

Here is the letter I wrote Dr. Jenny.

Dear Dr. Jenny,

Please look at the following lists of accommodations for the two procedures I thought you would most likely perform on me.

Also, the list of nurses that I am giving you that I have seen pictures of are the ones I feel like would be the ones I am most comfortable working with.

Please see to it that all my needs are met on my accommodations lists and the nurses I receive for my procedures are from the list of nurses that I have given you.

All this is important in order to keep my anxieties down and make me to feel less fearful of what is being done and be comfortable with who I get and get the comfort I need in the midst of my pain and fear during the procedures.

I am autistic, and Bertha is also planning on sending you a letter with this information I am giving you.

I may seem normal and some people that are not used to seeing me in the hospital setting may not think I seem like someone that would have the fear and anxiety over needles and the oversensitivity to pain that I have until they get me in there, and the people that cannot already see this are usually in for a shocking surprise when they get me in a position where I have to be stuck or have tubes inserted in me or ran through me and find out I was not joking about how I get and what I need.

I went to a clinic a long time ago where a girl thought I was joking when I asked her to comfort me when this other nurse did a Urodynamics test on me and then when the catheter was inserted and I screamed and nearly went ballistic on them the girl suddenly got shook up bad, patted me on the shoulder, and said, "It's okay. We're half way there. We're almost done. Please just try to hold on a little longer." It was too late, and the other nurse said, "I'm taking it out! I'm hurting him too much!"

When this lady said this, the girl's eyes welled up and she looked like she was about to cry but I could tell she was trying to hold back the tears to keep this lady from thinking bad of her.

I think the girl nurse that started out refusing to comfort me realized I wasn't joking after all was afraid if the head nurse that inserted the catheter saw her crying, who wasn't very friendly by the way, would think she was a crybaby. I think this is why she was trying to hold back the tears, because she felt humiliated in front of the other nurse for crying after she failed me.

Please do not make this mistake.

I have a vibrant personality myself, and sometimes it gives off a false impression that I am bold and brave, when in fact, I am a coward and a crybaby myself. I am terrified of needles, and I am very over sensitive to pain, and need my nurses to treat me like a mother treats her child when she tries to comfort them, like a mother and a baby, actually.

My nurses at Dreamer's Hope Hospital in Arkansas do the very things I am asking your nurses to do for me, and one of my nurses at my family doctor's office also meets these accommodations for me herself because she knows this is what I need.

I know there are some people in some places that may feel weird treating an older person like myself like a little baby but please understand this is really what I need and this is what helps me get through things.

Big City Hospitals Don't Like Cowards   Brian Evans

It's a win-win situation at Dreamer's Hope Hospital in PreOp and Inpatient care and they understand all my needs and they're okay with me.

My hospital, and my doctor's office, and most of the friends I have now consider me to be a special needs person, which is what I am.

I may seem intelligent, but that is because I went to vast amount of trouble to memorize books galore from the 8th grade on in all regular classes after leaving the Special Ed Department after the 7th grade level.

My mother spent hours on end drilling facts in my head for years just to pass my classes, then I took a Reading Comprehension Class my first year of college, and found out I only read on the 7th grade level.

One year later, I read on the 10th grade, 3rd month level.

By my 3rd year of college I made A's and B's like everyone else, finally, but there was always a subject lie College Algebra or some other subject that would blow everything and I had to change majors continually.

Plus, I couldn't get anybody to give me a job in my own field at the time.

I had no clue what I was doing on my Manuel labor jobs, and my bosses had to show me everything, and it aggravated them.

My social and performance intelligence lagged behind the intellectual intelligence, and if I hadn't been "booked" to death, I wouldn't be this smart, so, if I have an intelligent façade that make you think, "What's his excuse?" that's why.

Please have patience with me, and have mercy on me when I am in pain during the procedures you are liable to perform on me, which are invasive.

Please do not be upset with me if I fail you, and let your nurses keep trying until they can get an IV in me.

You will probably want to schedule me for your earliest appointment when you do your procedures on me, and tell your nurses to be ready to have a basket case on their hands, and do everything they can to help me as sweetly and gently as they possible can, because it will probably be hard to get an IV started on me because of my anxiety and oversensitivity to pain.

I have been to several different cardiologists and finally got one who did a Transesophageal Echocardiogram on me and a Heart Catherization Test and found an Atrial Septal Defect (Patent Foramen Ovale) that never sealed up, a Right to Left Shunt, a Trice Mitral Valve Regurgitation, and a Mild Tricuspid Regurgitation.

At least, a Cardiologist finally found the birth defects that I tried to tell people I had but unfortunately they were not very understanding about my fear of needles and got upset because I threw them off a patient. I told them I was sorry, but the very people who were doing what I needed them to do for me just quit meeting my accommodations and started acting mean to me and tried to hurt me. Then they griped about having to meet my accommodations after already promising all of them would be met. These people really scared me after this. I was afraid of these people.

Please do not be with me the way they were, but try to have compassion and have mercy on me and do the best you can, however long it takes.

Maybe your nurses can do better.

If it would be okay with you, I would like to meet your nurses on the Cath lab team and the Cardiac Care Unit so I can get established with them in hopes to help them understand me better so they know what they are dealing with before they even have to do a test on me.

If they are familiar with my personality and what I am like and what I need and feel, they can relate to me better before I'm just thrown at them one day for a procedure I think it would help them understand me and then they would feel more comfortable with me and I would feel more comfortable with them.

Out of all the nurses on the list that I have given you, I felt the best about Myra Sylvester and would like her to be the main one to comfort me through the procedures you are doing.

If I could meet Myra and the other nurses I liked, whom I named several of on the list, I feel like she and them would be more understanding of what I want them to do.

I didn't want anybody to feel like, "Who's he and what does he want?"

They need to understand this is really important.

It is very important that I get the people I need that make me the most comfortable of the bunch and that they do the things I need them to do to help me get through all this stuff.

Please explain to Myra and these other nurses that I am autistic, and it is very important that I get the people I ask for and that I have special needs I need them to meet and tell them to just follow my accommodations list I've given you and treat me like I was one of their kids because this is what I need.

Please try to understand. I know I'm different from most people but I do have a disability so I really need you to do everything you can to help me by fulfilling all my needs I have asked you to meet.

Please give me a chance and see what you can do, but please meet all my accommodations.

If I'm not given people that I like that I'm comfortable with, and they don't' meet the needs I'm asking them to meet, it's liable to scare me to such a point that it could throw me into a heart attack, so, please give me what I need by meeting my lists of accommodations I'm giving you.

It will spook me if I'm given *male* nurses, and it will also hurt more if they do everything, and I won't receive the comfort I need from the *female* nurses I need.

It won't help matters any to give me the straight faced, cordial acting *female* nurses either because they scare me, too.

In most instances, the straight faced nurses that act more serious usually get a power kick and think, "Why, if it isn't the little cry baby" What can we do to scare him now? We'll toughen him up. We'll be so rough it will make his life miserable." Or, "I think we're going to have trouble with this one. I hope he doesn't' give us any problems." Followed by, "Is there a problem? Are you going to do this for us or are we going to do it for you? If you're going to be difficult, we will make you do what we want, and we're going to make your life miserable, so, you better hope you don't give us any problems, or you will be sorry." Some of them are that mean. The ones that aren't still don't make me feel comforted and make me nervous.

The *bubbly acting female* nurses that understand me better have always been more compassionate, and said things like, "I'm sorry honey. We have to do this. I'm sorry this has to hurt. We'll be done in a little while; okay." or, "Come on buddy, come with me and let's get this thing done! You're going to be fine! You just wait and see! We're going to take care of you and you'll be just fine! We'll be right here for you!"

This is what I need and these are the type of nurses I like and do the best with.

This other cardiologist wanted to do a retest on the Transesophageal Echocardiogram in a year, and after what I went through, I wanted to find someone more compassionate, who would understand who had more living, compassionate nurses that cared for a person that had difficulty with needles and such and were willing to do whatever they needed to do to help this person get through.

This is what I felt like I saw in your nurses when I saw their pictures and this is what I hoped I was seeing with you also when I saw your picture.

I wanted more compassionate, more understanding doctors and nurses who would be more willing to meet my needs to the ultimate degree to be able to get me through all the scary things (scary procedures, needles, IVs, tubes, catheters, etc.)

Please be the doctor and team of nurses for me I felt like I saw.

I hope you understand.
                              Sincerely,

                              Brian Gene Evans

P.S. I needed to tell you that these heart defects I've had since birth that just now showed up on a test for the first time since age six years, nine months old will not show up on a less invasive test.

I figured you would feel sorry for me and say, "I tell you what. I can do a less invasive test" but several other cardiologists have tried this several times over, and so has the hospital, and not one has ever been able to find these defects on a Regular Echocardiogram (Transthoracic Echocardiogram), EKG (Electrocardiogram), CT Angiogram (which still involved and IV), or even a Cardiac Perfusion Test (which also involved an IV).

The only thing these defects have ever shown up on is a Transesophageal Echocardiogram and a Heart Catherization.

I think she just checked for coronary artery blockage on the Heart Catherization test and just checked for the valvular defects on the Transesophageal Echocardiogram.

Even if you just did a Transesophageal Echocardiogram, that would still involve IV sedation and a tube in the throat, and somehow, I have this feeling if I had to guess, you probably still wanted to do the Heart Catherization test even if you did find it on the Transesophageal Echocardiogram.

So, one way or the other, we're talking invasive procedures if you want to find anything.

I'm sorry. I know I'm difficult to deal with but I think this is the only way you're going to find it.

At least there's one good thing, Dreamer's Hope Hospital's nurses would tell you that, yes, this is difficult for me, but I am the kindest, friendliest, most well behaved patient they ever had. I hope you feel the same way.

Please do what you can to help me by meeting my lists of accommodations.

Thanks.

End of Letter

Because of the misunderstanding about the hugging thing at the other hospital, considering it was only on the Dear Physician letters, because I forgot to put it on my accommodations lists I made up, I revamped both of those lists to also include that to make sure nobody missed it this time.

Here is the revamped "Dear Physician Letter" Bertha wrote for me, which we sent to this lady:

Dear Physician,

I wanted to advocate for my sweet, dear, autistic husband Brian Evans who also has an anxiety disorder. He worries about everything and details are very important to him. Brian can talk but it is very hard for him to get what is in his head out of his mouth. It is much easier for him to write. Expect an extremely detailed letter each time he has something to tell you about. If at all possible make a way for Brian to meet the people who will be working with him before hand because he is terrified of medical procedures.

This is a summary of what you need to know about my husband. If and when you need to do any procedure on him please carefully read what he needs you to know about.

Brian is terrified of men in the medical field because he was traumatized by men torturing him as a child with needles in a Military Hospital. Please never use a *male* anything with my husband. It is very important that all the people working with my husband be sweet, happy go lucky, chipper, motherly *females*.

Most people with autism do not like to be touched, however, Brian is just the opposite. He needs to be able to hug his doctors and nurses in order to stay calm and know everything will be okay. Please find it in your heart to allow him to hug everyone. A hug to him is pressing his ear to the other person's check. He also needs to be given reassuring smiles.

The most important thing you need to know about Brian is that he has a MAJOR needle phobia. I would give him something to calm him down a bit, well before any needles are used.

He needs three happy go lucky *females* for anything involving a needle: One to hold his hand and gently caress the top of his head (just like you would comfort a terrified child), one to hold his arm or hand on one to insert the needle. You see, Brian looks perfectly normal but socially and emotionally he's a sweet little boy stuck in a man's body.

Thanks for your compassion.

In Christian Love,

Bertha Marie

<u>Accommodations for Transesophageal Echocardiogram</u>
(Revamped)

Brian needs you to know the following:

I need to be able to hug all my happy go lucky *female* nurses.

I need a very bubbly, peppy, chipper, happy go lucky *female* nurse to rub my head to calm me down and hold my hand.

I need another happy go lucky *female* nurse to do the IV stick.

Please spray a numbing solution in my throat before inserting the tube.

Please wait till I am calmed down from the IV stick before inserting the tube down my throat.

The happy go lucky nurse that comforts me through the IV stick also needs to rub my head to calm me down and hold my hand when you put the tube in my throat.

If you can, please put me completely to sleep before you even put the tube in my throat because I will be panicked if I am awake.

I also have a gag reflux, so make sure to watch out for this to happen.

Please slide the tube in my mouth and down my throat as gently as you can to keep from hurting me as much.

Please have patience with me over my anxiety and panic attacks over the tube insertion and the IV stick. This is a very scary procedure for me and I need your help.

All nurses must be very happy go lucky, peppy, *chipper acting females* that deal with me in this department and every department of the hospital.

They will all need to do the best they can to comfort me through the test and talk me through it when I'm being stuck with an IV or other instrument and try to keep me distracted when I am in pain.

It helps me when you all act like you're my buddies and you're going to help me the best way you can and encourage me through the procedure when I am scared and in pain.

It will be difficult for me not to jerk on a test like this one, so some of my nurse may have to hold me down to keep me from jerking.

You may have to have one of the nurse's hold my arm down for the IV stick to keep me from jerking.

Please ask these nurses to put me completely out with the gas and the IV.

At least make me as numb and tingly as you possibly can to keep me from feeling anything to make it easier for me.

The best kinds of nurses for me are the ones that act like someone a person dug up off of a Disney movie or something.

If you see how *bubbly acting* the Disney movie characters Anastasia, or Ariel, the Little Mermaid, or Barbie's Rapunzel, or Frauline Marie from the "Sound of Music" or Eliza Doolittle on "My Fair Lady" act, and notice the same personality tendencies in a real live person that's a nurse, this is the personality types I relate to the most.

Some people may think there is no such thing as a person that acts like this, but if you really think about it, there are some people that when you see the way they act might make someone want to say, "You know, you act just like Frauline Maria" or "You act just like the character, Aerial on the Little Mermaid" or "You sure act a lot like that girl named Anastasia on that movie. Have you ever seen that?"

Big City Hospitals Don't Like Cowards   Brian Evans

Ever heard people make these kinds of comments about people they've run into.

They may not be Anastasia or Eliza Doolittle or Frauline Maria or Ariel or Barbie's Rapunzel, but when you see the way they act in public you might think, "Boy, they may not be that person, but they sure do act like it. If I didn't know any better, I'd think it was them. Even though, they're not them, they just act like them."

I actually had a teacher once tell me, "You act just like Frauline Maria" and actually cracked jokes about me saying, "How do you solve a problem like Maria?" I had a boss once that kept calling me Gilligan and said, "You act just like Gilligan. Are you Gilligan?"

So, you see, it is possible. You just got to be able to be on the lookout for them and notice differences in their personalities that make them a little different from the average person due to their extravagantly vibrant personality that makes them glow and so cheery you'd think someone got them off a Disney movie or something.

Accommodations for Heart Catherization Test (Revamped)

Catheters feel like a sword is being run through me.

Dr. Scotty puts me completely to sleep when using urinary catheters because he knows it will be too excruciating for me to handle.

I feel like it would be even more excruciating if I had to have a catheter threaded all the way from my wrist to my heart or my groin to my heart, whichever of the two ways you chose to go, both would be overwhelmingly excruciating for me.

I need to be able to hug all my happy go lucky *female* nurses I get.

I need a very happy go lucky *female* nurse to rub my head to calm me down and hold my hand through the IV stick and the catheter insertion.

A very happy go lucky *female* nurse needs to do the IV stick.

A very happy go lucky *female* nurse needs to insert the catheter.

If Dr. Jenny needs to insert the catheter, because it has to be a doctor, that's fine too because she looks like she would be a very happy go lucky, peppy, chipper person herself from seeing the picture I saw. At least I hope so.

I need several other happy go lucky *female* nurses to assist with the procedure.

Please knock me out completely before inserting the catheter. If you refuse to knock me out, please, at least give me enough nitrous oxide to make me numb and tingly to help me not feel the stick and the catheter being run through me and put a lot of numbing stuff and pain medicine in my IV to keep from hurting me as bad.

If you do not knock me out to where I am asleep and can't feel what you are doing, you will need to be ready to do the following, because you will probably have a disaster on your hands because of how bad a basket case I will be and how much pain I will be in.

One very happy go lucky, *chipper acting*, peppy, *female* nurse needs to rub my head to calm me down while you stick me with the heart cath needle and when you insert the catheter tube from my wrist to my heart or my groin to my heart.

One happy go lucky *female* nurse needs to hold down my right arm.

One happy go lucky *female* nurse needs to hold down my right leg.

One happy go lucky *female* nurse needs to hold down the left arm.

One happy go lucky *female* nurse needs to hold down the left leg.

One happy go lucky *female* nurse needs to hold down both feet.

If they are unable to hold down both feet, you'll need to get one at each foot to hold my feet down also.

This is to keep me from jerking.

I am very worried I will jerk badly if I am the least bit aware of what is going on or feel anything when you do the heart catherization.

I guarantee if I am awake that this will be a problem because the pain will be so excruciating to me that they will have no other choice.

It will be very difficult not to jerk.

Please keep in mind, if I jerk on you, or panic, or scream all over the place, that it is not my fault. The pain will be that severe if you make me do this awake.

It is very important that you get me all happy go lucky *female* nurses.

No men and no straight faced, cordial, mediocre *female* nurses.

The *male* nurses and straight faced, mediocre acting *female* nurses will make me nervous and will only make the procedure go worse if I am scared of the person working with me.

I must be comfortable with the people working with me, and the nurses I do have will have to be willing to put themselves in a position to treat me the way a mother would treat their child or take care of their baby or this whole thing will not work.

It will work better for both of us if I get all the nurses I like, and they are willing to do what I need them to do and be willing to treat me as if I was one of their kids.

I know there have been some facilities I have been to that have a hard time understanding this, but this is what the nurses at my local hospital do for me and this is what works best for everybody.

Dreamer's Hope Hospital has never been upset about any of my requests and has always met them will full eagerness and complete compassion.

So, please meet all my needs and meet all my requests (my requests are what I need) because this is what I need to make the whole thing work.

I actually chose Dr. Jenny to be my doctor because I saw the Cardiac Care Unit picture, originally thinking she was one of the nurses and she was one of the ones I was happy with in the picture, and then I realized the picture said she was a doctor and I thought, "Great! This is perfect! This is even better! I get a happy go lucky *female* doctor and happy go lucky *female* nurses!"

I felt Dr. Jenny would be one of the most compassionate nurses I ever had and when I realized she was a doctor, I thought she would probably be one of the most compassionate doctors I ever had.

I really need this too because I am terrified of needles and need the most *chipper acting* nurses and doctors I can possibly get to help me through my anxiety and fear and pain because I have an oversensitivity to pain and a severe needle phobia.

Please do everything you can to help me and meet all my needs listed here. Thank you.

MY DEFINITION OF A HAPPY GO LUCKY NURSE
(REVAMPED)

PEPPY
HYPER
CHIPPER
COMPASSIONATE
FUNLOVING
SWEET
MOTHERLY
HUGGABLE
BOUNCY PERSONALITY (PERKY ACTING, UPBEAT,
VIBRANT)
KEYED UP, IN A GOOD WAY (PUMPED UP PERSONALITY
LIKE FRAULINE MARIA)
COMFORTING
ENCOURAGING
DETERMINED TO HELP YOU THROUGH AN INVASIVE
TEST THAT TERRIFIES YOU WITH A CHIPPER,
ENCOURAGING, APPROACH (TALKS TO YOU THROUGH
IT AND TRIES TO DISTRACT YOU FROM YOUR FEAR BY
MAKING YOU TALK ABOUT THINGS THAT MAKE YOU
HAPPY AND DO WHAT YOU NEED THEM TO DO AND
COMFORT YOU AT THE SAME TIME, IN MY INSTANCE,
RUB MY HEAD TO CALM ME DOWN AND HOLD MY
HAND THROUGH AN IV STICK, TUBE INSERTION, OR
CATHERIZATION PROCEDURE AND BE WILLING TO GIVE
ME LOTS OF HUGS AND LET ME GIVE THEM LOTS OF
HUGS)

HAPPY GO LUCKY NURSE VERSES MEDIOCRE/CORDIAL
NURSES

A CORDIAL NURSE (Or Mediocre Nurse) just walks in the room
casually, usually in slow motion and matter of factly says, "Hi.
I'm Jane. I'm here to take your blood. Come with me, please. We
need to do a blood test." This person may be nice and even smile,
but they are not much help.

A HAPPY GO LUCKY NURSE USUALLY WALKS IN PUMPED UP WITH A GO GETTER PERSONALITY THAT PRACTICALLY SHOOTS OUT THE DOOR TO GET YOU AND ACTS PEPPY AND FRIENDLY AND SAYS,

"Hi, I'm Jane. Come in with me and let's take your blood!" And then, when you act scared, they say, "It's okay. We're going to be just fine! Come on buddy! You just come with me and we're going to get you through this! You just wait and see! You're going to be just fine!"

When I start screaming and hyperventilating through a blood test, or IV, whichever one I'm having done, they usually say something like, "Breathe! Breathe! Take a deep breath! Try to relax, okay! Stay with me buddy! Try to hold on! We're going to get you through this! You just wait and see! You're going to be just fine!"

When I start screaming and hyperventilating through a blood test of IV, whichever one I'm having done, they usually say something like, "Breathe! Breathe! Take a deep breath! Try to relax, okay! Stay with me buddy! Try to hold on! We're going to get you through this! You just bare with me and we'll be done in a minute! I'm sorry this hurts but I'm going to be as gentle as I can, okay. It's going to be okay, buddy! You're going to be okay! Everything is going to be just fine!"

Then, when they're done they say, "See, we made it just fine. You're going to be okay. Now, let's set you up and you let me know if your dizzy or not and then I'll help you up!"

That, or, "Well, we're ready to go to surgery now. We're getting ready to put you to sleep. So, you just rest and have a nice nap while we do our thing and you'll never know anything ever happened. There you go. Goodnight!"

Along with this, I gave her the list of the 36 nurses I wanted them to choose from for who I got in the procedure room. They only had to pick four or five. There were several to choose from. There are very few people I said I did not want. I actually picked at least 3/4ths of the people on their list and maybe even 90% of them. I didn't think it would be that hard to chose from that list and get me a group of nurses I was happy with.

After we gave Dr. Jenny these revamped lists of accommodations for the most likely tests she would do on me, a lady from her office quickly called an hour later and set me up for an appointment that would occur on a Friday two weeks later.

Everything sounded like it was going great. Dr. Jenny gave the accommodations lists to the Wanabe General Hospital's Heart Cath Lab and seemed to think she could meet my needs.

On Monday, I faxed Dr. Jenny some additional records on my heart condition from other doctors who previously found stuff, mainly the childhood heart defect records, a couple of borderline EKGs, a heart murmur my hernia surgeon noticed on auscultation and some notes I had on symptoms I had in the past year and some blood pressure readings.

I didn't mean to overwhelm her. I know it was a lot, but I thought if she already had her hands on all of it, she could look at all of it before I even got there and have a really big head start on how to treat me after that.

I actually had a family doctor I did that to a few years ago that thanked me for it when I did that to him because he said it really helped him diagnose me better to know the full of what was going on.

Most doctors have got aggravated to death with me over things like that so I hope she didn't get aggravated about it.

Then Jane Lee from the Wanabe Hospital Cath Lab called me on the phone the following Monday.

Jane Lee said, "I wanted you to know that I am going to talk to our group nurse and she is out of her office for several days. I don't know that she will be willing to accommodate you due to scheduling with the nurses you're wanting because they have a certain schedule they meet but I'll talk to her.

I'm not sure about some of your needs either but it's mainly the scheduling. I'm not even sure Dr. Jenny is taking new patients." I said, "I just looked on her website and she is taking new patients. I just got an appointment last Friday for two weeks later."

Jane Lee said, "Well, I don't think Dr. Jenny knew that it wouldn't be easy to meet your needs and we wouldn't just be able to schedule whoever you wanted to work on the day you come in."

I told her, "My hospital does it all the time. They just schedule me when that person or group of people I'm asking for is working to start with, then there's no problem."

Jane Lee said, "I don't know. I just don't know if we can meet your needs. It's mainly the scheduling but I'll have to talk to our group nurse the next time she comes in. Didn't you say there was a hospital that normally does this kind of thing for you?"

I said, "Yes. There is. They do it all the time and I've been going there off and on for years and always get who I ask for and they always do what I need."

Jane Lee said, "That's what I thought."

I said, "But they don't do Transesophageal Echocardiograms and Heart Catherizations. That's why I went somewhere else to begin with and that's why I'm coming to you. The nurses did not understand me at the hospital I just went to and I was hoping your nurses would be more compassionate."

Jane Lee said, "I'm just afraid they wouldn't be able to meet your needs here and you may need to find a different Cardiology.

I'm going to talk to the group nurse and do everything I can to get her to work with me but I just don't think she'll work with it. I just don't want you to get traumatized again because I'm afraid after what already happened if you come here you'll just get traumatized all over again."

I said, "But the nurses looked really nice and I only left out the ones I didn't think I'd hit it off with, which were about 3 or 4 people in each of the pictures with several people in them."

Jane Lee said, "I don't know. I just don't want you to get traumatized again. And I doubt will be able to work out the scheduling but I'll see what I can do and call you back after I talk to the group nurse."

Two days later, Jane Lee called again.

Jane Lee said, "I talked to the group nurse and she just can't meet your scheduling needs. I'd cancel your appointment and just try to find a different Cardiology. There surely is someone out there that can help you.

I wrote Dr. Jenny another letter telling her about all the doctors and nurses at the hospital and everything they did for me to accommodate me and also explained this is why I was so set on this Myra Sylvester lady and hoped that wasn't what the problem was.

I said, "You do work with her don't you? Can't you talk to her? All I want her to do is do for me what my PreOp nurse at my local hospital does. I don't mean anything bad by it. I just need her to rub my head to calm me down and hold my hand while someone else does the IV stick, and these other nurses I gave the names of they could help comfort me too and also help brace my arms and legs down if someone had trouble with the heart cath if I happened not to be completely asleep and needed them to help me, or at least help with the IV, and brace my arm down for that if need be."

The following Friday evening around 5:00 pm Jane Lee called from the hospital again and said, "Is Bertha there?"

I almost didn't recognize who it was but figured it out after Bertha had talked to them.

Jane Lee said, "I just don't think we can meet his scheduling needs."

Bertha said, "Oh, I need to explain that to you. He didn't mean for you to give him all 36 nurses at once. He just wanted you to choose the three or four or five nurses you needed to get him through his procedure. He didn't mean for you to give him all of them, just chose from them."

Jane Lee said, "I know, that's not the problem. We just can't."

Bertha said, "What's wrong?"

Jane Lee said, "We just can't meet all his accommodations and

I just don't have enough confidence in my nurses to meet his needs."

Bertha said, "So, you don't think you can help him with this."

Jane Lee said, "I talked it over with the group nurse and neither one of us feel confident our nurses will meet his needs. I just don't want him to get traumatized again. I'm afraid if he comes over here he'll just get traumatized all over again. I just don't want that to happen. We just can't. I suggest you cancel your appointment with the Cardiologist. We're just not going to be able to do it. I just don't have enough confidence in my nurses. I'm sorry. I hope you can find someone to meet his needs."

Neither one of us, Bertha or I could understand why these people could not control their nurses.

These ladies acted like she didn't even trust her own nurses to behave themselves and they might not be nice, either. They're supposed to do what I want and they're supposed to give me what I need.

They need to be able to control their nurses and make them be nice, and they ought to be willing to accommodate me, instead of thinking their above comforting and consoling their patients because they probably think their all professional, like one other place I ran into.

Like I said, they're not your business executive; they're your nurse, which means they are your caregiver, which also means they are required to treat you like a mother treats a child with tender loving care in their dealings with you. I believe it's in their creed or oath to do so too.

I tried to call and cancel the appointment and got a calling service because the office people were gone. They suggested I wait till Monday to cancel.

Then when Bertha called them on Monday to explain things and to cancel the appointment they said, "It's already cancelled. Would you like to reschedule?"

Bertha said, "No."

They talked like they didn't know how it got cancelled but they looked on their computer and it was cancelled. Bertha thinks the hospital cancelled it for me, even though they weren't the doctor and should not have had authority over the doctor. The doctor should have had authority over them but, oh well, I lost out on that one.

Chapter Thirty Two
My Experience at What a Relief General Hospital

We were fishing around for a different Cardiologist and hospital that would understand my emotional needs and not hold it against us like what this other facility had just done to me. We told this place about our bad experience with the Cardiologist and her team of nurses that did my test at the Heart Cath Lab and about my book I previously wrote before this revised edition of the book.

The *male* doctor there, Dr. Plumber was nice and said, "If you ever need anything like this, you've come to the right place. I'm a plumber and I specialize in Transesophageal echocardiograms. That's my specialty."

He checked my heart over, did an EKG and looked at the previous test results and said, "Well, there is a hole there yes but it's small. You probably never had a problem with it in your life and you probably never will. You probably won't even have to worry about it until your 70 years old. If you have a stroke let us know and we'll retake the test. This kind of thing affects the pressure of the heart after while and it can grow bigger but it probably won't. But sometimes we have to recheck these things to make sure, so if you ever do start having stroke symptoms, let me know."

I wasn't really wild about how complacent he was about the whole thing but at least he was nice and he was more than happy to meet my emotional needs.

I gave this place a list of my accommodations and asked for "*chipper acting*" *female* nurses only and that I needed hugs from everyone and needed a *chipper acting female* nurse to rub my head to calm me down and hold my hand while another *chipper acting female* nurse does the IV stick, blood test, or shot. They said they were totally fine with this and this would not be a problem.

When I first got there, they told me this guy had a *male* nurse and I'd get him, even after they said I'd get a *female* nurse on the phone.

However, the receptionist told Bertha, "Oh, that's okay. We can get him a *female* nurse. We'll look around for one."

They got one, and I sort of liked her, but I wanted someone a little bubblier than she was.

I think they all figured that out and then made plans to get me a better nurse the next time.

On my follow up visit, I was told my Cardiologist was having a meeting that day, and they wanted to set me up with his APN nurse, Stacy. She did really well with me and gave me hugs, and she even had an even more chipper nurse go in there to do my EKG than the one she got the last time for me. She told me she saw the book and read some of my book and liked it. She said the Cardiologist left it on his desk to read it and he's been passing it out to all the nurses to read.

I said, "He has?"

She said, "Yeah. Several people have read it and really like it."

I told her, "I'm glad I got you. You're my favorite nurse here."

She said, "Really? I always wanted to be the favorite. I've never been anybody's favorite nurse before. I'm your favorite one? Really? You just made my day!"

I asked her, "If you do decide to do another Transesophageal Echocardiogram or a Heart Catherization test, you're not going to send me back to that other lady are you?"

She said, "No! You're my patient! You're my patient now! My patient!"

I said, "So your nurses will meet my needs if I have to have another test like this and not be mean to me like they were at the other place."

She said, "No! There not about get by with that at my hospital! If anybody ever does this to you again, they'll be talking to me! They're not about to pull that kind of stuff here! I won't let them!"

I was really relieved because she had all my accommodations I always give to all the other hospitals and promised to meet them and said that she was going to make sure her nurses treated me right at this place and if they didn't they were in big trouble. I really like this lady.

We went to the desk to make an appointment for my next Cardiology appointment and this lady said, "Make him another appointment for November 2nd, and make it with me!"

She made me really happy. I hope everything continues to go well with this *female* APN.

Chapter Thirty Three
My Last Wonderful PreOp Experience Where I was the Patient

I was having swelling in the ankles and busting veins in the legs and feet at this time and mainly the feet. I told doctors about this but they did not believe me. I felt like my nurses thought I was just being inappropriate for trying to show them this. I felt like my nurses acted like they thought I was just trying to be naughty by showing off my feet to them so they'd have to look at them. It seems like if you want to uncover anything to let them look at something that needs to be seen they get the wrong idea.

They're nurses. They're supposed to expect to have to look at things like this. It would be one thing if I had to pull my pants down to show them something that's wrong, but this was my feet. All I had to do is take my shoes and socks off for them to look at them. I may be in my bare feet when they see me, but that's their job. They're nurses. And even if it would have been something like a rash I had to show them or knots on the legs, or a boil, or a bite or something like that and I really did have to pull my pants down in front of them in order for them to see it, which has happened before, by the way, they need to look at the situation in the right context. I may be someone they really don't want to see uncovered, but a patient is a patient, and when you're a nurse and a patient asks you to look at things like that, they are not being inappropriate. They are coming to you to be treated for things that need to be treated because you are a nurse and that is what you are there for. Nurses have to do this sort of thing for their patients all the time.

So if I ever do have to uncover a certain area of my body for them to look at something that needs treated, they need to look at it like, "I'm a nurse, and I need to look at this, and it is my job to do what I can to treat it."

That's just the way it is. When it comes to hospitals and doctor's offices, these people have to remember that dignity is thrown out the door when you take care of a patient.

338

You are going to see things you normally wouldn't have to see, and they will have to show you things they normally would not let you look at.

They only do this, because they need treated for what's wrong with them. You're the nurse and you're supposed to do something about it when patients need things taken care of and not judge them for showing you what's wrong with them in the first place. That's just the way it is. Besides that, there are instances where these nurses make their patients change into hospital gowns for them and get to see them even more undressed than this. When they do make them change into a hospital gown they make them run around in their bare feet anyway. In some instances, there are nurses that let you wear your socks with your gown, but when I was a kid it was very rare to be allowed to wear your socks with your gown in the hospital. Back then, they didn't even give you those hospital surgery socks to put on your feet, like some people do now either. There are even some people now that don't even give you these, but some people do depending on where you go. At the military hospital I had to go barefooted in front of everybody and they got to see my toes and everything whether I liked it or not. And I noticed recently, nurses are steering away from letting their patients even wear their socks. And now, where they were able to wear their underwear with a gown before, they're starting to tell them even that has to come off, even if it is a simple procedure where they probably aren't even going to do anything down there. So, since some nurses are starting to not allow their patients to wear their socks again, if I would have been asked to change into a hospital gown instead of just trying to show someone my swelled ankles, chances are they probably would have seen me in my bare feet anyway if they told me to put on a hospital gown. That's because more and more people are requiring their patients to go barefoot in their hospital gowns again. So if they did make me take my socks off when they put me in a hospital gown, they would get to see me in my bare feet anyway. And if nurses can handle something like that and it not bother them, they shouldn't be complaining about other things, when they just have to see other parts of their body uncovered individually, rather than all at once. Like I said, it's their job, and they do this all the time.

If they can't handle that, they don't need to be in the nursing profession. Besides that, I'm not going to show you something if there's not something wrong.

If there's not something I need you to look at that I want you to look at because I think you need to check it out, I'm not going to ask you to look at it in the first place. The whole thing is ridiculous. I wish people would just take me for my word when I say something is wrong and I need them to look at something. If it's not there, I'm not going to show it to you. If I tell you there's a knot, there's a knot. If I say I've got a rash, I've got a rash.

If I say I've got a bite, I've got a bite. If I say I've got busted veins behind my ankle in my left foot and ankle edema, then I have busted veins behind my ankle and have ankle edema.

If I tell you I have a square place at the bottom of my left leg above my foot where a bunch of hair disappeared in one day and there's a bald spot there now, you can be assured there is a bald spot there and the hair disappeared in one day. This is most likely because of a thyroid condition, which I was trying to tell a nurse I had and showed them this because nobody believed me and I thought she would. I was hoping she'd tell someone else, but instead, it ran her off. Luckily, she figured out I was just being informative and then came back and started nursing me again later when she figured out it was all a misunderstanding. One nurse thought I was joking once when I said an EKG lead was loose.

I showed my wife Bertha and she asked, "Does that really matter, since it's still on there?"

I said, "I just thought they might have trouble reading my heart monitors if it was loose."

She went to get a nurse's attention to come have a look.

The nurse said, "Oh, I guess you're right" then fixed the EKG lead.

So please, if I tell you something like that is wrong, just take my word for it. I'm not going to tell you something that isn't true. If I want you to look at something so you can take care of it, I guarantee if you take my word for it, you will see what I'm talking about and see that there really is a problem that needs taken care of and fix it for me.

A *Female* APN nurse at my last doctor's office believed me about my swelled ankles and looked at it anyway.
I was apprehensive about taking my shoes and socks off because I'm a very shy about my feet but I still wanted her to see what I was talking about.
I asked, "Is it okay if I take my shoes and socks off so you can look at it?"

She said, "Are your feet dirty?"

I said, "No."

She said, "No. I don't mind. Go ahead."

She looked at my swelled ankles and said, "Well, it's not too bad. Hold on. Let me look at your legs. I'm setting you up with a Vascular Surgeon."

Then another nurse walked in to ask her a question for just a minute and I pulled my feet back because I was kind of embarrassed. The APN nurse that examined me noticed my apprehension.

When she was done looking at my feet and examining me she said, "Well, you can get dressed now? Or, put your shoes and socks back on."

She didn't come out and say it but she kind of looked at me like she thought, "Goodnight. A guy embarrassed about his feet. How ridiculous can you get?!"

She started to set me up with a surgeon that used the same hospital I had the heart cath test in. We asked her to pick someone else. She knew someone else in another town, but we had a fall out with the hospital in that town too. They didn't act mean or get me in trouble like all the other hospitals did that gave me trouble. They just shewed me away because they didn't think their nurses would meet my needs like my own local hospital did. She then decided to send me to my favorite *female* surgeon in town, Dr. Wonderful.

I went to see Dr. Wonderful to have her look at the problem. I also had a problem with big cysts in my upper legs and on my side on my chest. She also checked this out. She did a vein test on my legs and didn't find anything but was a little concerned about the knots on my legs and my side. My mother wanted that checked out the worst anyway. She decided to do surgery and was nice as usual. I told her what happened at Transylvania Regional Hospital with those girls.

She said, "Well you know what I think? That place has so many nurses in it and so many patients that these girls that did this to you probably felt like they were hid in the crowd of nurses and they could basically do anything they wanted to you and not get caught. I think they did it on purpose my self and it's not right. Since they treat you so well at this hospital, why don't you have PreOp at this hospital do all your IV's from now on and they can do your sticks and send you to these other hospitals so they won't be a problem to you anymore, then you won't have to put up with all this stuff."

I thought, *"I really like the idea, but I'm not sure, but if I think these places are going to be mean I like that. If they are going to be nice, I'd rather they do it. I wish I knew which way to think. I'd hate to miss out on a new wonderful experience. If they were going to be nice about it I'd just want to let them go ahead and do the IV themselves but if they were going to be mean about it I would rather go this route with it."*

I thought, *"I'll have to think about it and see what I think. I'd like to see how these other places are going to react to me first before I decide for sure."*

342

If I would have thought a certain hospital was going to be mean about doing the IV I might be able to have my own hospital do the IV for me and then send me their way just to keep from being harassed.

This lady surgeon I liked, Dr. Wonderful along with Rosie and my other nurse friends comforted me the way they always did, and that included rubbing my head to calm me down through an IV stick and holding my hand to keep me from being scared. I did really well this time. The Lidocaine/Prilocaine 2.5% cream worked really well this time and unlike anytime before Anna, the nurse got the needle to slip right in like a knife through butter and it barely hurt me this time. It was the most wonderful experience I ever had, and Rosie still comforted me anyway, because I need the comfort no matter how much pain I feel. I need it worse if I feel a lot of pain. I sure need it then. But I still need it even if I don't feel anything, and I never know when that's going to be so it's best to comfort me anyway.

It has happened before, a nurse did a real good stick on me and it looked like things were going to be like a bed of roses, but it didn't work out that way. They couldn't get the needle to stay in that time and had to start again and when they picked the vein right next to it I screamed to high heaven and everyone in the building heard me.

When that happened back then I said, "I'm sorry Rosie. I didn't mean to cause so much trouble. It just hurts really badly."

Rosie said, "Don't worry about me. I'm here for you."

They need to understand the reason I have been doing so well is because they are meeting these needs and I feel like they are my friends. But, take that away, and not be friends anymore, but make me be like everybody else then disaster happens.

Chapter Thirty Four
Nightmare Arena
The Day of the Opposites

This story is rewritten with fictitional names. None of the names here are the real names of the real people involved. Everyone was given fake names to tell about an actual account where I had some bad run-ins in the Emergency Room.

Since the incident with the heart cath lab at Transylvania Regional Hospital took place, Dreamer's Hope Regional suddenly started acting strange, mainly in the Emergency Room. The people in the ER window were continually great with me, but the actual Emergency Room kept getting new workers in it and everyone acted so different since the last hospital experience I had out of town, that regardless of everyone sticking up for me and taking my side about what happened at the other hospital, strange things began to happen. I told this hospital how the nurses at the other hospital thought they had their rights, which it's not about their rights; it's about the patient's rights.

They said, "They did huh. Well that's not right."

I turned the last place in; they did get in some trouble, just not as much as they should have. Now the newer nurses at the hospital I normally went to starting acting like they were picking up on this *nurse's rights* thing I told them this other hospital complained about. This has never been a problem at this hospital ever before, and there are still some people in this area that still think it's about the patient, but many more are leaning toward the nurse. They're not considering how the patient feels all of a sudden, because like the other place, now many of the new people act like they are just there for the paycheck. I'm like really shocked. This is never how nursing was meant to be. To nurse means to nurture and any nurse that is unwilling to comfort their patients like a mother comforts their child or baby does not need to be a nurse and needs to find a different profession to work in. If you're not a touchy feely person in the first place, you really shouldn't be a nurse.

Your patients need all the affection they can get from you to help them through their crisis. That means, not just me, but everybody. But nurses should especially be willing to be this way for me because I am mentally disabled with Autism and have sensory issues and have special needs. It should be especially important to do this for me because of my disability and not doing so is really a type of disability discrimination.   It's not right and any form of comfort a patient needs, no matter how different it feels to you, should not be withheld from those who need it. That's especially true for special needs individuals with autism and other disabilities.

I met a disgruntled girl in a blue outfit, Jackie on a Saturday evening that was working both in the front window of admissions and taking patients to their room in the actual Emergency Room behind the double doors. This girl acted hateful when we asked her for a hug. Then we saw a stoic acting *male* doctor, Dr. Base came in to talk to Bertha that was kind of blunt and proud acting and made you feel kind of low. Then a *chipper acting female* nurse, Stacy I liked that liked me back finally came in the patient room and Bertha asked her if she could give me a hug. Bertha told her that I was autistic and she was very friendly to us.

She said, "Sure."

We told her how uncomfortable all the other people were making us that evening.

She said, "I'm sorry you had to deal with that."

She felt bad about it. Bertha asked her what her name was.

She said, "I'm Stacy."

I said, "Am I ever glad we saw you! I'd like you to be my nurse the next time I come in here. Would you be my nurse the next time?"

She said, "Sure, if I'm working."

She was very compassionate about everything and I really appreciated it. That girl in the blue outfit, Jackie that also worked in the admissions window that night may have been hateful about my wanting to hug her, but another girl in a pink outfit, Lacy smiled at me and acted like she really liked me and thought I was sweet. I almost went to give her a hug but Bertha didn't think we had time because she thought they were about to come get us.

I really think Lacy would have been more than happy to give me a hug herself but I lost out on my chance and wish I would have asked her. I really think Lacy would have hugged me.
Last year, several men came to get Bertha in the ER. I was really nervous and started breathing thin to the point that I was tight in my chest from fear of the men that came to get her.

Bertha was worried and said, "They're not coming for you. They're coming for me. It's okay."

Then, I said, "I hope they send a girl in here. All those men make me nervous. I really wanted girls in here."

I got the feeling they might have overheard me.

The young girl, Lucinda who had seen me before spotted me from across the Emergency Room and noticed something was wrong. She immediately came into the room when she noticed.

I said, "Am I ever glad to see you! I was hoping they'd send a girl! They keep sending all these guys in here!"

Bertha told Lucinda, "It's a good thing you came in here. He's about to croak. He's afraid of men, especially *male* nurses. They tortured him when he was a child."

Then Lucinda said, "Yeah there's a lot of guys out there, isn't there?"

I said, "Yeah."

After that Lucinda came in there three times in a row before we left to keep me from being scared and I thanked her for it. I also asked her if she would rub my head to calm me down and hold my hand through an IV stick if I ever had to have an IV.

She said, "Sure. Just let me know when you have to have one and I'll be there for you."

On a different day, I also asked Renee (the lady) ER tech that takes patients to the ER if she would do the same thing for me and she also said, "Yes."

Recently Misty came in the ER room to hug me when Bertha was in the hospital because she knew I liked her when Bertha was there. A young blonde girl came in the room after she left named Tracy.

She said, "Do you need anything?"

Bertha said, "No."

I wanted to say, "I want a hug."

I didn't ask and she left the room and walked down the hall. I wanted to catch her coming down the hall on the way back to the room so I could catch her to ask her for a hug, but every time someone came back it was someone else.
I still said "Hi!" to Misty two or three other times.

Misty acted like she was wondering what was going on when I kept looking down the hall for this different girl with blonde or light brown hair in her 20's who came in the room the first time and asked if we needed anything.

If it would have been the young girl, Tracy I would have said, "Wait! Please! Can I have a hug?"

I think she was the type of person who would have given me a hug cheerfully.

I just wasn't able to catch her but she was very friendly. Because Misty was the one that showed back up every time instead of her, I was very disappointed.

I even looked and took a peak at the nurses' station. Tracy still wasn't there. Just Misty was sitting there.

Next thing I know, a *male* nurse comes in the room to check on Bertha.

I thought, "What did they do that for? Did Misty think I was after her? All I wanted was a hug from Tracy. I wasn't even looking for Misty. I was looking for the blonde girl that came by earlier I was desperate to get a hug from."

An ER experience can be scary if you don't see nurses that make you feel better. I need as much love and affection as I can possibly get from all the *chipper acting female* nurses I can possibly find. I know this sounds strange to people, but you know how in Special Ed people with this personality type will act like your buddy and do everything in their know how to make sure you are okay and try to make your day?

That is how it was with me when I did used to be in Special Ed. Most of the time I get that kind of buddy system with the nurses in PreOp and Radiology that deal with me and it works out really well because of this. If we could get that same buddy system of *chipper acting female* nurse going on in the ER and Inpatient Care that I had in PreOp and Radiology, like I did back in 2012 everything would be a whole lot better. That's because these *chipper acting female* nurses were the ones that I got and they all gave me hugs and comforted me the way I asked them to through all my needle sticks and any other scary procedures that may come about in the ER. It's really important my nurses do this for me. I just can't seem to get them to understand this.

I need them to do what I'm asking them to do for me to comfort me and I need them to be like mommies and buddies to me.

Big City Hospitals Don't Like Cowards   Brian Evans

The people in the ER admissions window understand this very well that know me and know I mean absolutely no harm. They know that I require a lot of affection and need lots of love and cheering up to keep my anxieties down to keep me from being scared of what is happening to me or Bertha. It will still be scary, but just not near as bad as it could have been if they would just do this for me. PreOp and Radiology did this for me, so why couldn't they?

The last three times in a row Bertha went to the ER they sent "all *male* nurses" in there again to see her. At least they were nicer than that set I saw the day Lucinda walked in to save the day, but still men make me nervous and even if they are nice. I feel much better when they send the *chipper acting female* nurses in there because I get the environment I need from them being there to keep me calm even when Bertha is the patient being seen.

This last time they sent all men in there to see Bertha, I saw Dana, who I thought understood me because I told her the year before I wanted her to do the IV stick on me if I ever had to have one and Lucinda to comfort me and back then she acted like she understood. This time Dana acted kind of different. She was kind of nice, but she was more matter of fact than normal. I couldn't understand what was going on. I really wanted Denise to go in there with Bertha. She should have known from an earlier experience that sending a bunch of men in the room would make me nervous. Lucinda understood that, but Lucinda was not working that night.

Dana should have come in there herself knowing how scared I was not having any *female* nurses go in there and only seeing *male*s. I don't want anyone doing that to me, and when they send them all in like that for Bertha they make me afraid if I go in their as the patient they will do that to me.

I was telling my Radiology Tech Karina, who normally understands me that I was scared of this happening. I told her how ever since the incident at a hospital out of town I went to recently that treated me horrible, I felt like everybody's punishing me in the ER and Inpatient departments, but especially the ER.

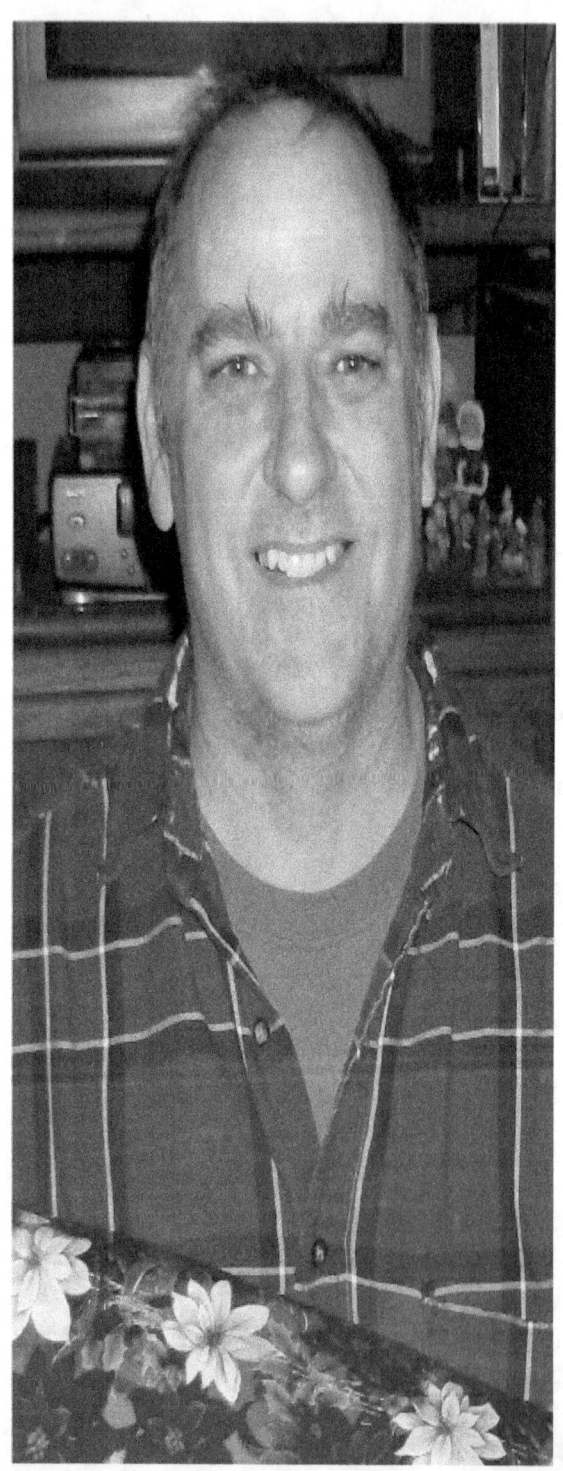

Most of the people doing this to me however are new. Karina thinks that no one is mad at me and that they just don't understand me because they don't know me yet like everyone else does. She also said I don't understand them because I'm not used to people like that that act so stand offish after having such loveable nurses everywhere back in 2005 and 2012. I used to love Inpatient and hate GI and even liked some of the ER people. Now all of a sudden the GI people are better and the inpatient people are all new and don't understand me for anything. I wish they would have kept the ones they had back then or they hadn't have quit. Maybe they wanted to hire people they thought would stick around longer, but I would rather wonderful nurses stick around two or three years and then quit and more wonderful nurses take their place that may only stick around another two or three years, than for wonderful ones to stick around two or three years quit and be replaced by a bunch of standoffish, stoic people that will stick around longer. Why can't they hire more nurses like my ex-nurses? They had a good set of *cheerful acting female* nurses I liked that liked me back in 2005 and 2012 that understood me really well. I did wonderful with them and they all loved on me and hugged me and comforted me if I asked them to and everything and were wonderful with me. If they would just hire more nurses like that again, I'd have it made. I know some of these new people may think they like their space, but you guys need to be hiring more touchy feely type nurses that are *chipper acting* that don't mind comforting their patients even if that means hugging and loving all over their patients in a motherly fashion. That's what nurses are supposed to be there for.

It's not just a job where you say, "Hey, I think I'll be a nurse and go poke some people to death with needles and take vital signs."

That's the wrong motive. If you're going to be a nurse, you need to think about the patients' needs before you even think about becoming a nurse and be willing to meet them. That includes their physical needs and their emotional needs whatever they may be.

Your patients are supposed to be like children to you even if they are adults and you should treat them with the same love and compassion as you do your own child and comfort them in the same way as you do your own child.

You're supposed to do all the scary stuff you have to do to them and still comfort them. You're also supposed to cheer them up in the process because you feel bad that you have to do something that hurts them. How would you feel if you were the patient and they hurt you with needles or you were in pain and they said I'm just going to stand back here and smile while I stick you to death to cheer you up and hope you handle it okay? I don't want to get too close. I'm just doing my job as a nurse." I don't think you would be very happy about that would you? I'm not. I've had people pull that kind of stuff on me before and it doesn't work. And in my opinion it's a cop out on their part because it's part of their job to meet their patients' emotional needs. If they're not meeting their patients' emotional needs they are not fulfilling their purpose as a nurse like they ought to be. They're just there for the paycheck and that's not right. No matter how nice you are, if a patient has needs and you refuse to meet them because you're standoffish and don't want to get too close, you are actually hurting the emotional state of the patient. You may even make them worse off than they would have been in the process. Columbia State University recently started requiring a class for nurses where they had to go to a hospital and go to each patients room one by one on an inpatient floor or ward and not nurse, but only meet the emotional needs of the patients they saw and learn what they need and meet their needs.

At the end of the semester, they would ask each of their students that took this class, "Are you wiling to meet the emotional needs of your patients? Is what you just had to do this semester going to be something you are willing to do? You need to decide now."

If the answer is no they will suggest they find a different major.

If the answer is yes, then they will tell them to continue on in their pursuit to become a nurse and wish them good luck.

352

Big City Hospitals Don't Like Cowards   Brian Evans

I'm not sure where the hospital in this story is hiring its new workers from. If it is the college nearby you might suggest they also require their students take a class like this one where they make them only meet the emotional needs of the patients in the hospital for one semester.

Then ask them, "Is this something you are willing to do?"

If they're answer is no I think they ought to ask them to find a different major.

If their answer is yes they should be encouraged to continue on.

This is a very important part of nursing that is being grossly neglected. If you are not willing to meet the emotional needs of a patient it is a detriment to the emotional well being of that patient. This will hinder their life, it has mine. Not meeting the emotional needs of your patients can scare them like it has me. They may even loose their will to live like I nearly did myself. When people do this to me, this is what happens to me.

Have you ever seen the movie, "Cipher in the Snow"? When you do this to me you are doing the same thing to me they did to this boy. This boy felt ignored by most people and felt unimportant and he felt like his emotional needs were not being met by his peers and teachers. So, am I saying this boy committed suicide? No. Watch the movie. He didn't have to.

He was so overwhelmed with emotional disappointment and sadness that when they stopped the bus on the road one day, this kid said, "Could you let me off the bus? I need to take a break."

The kid stepped off the bus and passed out in the snow and died of a broken heart. This is a true story movie. This is what you are doing to me when you refuse to meet my emotional needs and it has already come very close to this point in many instances. Like him, I have never attempted suicide. I just suffered from a broken heart and wind up moping around in a horrible emotional state.

I was so discouraged with the way things were going when I didn't get hugs from everyone, like I needed, when Bertha was in the hospital for a surgery herself. After while I started getting tremors, almost dropped my tray and nearly passed out.

I never passed out, but I casually walked back to my patient room broken hearted shivering in the process and when I got back to the room I barely ate a thing.

The RN, Fanny that knew me from years before saw the look I had on my face and knew something was terribly wrong.

She kept saying, "Are you okay?"

I kept walking around with a sad countenance and sitting around with a sad countenance.

She said, "You need to eat something. I'm really worried. Please eat something. Okay. Are you okay?"

I think I kept saying "Yeah"

In reality I was never okay to start with the whole time. It is very important that they do this for all patients. And technically they are really actually required to do so anyway. I don't know if the teachers quit teaching their nurses this or if they just overlook it somehow, but I have medical school books that say they are required to comfort their patients. I have also found internet references and encyclopedia references that make the same claims. If they found out what a nurse really was, they would be shocked.

Nurse means "nurture" and I even got a spelling thesaurus gadget from a senior at bingo and guess what it says it means, "To act as a parent to."

I even found a quote from someone in the medical profession that said that "Nursing is a good training ground for raising a family."

Believe it or not one of my Medical Assisting Books even has a quote that says, "They can and must comfort their patients." There's an eye opener for you. When I took a college course in Abilene, Texas, a Director of Medical Assisting from California made this quote too. We're talking about someone in charge here making this quote. Plus the Glenco Health Book says that Certified Surgical Technologists have to learn to be willing to comfort their patients as part of their completion. You'd be surprised what I know about all this. You're going to love Chapter 39. I already knew a lot and I researched it to confirm it and proved it all the more when I did.

Another thing that has worried me is every time we go in on a night or weekend to the ER I ask if Lucinda is there because most of the weekend people scare me, especially the night ones.

I've asked so many times that people act like "Why does it have to be Lucinda? Can't he take someone else and be happy?" They don't understand that Lucinda understands me and does what she can to keep me calm when she's working and she agreed to help me through IVs and she's very friendly and loveable and cheerful and compassionate. She's like the Rosie Ferry of the Emergency Room. This is what Rosie does for me in PreOp. I need someone like Rosie to help me through the scary stuff and Lucinda passes the test. I wish these people understood that. Lucinda understands. Why can't they?

Last year we asked for all women and no men in the Emergency Room. That day I got sent to express and Juanita Corning, APN took me back there and I didn't get to be with the girl nurses I was happy with in the ER. Juanita Corning, APN is not a chipper person at all. Juanita is a *serious trended female* nurse who is very blunt and right on the brink of being a crank. I'm sorry if certain people may like her if I am offending anybody. I just have to be honest. Juanita Corning, APN scared me to death. Then her assistant lady, that was tall, hefty, and manly, that seemed more like a guy than a girl and had incredible strength when she was testing the reflexes in my legs and pounded me with her hands. I knew she didn't mean to hurt me.

I thought, *"Good Night! This lady is rough! I felt like I was being karate chopped! That's the hardest anyone has ever checked my reflexes!"*

I was scared Juanita Corning, APN would decide to do an IV and put me in the hospital and I wasn't about to let her do it. I was about to cringe. Juanita decided to give me a prescription and suggested Physical Therapy instead. I was relieved. That lady was scary.

A *chipper acting female* nurse, Jay Lynn finally came in the Express Room and I was incredibly relieved. She wanted me to sign papers and I sighed and said, "Am I ever glad to see you! That other woman makes me really nervous! I was so scared!"

Bertha told her, "He's scared of those other two ladies. He's really glad you came in here. He needs *chipper acting female* nurses like you, not serious acting ones like them. Serious trended *female* nurses scare him."

You want to know what I was scared would happen if Juanita Corning, APN would have decided to do an IV. I feared she'd start coming at me with one and said, "I'm going to do an IV." I would have said, "Can we get someone else please?"

I have a feeling she would have said, "No. We can take care of it. We won't need anybody else. We've got it under control ourselves."

If this would have happened I would have thought, "You've got it under control alright. You have me trapped and you're about to torture me and I know you're not about to comfort me because you probably think I'm just a big baby."

This part never happened. I didn't have to have an IV. I just had a sick sense she would be this way if I did. That was really scary.

I told Cindy about it and she said, "Yeah, I know. I'm really sorry. I had no idea that was going to happen or I would have done something different."

Bertha said, "Next time I'll be sure to say, not just a *female* nurse, but a *chipper acting female* nurse. I'm sorry I didn't tell them that. I'll make sure to tell them the next time, because I don't want you to have a scary experience like that again. I'll just tell them the doctor can be a man, but all the nurses have to be *chipper acting females* and then you should be able to go to the regular ER again the next time."

That's all my horrible experiences I had in the past year in the ER anyway.

Then after that this Juanita Corning, APN lady wanted me to go to Physical Therapy and Dr. Benny's nurse, Jacquelyn called the Physical Therapy and the girls in there said they weren't going to be my therapists anymore because they felt like they had to be too intimate with me when they did therapy on me and wanted me to have a guy instead so they told her you'll have to go to Zack if you get therapy.

They asked me, "Do you still want to go?"

I said, "No."

She said, "That's what I kind of thought. I tried anyway. That's the only option they gave me."

Bertha just had a bladder tuck surgery and things did not go very well. Bertha did fine except for throwing up several times and being in a lot of pain, but that's not what went wrong.

The PreOp experience went wonderful also.

The inpatient ward experience was not that great. What went wrong was, when Bertha got to the inpatient care unit about 95% if the *female* nurses working in there were new people I never met before. All of these nurses refused to give me a hug and badly hurt my feelings. There were a couple of people I got that hugged me. Betsy and Riana were good with me and Janice, the RN was good to me during the day shift. Lynne was too, but I only feel so-so toward Lynne. I don't mean to hurt her feelings. I like her alright, but I just like Betsy and Riana much better. The night nurse Ariel, which also took care of me in 2012 gave me several hugs and was receptive to me. These were good.

Everywhere else I turned it was "I'm not a hugger." or, "No thanks." Or they wanted to run off somewhere. They all acted like "We'll be nice but we're not going to go out of our way to meet his emotional needs." They never came out and said that but they acted like that was their attitude, and it severely hurt my feelings. I felt very out of place and felt like I could have no comfort for my situation or have my emotional needs met I needed met because of it. I barely ate any of my food I got in the cafeteria, either time I went there. My nurse, Janice was worried about me and kept asking me if I was okay. Janice said, "You need to eat something. I'm really worried. Are you okay?" I kept saying, "Yeah." I really wasn't okay at all the whole time I was in there. I felt like I couldn't get any hugs from anybody anywhere and I was incredibly heartbroken and felt insecure from feeling out of place. Being able to hug people I like, especially my nurses is one of my emotional needs. I felt rejected everywhere I turned.

I was crushed and I felt trapped because Bertha was the patient and not me. I couldn't just leave when I didn't like the way I was being treated. I was stuck. It's not like the GI Department where a couple of hours and it's over and if I don't like the people in there I can have Karina or Rosie come in there and help me.

No this is 24 hours. If Bertha would have been having a more serious surgery than the one she had, it could have been 24 hours a day 7 days a week too. It could happen.

But this time it was a one day stay only. Twenty Four hours is way too long to be stuck in a place where you are nervous where people refuse to meet your emotional needs and you can't leave because you're not the patient but your wife is. This is traumatizing to me when no one is meeting my needs and I need them to comfort me and give me hugs.

It's extremely traumatizing to me when all of them just want to shirk away and just act like, "Oh, I'll be nice. I'm just not going to give this guy a hug. I don't want to have to baby this guy. He can just stay away. I'm not going out of my way to pamper this guy just because he wants to give everybody hugs. Who is this guy and what's wrong with him anyway? How did I get stuck with having to deal with somebody like him?"

Their attitude, even though they did not say these words, but showed this is how they felt toward me with their actions has ruined my reassurance of any possibility that if I'm the one that was a patient that had to go to inpatient care and needed them to comfort me and give me hugs that I can depend on them to pull through for me when I have to go in there. If there ever is a next time I have to go in there I don't want to have to feel like I have to worry my emotional needs will not be met and I will be shunned away if I'm their patient next and then have to fear that none of them will ever give me a hug. I don't want to have to fear I'll get a serious acting *female* nurse instead of a *chipper acting female* nurse because they don't want to deal with me either. I don't like mediocre nurses. I wish the nurses I saw were huggable like the last set of girls they had in there in 2012 were.

I don't want to be thrown off on a bunch of men either because they think, *"I don't want to deal with him. He can have a guy nurse take care of him."*

No I never want a *male* nurse to take care of me anywhere in any department of any hospital anywhere. I will always insist on happy go lucky *chipper acting female* nurses only. I cannot have it any other way.

Then to make it worse I went in the kitchen to get breakfast for me and Bertha and I asked the nurse in there for a hug and she said, "Why don't we just bump?"

I said, "I guess." And the lady bumped arms with me but this made me really upset.

That was not what I needed. When somebody refuses to give me a hug and wants to shake hands or bump arms I do not feel comforted by this at all. I feel crushed. When the lady that backed out of giving me a hug continued down the line and then finally left, I just stood there in one place and almost didn't move because I was hurt that bad by it.

I then moved very slowly in slow motion from one food item to the next and went forward. I suddenly noticed there was a guy behind me in line that noticed something was wrong and waited generously for me to move. I got the feeling he knew something was wrong and did not try to rush me knowing something was bothering me. When I got to the part of the line where the drinks were I got two waters and a Pepsi I started crying really hard and I think the lady in front of me noticed. I touched this other lady nurse on the shoulder, really wanting a hug and cried even more. This middle aged nurse, about 30's or 40's, had a look on her face like "What does he want? I hope he doesn't want a hug from me too."

She never said anything. She just looked at me like she thought, "Oh great! He doesn't want me to hug him too does he?"

I turned part of the way back around and tried to hide it and cried even more.

Then I went to the register and said, "I got a variety of stuff." All this is for Bertha and this is what I got for me. And I got two waters and a Pepsi."

I had a hard time containing myself when I got to the register and could barely talk to the cashier at first but then was able to tell her what I got and who it was for so she would know what to charge me.

Somewhere around that point in time when I was at the drink machines I spotted Brandy from Radiology and MRI. I gave Brandy a hug and she started talking to me and I told her about Bertha being in the hospital. I think it was when I first got to the drink machine. I wasn't sure if she noticed something was wrong. I didn't think she noticed I was having an emotional breakdown, but she may have noticed more than she was letting on that something wasn't quite right and just didn't say anything. I think Brandy stopped to talk to me to cheer me up, but she probably just stopped to talk to me to let me know she was there because she knew I would want to talk to her and give her a hug and was just trying to give me the opportunity to catch her before she walked off so that I wouldn't miss out. I really didn't think Brandy noticed anything was wrong because I must have hid it really well.

After she walked out the door and I continued with my drinks at the machine, I lost it and cried like crazy because of that first lady nurse that wouldn't give me a hug that I really liked. After I got the Pepsi and two waters, and cried and touched the other middle aged *female* nurse in front of me in the line on the shoulder I started crying again.

Instead of asking me what was wrong, she just looked at me like she was thinking, "What does he want?"

I got the feeling she thought, "Oh great! I suppose he wants a hug from me too."

I wasn't sure if she noticed something was already wrong or not but she may have noticed something was bothering me, I'm not sure. After that, I had trouble with my food and drinks at the register when I told the cashier what I had so she would know what to charge me and cried again.

When I picked up my food and drinks to walk out of the cafeteria back into the hallway again I began to get a tremor in my hands and felt really shook up.

I even thought I might pass out but I never did. I think I may have come close to it but I don't think the cashier noticed. The cashier actually kind of had an unenthused look on her face too.

She gave me the feeling she was probably thinking, *"Oh boy, I'll be glad when I get this guy rang up so I won't have to be bothered with him. Let's get this over with so I can be done with this."*

She never said anything either, so she didn't say this. She just had that kind of look on her face like she felt like I was somebody she just had to put up with that she wished she could get rid of.

I think the cashier just noticed I was a little upset and was having a hard time holding on to my stuff.

If she did notice I was having a breakdown I got the feeling she was probably thinking, *"Oh brother. Does he have to be such a crybaby? Why can't he just be like everybody else?"* from the look she had on her face.

I think when she saw how much trouble I was having she finally said, "Would you like a tray for all that? It might be easier to carry."

I said, "Yeah. I guess so."

I was right on the brink of losing my balance and my sense of direction but I managed to walk the rest of the way back to the room where Bertha was. I was all shook up. Janice even acted like she was worried about me too.

Janice didn't know that this happened, but I could tell that she could tell that something was wrong. She knew that I didn't seem like myself and was really worried about it. She constantly asked me if I was okay with an extremely concerned look on her face.

I could see it written all over her face that she was thinking, *"Something's wrong with Brian. He's not acting himself. Something is bothering him really bad and he looks really sad."*

She was right too. There was something wrong. One of the things that was wrong was her girl nurses I liked not being willing to give me a hug and hurting my feelings. The other thing that was wrong was the two lady nurses in the cafeteria I saw that I liked that wouldn't give me a hug, especially the first one. This was really bothering me and I really was extremely sad and very disappointed and depressed. I felt rejected by almost everybody.

I get like this when people consistently refuse to meet my emotional needs and this is the real reason I start losing my will to live. I was incredibly crushed by nearly everybody. I don't think all these people realize that not giving me what I need like this actually traumatizes me this bad. I can't handle not being able to hug people I like, especially when I am in a hospital based situation where something medical is going on. It doesn't matter who, it can be either me or Bertha. If I'm the one going through the experience I need to hug people I like even more so. If it is Bertha, she is my security and I am very emotionally distraught, I need the comfort of others to feel at ease. I can't handle being treated like I'm some stranger over here that you really don't want to get to close to, and just want to shun away. I don't appreciate being greeted like I'm someone at some firm somewhere. I have a sensory issue it my right ear where I need to put my ear on people's cheek or the sensation drives my crazy and I can't function. I have always required a lot of affection my whole life. It's not my fault I make people feel like I'm a nuisance to them. Autistic people have sensory needs that have to be met a certain way in order to offset the uncomfortable sensation they are having. It's like pouring water on someone's burning tongue, or putting anti-itch cream on someone's arm that itches, or putting someone's hands under water in the sink after they've burned themselves on a stove, or someone cooling their face in front of a window air conditioner after being out in the extreme heat for a long time. It's also like someone brushing their teeth to get the yucky sleep taste out of their mouth.

Or even someone taking Pepto Bismol or Mylanta to soothe the stomach after experiencing indigestion, inflammation, or ulcer pain. Giving someone a hug and placing my right ear on their cheek is like taking the Pepto Bismol to soothe the stomach when it's irritated. The Pepto Bismol soothes the stomach and tames it down and that's what getting to hug somebody does for me.

If someone asked you, "Could I have a piece of chocolate cake?" would you say, "Here, have a cracker." when it is in your means to be able to give them a piece of chocolate cake. I wouldn't think so.

When people try to force me to shake their hand or bump arms instead of hugging me because it's the way they want to do it because the hugging thing doesn't seem normal to them, they don't realize that when they do this to me, that it would be like you wanting to brush your teeth to get the yuck out of your mouth and then someone give you some Listerine.

You say, "But I want toothpaste. I know Listerine freshens up your breath, but I need a toothbrush and toothpaste to get that yuck out of my mouth."

 And they say to you, "I'm sorry. You can't have toothpaste and a toothbrush to brush your teeth with. I'm only giving you Listerine."

If they did this, they would think they were justifying themselves for making you do what they want you to do instead of meeting your actual need, because the Listerine, in their mind is supposed to freshen your breath. But that Listerine is not going to be able to get that stuff off your teeth to make you able to feel clean and refreshed and be totally rid of the yuck taste feeling in your mouth until you get your toothpaste and brush your teeth with a toothbrush and toothpaste. Without the toothpaste, you're need to get that gunk off your teeth will never be met, because you need to get that yucky stuff off your teeth without it.

You may be able to temporarily keep your mouth from stinking someone else out, but you will never get that gunk off your teeth until someone gives you the toothpaste you ask for to get it off of there.

So when someone refuses to give me a hug and asks me to shake their hand instead, it's like making you settle for Listerine instead of giving you the toothpaste you asked them for. You may have asked them for the toothpaste because it is what you wanted, and they may see it as a want, but in reality what you asked for is really a need. You may want it, and it is true that you were asking for something you wanted, but what you wanted was also what you needed, and that was the toothpaste you asked for that was going to get that gunk off of your teeth. Without getting the toothpaste, the Listerine is of no use, because the Listerine is only a breath freshener, not a gunk remover, and without the toothpaste the gunk will never come off your teeth no matter how much Listerine you used. This is what people do when they refuse me a hug, but it is even worse than this; it is so horrible that it is like refusing to give someone a teaspoon of Pepto Bismol to soothe their stomach pain. Without it their stomach will ever be inflamed and in pain and agony. When they receive it they get relief and it tames their stomach down and makes it calm and at ease. When someone gives me a hug, it calms down the sensory output that causes me to need a hug and tames it down in such a way that it is like soothing a person's stomach with Pepto Bismol. If this confuses you as to what it feels like, a hug doesn't feel like a bottle of medicine if you're taking it that literally. A hug just has a medicinal like affect on me when I am able to hug someone. When I press my right ear on your cheek it feels similar to what it feels like to lay your head on a feather pillow, especially the part of your face I put my right ear is on when I hug you. It is very soothing and very calming and helps me to stabilize myself. I was born like this. It has never been any other way. I have been like this and had this kind of sensory issue all 48 years of my life that I've been alive. There is nothing new about it. It has always been this way and always will be this way.

I have always needed this to be this way and will always need this to be this way, and unfortunately for some people who get tired of it, I actually need several hugs a day from every person I meet that I like. It is that serious a thing. I actually have to have this or it will send me into a physically chaotic state of some kind.

I'm not sure how to describe it, but like I said, it's like putting someone's hand under cool water after they accidentally burn it on the stove; you have to put it under cool water several times throughout the day, especially the first few minutes or few hours after the burn accident occurs. You have to do this, no matter who you are, or you will be in serious trouble from your burn and it will get detrimentally worse if you don't. You have to cool it under water several times or you will be in trouble. You have no choice. You have to do this because it is detrimental you have this done.

Not cooling your burned hand under water will only throw you into physical chaos and could cause very serious damage that could have been prevented had you let yourself put your burned hand under cool water several times. You don't and the burn only gets worse, and the damage from the burn magnifies the less you take care of it. This is the same way it is with my needing several hugs.

Not being able to do so is physically detrimental to me and physically and emotionally chaotic and is too much for me to bear.

I have to be able to hug people I like and I have to be able to do it often. It is the only way I can handle it. I can't have it any other way. I wish there was something you could do. I wish you had all your 2012 girls back in inpatient care again. They understand and their being back would solve everything. The hospital is supposed to be a place of comfort anyway, not a place where you feel like someone is pushing you into feeling like you have to act like your business associate or something at some big firm somewhere. None of my other nurses were ever this way to me except what very few I run into that don't understand but this go around. It felt like the people in GI and the people in inpatient care might as well have switched places with each other.

In 2012 the GI people were treating me like these people are now, and in 2012 the inpatient care people were more like the people in PreOp in radiology than like those that were in the GI lab at the time. Now, in 2015, the GI people act almost as nice as the 2012 inpatient care people and the 2015 inpatient care people now act almost as horrible as the 2012 GI lab people that were originally in GI before they got better people. If there wasn't so many new people in here with totally the opposite personality of those that were in here in 2012 I wouldn't have this problem.

The hospital needs to hire more *chipper acting females* that act like their crew acted who are lovable and huggable and caring and compassionate instead of these people they're hiring that are cordial and nice but don't get too close personalities. The Radiology people have treated me from 2002 to the present, and especially 2005 to 2015. It was because everybody gave me all the *chipper acting female* nurses I asked for when I did and they all gave me several hugs. When I had to have an IV done a *chipper acting female* nurse would rub my head to calm me down and hold my hand while another *chipper acting female* nurse does the IV stick that I did so well. And it is because everybody gave me the nurses I needed and were willing to do this for me that I called this hospital Dreamer's Hope Regional Medical Center. That's supposed to be a good thing. Without all this there is no dream, because this is what the dream is. I wish they could get more people like you guys. They just hired Sherry Ann and Jillian in your department and they're the perfect personalities. If they hired more people like them in inpatient care and the ER, since they are also getting new people that don't understand as well as the originals things would be better.

In the ER a few of the new ones are good with me, but most of the new ones are not. At this rate, if they keep hiring all these untouchables and stoic people the dream of having nice loveable people that understand me will be more like a shattered dream and only qualify for the PreOp and Radiology people. I hope they get more people in these other departments like my other favorite nurses in case me or Bertha either one have to be in there again. I can't handle these other people.

If I would have been the patient, I would have said, "I'm out of here!"

They would have said, "Wait! You can't go! You're sick! You need us to help you!"

And I would say, "Not without *chipper acting female* nurses that will hug me and rub my head to calm me down through needle sticks."

If I don't get that, I'm not sticking around for anybody at any department of anybody's hospital in any town.

If all the original workers that are nurses and nurse's aides at the hospital that understand me and are willing to meet my emotional needs keep quitting their jobs and they keep hiring people like this who are cordial but not huggable and lovable then the dream of a hospital with nurses that understand my emotional needs is lost forever because all the original workers that understood me that are willing to meet my emotional needs are gone and all the new ones don't have a clue and treat me more like a business associate than they do a patient and my needs will never be met again because all the people that were there that understood are gone. I was worried when Rita Sullivan quit her job in PreOp and she stated Jan Sift might also quit her job in the next few months I got worried Rosie might quit too. I thought if these people quit, they're going to have to find a new set of *chipper acting* nurses to stick me with the IV and rub my head to calm me down. Luckily I have now met the new workers Jessie and Sharon who I like very well and I think if this should ever happen where all three of my helpers are gone, if these two girls will just stick around, I think I might have another good match if they will just have mercy on me and Sharon rub my head to calm me down and hold my hand and Jessie work with her, but I don't know if Jessie does sticks or not. Jessie could do the stick if she does sticks, but if not; they'd have to find another one I'm comfortable with, a *chipper acting female* nurse. While Rosie is still there, though, I'd like her to do it.

Hannah and Mara were acting like they wanted to throw me off on the guy anesthesiologist to do the stick if Rosie and Jan left.

I said, "No, I don't want a guy doing anything on me. I need a girl. You need to find somebody to take Jan's and Rosie's place if they retire. I'm not letting a guy mess with me. I need the tender loving care of a happy go lucky, *chipper acting female* nurse to do the IV stick and comfort me through the IV stick the way I want comforted, rub my head to calm me down and hold my hand. That's the only thing that will work and I will have it no other way."

I hope if these two ladies ever retire in the next couple of years or so that someone will take their place I like as much as them.

If Sherry Ann and Jillian can take over where they left off when they retire, that would be great, and it would be very wonderful too. It would mean the world to me for them to be the ones to do this for me if Rosie and Jan ever left. I hope they can work this out for me when the day comes for this to happen.

Recently, my mother and sister were visiting us and my mother had to take my sister to the ER. I saw a Janitor I thought I remembered giving a hug a couple of weeks before when we were walking down the GI hall toward Radiology, probably for a shot, or one of Bertha's procedures.

This lady I thought to be the same janitor that day shrugged up when I walked up to her and told the lady next to her, "We're not allowed to touch anybody?"

I was shocked and thought, *"What?"*

I told this lady, "I'm sorry. I thought you were the janitor we hugged two weeks ago. Are you not the same janitor?"

She said, "No, that was somebody else. I don't know who that was."

Bertha said, "He wants a hug. He's autistic."

The lady then opened up and said, "Well everybody needs a hug. Sure. I'll give him a hug. Here." And she hugged me.

I was confused and thought, *"What is going on here? What's wrong with everybody? Is there something strange going on here? First the inpatient girls refuse to hug me as well as the nurses in the cafeteria that day when Bertha was in the hospital over night after a bladder tuck surgery, and now this janitor in the Emergency Room Lobby says, "We're not allowed to touch anybody?" What's going on here anyway?" I wanted to walk to Radiology to see if Karina and all my other Radiology friends were still okay. I was afraid something strange was going on and they would never hug me or comfort me again. I thought, "What on earth is going on here? What just happened? And why are people acting so strange all of a sudden? Is there something strange going on here or something? What's going on here anyway?"*

I wanted to leave but I had to wait for my mother and sister to come out of the main ER room. I couldn't figure out what was going on and I wanted to get out of there.

I was scared and panicked and I almost got mad because I felt trapped but no one knew I was mad. I just walked out the door and wanted to never come back. I never felt like that about this hospital ever before and all of a sudden all hell broke loose. I couldn't figure out what was going on and it had me spooked.

Next thing I know I had this weird dream about the radiologist that normally helps me with my shots, Karina because of all the weird things that just happened. It really had me spooked and then I wrote her and told her about it and told her I had the dream, scared to death.

I never thought she would do the things she did in the dream before, but now that this happened I didn't know what to think and I was spooked.

Big City Hospitals Don't Like Cowards   Brian Evans

Here's the letter I wrote about the dream I had.

Dear Karina,

I had this horrible dream last night that you were upset with me because of the letter I gave you about what happened on 1st floor when Bertha was in the hospital. In this dream you were upset with me as I said and I wanted you to comfort me through a blood test. You took me to a different end of the hospital and didn't tell me what was going on. You acted like you didn't dare tell me what was about to happen to me. We waited several minutes for a couple of nurses to come get me for what I thought was going to be the blood test. You decided you needed to leave for a minute and you'd be right back. I got tired of waiting and went to the bathroom. When I was done using the bathroom, on my way out, you knocked on the bathroom door and said, "We need to go." I said, "Okay." Then, you had this grim look on your face acting like you were upset with me and you also acted like you were hiding something you didn't want to tell me about. You told me to walk down a certain hall with you in a part of the hospital I was unfamiliar with and walked me to some room I'd never seen before. There were these two nurses there. One of them said, "We decided the blood test Karina does for you was not enough. We have something even better we need to do for you."

Then they showed me the needle from an injection and said, "You see this needle. You want to know how Karina made this less painful for you. This is how she did it." She put the needle in a napkin and placed it under a pillow to the side of the bed.

Then this nurse and another lady nurse with her proceeded to stick me with a needle to do what I thought was a blood test. You were at the head of the bed and I begged you to comfort me. I was scared and I kept saying. "Karina, please help me! Karina, please comfort me!" but you kept looking at me with this grim look on your face and acted like, "I really don't want to deal with this."

The next thing I know there were four or five other nurses toward the back of the room against the sidewall that walked over to the bed. Now, I was surrounded by about 5 or 6 or 7 *female* nurses that circled the bed all around me. Then the first lady started poking me with injection needles in several places in the arms and in the legs and I was screaming in pain. I'd only put enough Lidocaine on for the blood test. I wasn't expecting this and they were sticking me everywhere you could think of with needles where there wasn't any Lidocaine to numb the area. I thought they'd never stop. I kept begging and pleading, "Please Karina, help me! Please comfort me!" I was saying, "What are you people doing to me? Why are you doing this? Please don't hurt me!" You kept trying to get out of comforting me and just kept standing back behind me acting upset with me. A couple of times you just barely gave in and only comforted me for a second and then quit just to keep me quiet, but then you wouldn't do anything else and I needed your comfort the whole time they were doing this. I was scared to death. These ladies were saying, "We're trying to see if you really need comforted or not?" I kept thinking, "Can't you see it? Isn't it obvious? Please, don't do this to me." One of them finally said, "Well you actually have a genuine need to be comforted. We know that now." I remember thinking, "Thanks a lot. Now you decide that after you tortured me to death beyond end. Why couldn't you just believe me that I needed comforted? Did you have to do this to me?" I looked up and I said, "Where's Karina?" and the second lady on the side said, "She's gone. She left." I felt abandoned and scared to death. I suddenly woke up and remembered, "I forgot to tell Karina to be there for my B12 shot on Tuesday." Please tell me you would never do this to me. I don't think you would. I hope I haven't done anything to upset you. Is everything still okay? I think it was just a bad dream. I hope to see you Tuesday. Thanks. Your friend, Brian

After I had this dream and told her about it, I was afraid Karina would be upset with me for thinking such a thing if she didn't already feel this way. We had my shot scheduled for that Friday and I backed out and rescheduled it for Tuesday.

Bertha talked to her on Friday when she was out running errands and handed her a letter I gave her explaining what led me to think all this. I almost didn't go back.

Bertha handed Karina the phone and said, "You have to talk to him. I'm really worried. He had this horrible dream and he's afraid you're not going to comfort him."

So Karina talked to me and said, "Did you have a bad dream? It's okay. I will never do this to you. So do you still want to come? Are we on for Tuesday?"

I said, "Yeah."

Karina said, "Good. I'll see you then."

Tuesday came and Bertha went to have carpal tunnel surgery and I was trying to get us both breakfast and get tagged at the ER and go to the place that does shots, but they weren't open yet and I told the Radiology people to tell Karina we were here, that I'll be in PreOp Waiting. After I went to get my money and breakfast, I saw Diamond in the hall, who I really like and I wanted to give her a hug.

Diamond said, "That's okay. You don't have to worry about your breakfast boxes. I can still give you a hug. I'll just maneuver them."

I said, "Thanks."

And I was very happy. Everything went wonderful with the PreOp people again, and the doctor was fast, so Bertha was already ready to go when I took the breakfast boxes in the waiting room. Because I was supposed to have a shot, Dana wheel chaired Bertha to the room they do shots in. We waited for Karina and at first it looked like she was going to help.

I asked her, "Can you rub my head while they gave me the shot?"

She said, "No. We're going to try something different today. I
need to teach you that sometimes we can't always get want we
want. It's not going to kill you if I don't do this for you. It's okay.
So, when you run into someone else that does this way, its okay
and you just need to let them stick you without doing this if that's
what they want. Next time I may do it the other way again but this
time we're doing it this way."

I was upset and kept saying, "Please, please, do it the way we
always do it. Please. Will you do it the next time?"

She said, "We may do it the next time but not today. I need to
show you its okay if people don't do this for you because you
won't always have me or Rosie here to do this for you and you
need to be able to do this if someone else don't want to do this for
you."

Next thing I know, when Karina leaves, this other lady hands me
an appointment card and I felt like it was being shoved on me.

I felt like that was her way of saying, "You are going to do this and
you are going to do it my way! I'm not letting you out of this!
You will come back!"

She never said this, of course. That's just the impression I got
from what she did.

I feared the next thing you know if I went for something involving
an IV and I tried to walk out on one of the other girls, she might
say, "Now you march right back in there and do what they ask."

Then, I thought, *"If that don't work, she may even have someone
lock the door behind me so she can force me into having to do
what they want, but I wasn't sure."*

She just came across that way unintentionally, I found out. Bertha
told her I feared she would do this to me if I walked out on her and
she said "No. He's free to go." We went back to talk to her Friday,
but she was not working that day.

I had already asked all the Radiology girls two months before if they would rub my head to calm me down and hold my hand if I had an IV and every one of them said, "Yes."

On Friday, I saw Diamond in the cafeteria.

She acted strange like she didn't want to talk to me. She acted like she already knew what I was going to ask.

I asked, "Can I ask you something?"

She said, "I'm at lunch right now."

I said, "Please."

She said, "Okay. What do you need?"

I said, "If Karina doesn't rub my head to calm me down when they do my shot can you do it for me?"

Diamond said, "I'm sorry. I can't."

I gave her a hug as usual. I suspected Karina told her not to cave in and baby me if she didn't.

Bertha said Diamond was almost in tears because it crushed her to have to say no and hurt my feelings. Bertha felt like Diamond really wanted to and would have actually done so, but that Karina must have told her not to. We saw Brandy and Macy in there with another nurse friend of ours sitting at a table to eat lunch. They were excited to see me and all gave me hugs.

I asked Brandy, "If Karina doesn't rub my head to calm me down for the shot can you do it?"

Brandy said, "No, I'm sorry I can't."

I said, "If I'm ever sent to have a CT or an MRI could you rub my head while Macy does the IV stick?"

Brandy said, "I can stick you. I can stick you."

Macy acted like she wasn't going to play this game.

She said, "I'll do it. I can rub your head."

I said, "Thanks."

I saw other people in the hallway on the way to the car and thought everyone was acting strange.   Sarah turned her head when I tried to hug her and then walked away.

I was shocked and thought, *"Sarah. You never did this before. Is something wrong?   Why is everybody acting so funny? Is something wrong?   What happened?"*

Then we walked down the GI hall to the elevator and I saw one of my GI nurses and asked her for a hug and she acted strange.

I finally said, "Please."

That girl gave in but turned her head away also.

I saw another *female* nurse in the same hall after that I liked and asked, "Can I have a hug?"

She said, "No." and walked on.

Then a *male* nurse joined her walking side by side with her.

He acted very hateful, "That's invading her space!" in a very angry tone of voice.

I was really spooked and thought, *"What's going on here? Why is everybody acting so strange? No one's ever acted like this before. Is this the day of the opposites or something? What's going on here, anyway?"*

Bertha wanted to talk to her but she said she needed to wait till Monday. She felt bad this had to happen on a weekend. She left me in the car on Monday when she went to talk to Karina and she talked to her and three other people in the waiting room.

They all said it was unfair to me that it had to be this way but they couldn't do this for me anymore. We couldn't go in there just to give our friends hugs and they were not trained to deal with autistic patients. She told them they needed to read the last chapter in my book.

Bertha said, "You know you are supposed to comfort your patients don't you."

Karina said, "Yes, to a point. But we can't give him hugs and we can't rub his head through an IV stick or other needle stick ever again. It's too intimate a thing."

Bertha explained to Karina that I had the mind of a child and I needed all those things.

Karina said, "Unfortunately, we cannot meet those needs here because if someone sees him hugging them whether he means it or not they could report it and get him in trouble. We just want to protect him."

They all told her, "We know Brian has all these needs and he needs to have them met but the nurses at this hospital are not trained to deal with someone like Brian. He needs to find a special needs doctor and a special needs hospital that deals with people with special needs like him because we just don't have that here. We know he is just sweet and we don't want him to get in trouble."

What I was thinking is, if someone did say something or try to report something, why couldn't they say, "Maam or Sir, he's autistic, he can't help it. He has to have this to meet his needs because he is autistic. He's not like you and me."?

That's the way the normal person that even half way understands this whole situation would handle this. Instead they put me in the same frame as everybody else. They told Bertha they would not be able to meet my special needs so we are not going back.

Regarding a special needs hospital and doctor Bertha said, "How do you even find them? Where are they at? I've been trying to find one?"

They said, "It will be hard to find. It will take a while but we will make some calls and get back to you. We think he would do better at a Children's Hospital if they would take him but we are afraid they won't take him because of his age. If he can just find a doctor that takes care of special needs people and a hospital that takes care of special needs people he should be good to go because then they could meet all his needs and he would never be misunderstood ever again if he does."

The problem is Bertha has also been researching it and can't seem to find anything, and everything seems to be only for kids because everybody thinks kids outgrow autism which they do not. They will always be that way, and they need a medical hospital for special needs adults as well, so people like me can get their needs met and be understood and they realize they are true needs and not just wants, but genuine needs.

One of the ladies said she would do some researching for us to find doctors that deal with special needs patients and a hospital for special needs patients.

A couple weeks later we actually got something in the mail with four phone numbers all except for one was disconnected or out of service. The one that was still in business was a development center for children.

We have a nurse friend who has an autistic son herself. We were telling her about the hospital not wanting to comfort me or give me hugs.

She said, "Well, what do they think comforting is anyway?
They're a friend. Friends hug. They're supposed to hug you.
And, how do they think they're supposed to comfort you if they
don't want to rub your head? That's like what you do with a baby.
There's nothing wrong with that. You're supposed to comfort
your patients if you're a nurse. That's your job. That's why I
don't like this place. When my kid turns 18 I'm going to leave.
There are autistics out there who are kids now that will grow up
one day and what are nurses going to do when this happens? They
need to be ready for it now and be willing to be there for them.
That's ridiculous."

The hospital that was once a dream for meeting my needs so well
is now a shattered dream and going anywhere without having my
special needs met is a nightmare in and of itself.

I need my needs to be met and when they are not, things are
downright spooky out there. That's why I get excited about
chipper acting cheerful nurses in the first place because in the past
they were willing to comfort me and cheer me on.

Just because I have a vibrant personality my self and I thrive on
cheerful acting people does not mean I'm not sick. That's just my
personality. Plus, it helps me deal with my anxieties over
upcoming procedures when I am able to be cheerful over receiving
cheerful people for my nurses.

We have a friend whose dad was in the hospital a couple of years
ago. He kept getting out of bed consistently regardless of the fact
he was a fall risk. He wasn't about to let that stop him, when he
decided to go to the bathroom he was going to go to the bathroom.
If he decided to take a walk, he was going to take a walk. This
man was also medically sick with something or he wouldn't have
been in there in the first place. Do you think that stopped him
from wanting to roam around all over the place, though? No. But
just because he did that didn't mean he wasn't sick. That's just the
way he was, and he was that way no matter how sick he was.

You think I'm bad, wanting to run give everybody hugs all the time when I'm supposed to be sick in bed. This guy was unstoppable and he didn't care if he got hugs or not, but he did like to visit and when he wanted to walk somewhere, he jumped at it whether he was capable of it or not. It was so bad to the point that they had to have a *female* nurse stay in his patient room with him consistently to babysit him so he wouldn't hurt himself. So do you think that meant he wasn't sick? No. You figured that one out, huh. Have you ever been in this situation?

The same goes with my wanting to go on a hug run because I'm so excited to see everybody and act all cheerful about seeing cheerful nurses. Just because I do this doesn't mean I'm not sick. I'd probably still do this even if I were deathly ill. To me, I'd rather get hugs and be able to be cheered up by those around me and talk to them so they can cheer me up than be completely confined myself. Now you see why I am the way I am.

That's just me. One day, you will see what I mean and see for your self. It was nice knowing you while I did.

We left this hospital never planning to go back again but we were afraid we still needed to further challenge these people and talk to someone to straighten it out in case there was an emergency that caused me to have to go there anyway since it was the closest hospital to where I live.

Bertha had written the President of this hospital to see if he could straighten it out because he seemed to be understanding of us but for some reason the compliance officer got a hold of our letter so I don't think he even ever saw the letter. Even if he did, he probably didn't want to cause a riff between us and him due to being sort of friends. He may have told his administrative staff to take care of it. Either way, I don't think he intended for all this to happen. If he did, he probably didn't want involved because it probably made him feel guilty to have any part of how these people were acting.

Instead of him, the compliance officer wrote Bertha an ugly letter admitting that "Yes, they were supposed to meet the emotional needs of the patient as well but that did not include any physical contact, no touching, and no hugging." He said, "I cannot and frankly will not make my nurses do this for him because it is unwelcomed and unwanted. We cannot meet his perceived needs."

Get ready for what I am about to say at the end of this book because in Chapter 38 you will see comments made by various nurses, doctors, and other medical professionals in the field of medicine that completely contradict everything this man is saying here. Not only do they state nurses are to comfort their patients but they actually tell their nurses to "touch" their patients and use "touch therapy" to comfort them by do the very things I am asking them to do myself. I even took notes from Nurse Education DVDs where they showed the nurses rubbing their patients' heads and holding their hands. I think you're about to be in for a shock.

Please read the rest of the book and it will help you see why I am the way I am with all my pickiness over which nurses I get and what they do. Thanks. I think you will be enlightened. Thanks for reading.

Chapter Thirty Five
Why I Look Smart, My Need to Hug:
I am Really a Special Needs Person

The only reason I am smart is because my mother drilled me to
<u>death</u> <u>from</u> <u>the</u> <u>8th</u> <u>grade</u> <u>on</u> when I went into all regular classes,
hoping that if one day I made A's and B's like everybody else
which did not happen until my third year of college that somehow I
would be able to do any job every one else was able to do. This
was after I took a Student Achievement Test in my 7th grade
Special Ed English class and my teacher thought I was ready for
the regular classroom. What my Special Ed teacher in the 7th grade
didn't know was that half the reason I was doing so well is because
I thrive on people with excitable personalities, and if they get me
pumped enough, they can cause me to figure out things I normally
would have not been able to figure out. This may sound crazy, but
I can be absolutely stumped about something and then accidentally
figure out the very thing that stumped me just because I saw Eliza
Doolittle sing "I Could Have Danced All Night" on TV. My ex-
Special Ed English teacher from the 7th grade had that kind of a
personality, so the more she got me pumped the better I did, and I
probably only did so well on the Student Achievement test because
my teacher had me so pumped already that I was thinking on a
higher level than I normally do. Without the extra excitement I go
brain dead on people. I actually have a problem that is backwards
of someone with ADD. They usually have difficulty doing well
because they are hyper. I have to make myself hyper on purpose to
think straight or I'll be a dope head about everything and not get it
about anything because I will go brain dead if I don't hype myself
up to catch things other people catch. As a result of this, when I
went to all regular classes, all the festivity disappeared, and reality
kicked in as I struggled to pass my classes with teachers and
students that did not have upbeat personalities like she did. I think
I only did well on that test because I was so pumped I figured out
things I normally would not have figured out, and just did
especially well on the test that time.

Big City Hospitals Don't Like Cowards   Brian Evans

My first year of college I was told the shocking news that I only read on the 7th grade level and after taking a Reading Comprehension class for a year I got up to the 10th grade, 3rd month reading level and never got much further. Seeing this fact, I can't see how I could have possibly done well enough on the Student Achievement Test in the 7th grade to qualify me for all regular classes in the 8th grade. We're talking my first year of college and I'm just then reading on the 7th grade level. Try explaining that one. It doesn't make sense to me. I think I only did well on her test because of how hype up she got me before I took the thing. I think if she had not hyped me up, I would have blown it dramatically. My 7th grade Special Ed teacher thought if I was drilled long enough for enough years, I'd eventually make the same grades as everybody else and as a result be able to perform any job anyone else could perform. She even got my mother to believe this would happen. Well, it didn't work. I was fired from three jobs and let go from seven jobs because I wasn't fast enough and I didn't get it about anything.

My boss at Dollar General in Abilene even said when I worked for him, "You mind if I tell you something. You're book smart but your not street smart."

Every employer I ever had said, "Can't you figure anything out? It took you six months to learn what everyone else learned in one week."

It never failed.

It was my life story, and people think I'm smart because of my book knowledge. It has also been suggested to me through my adult years by people that know I have a language learning disability that I am intellectually smart and sociably retarded. In revealing this shocking truth, I wish people would lay off and let me be the airheaded, special needs person that I am, and not expect me to be like everybody else, because it was not my will to be normal. I've resented it my entire life. I wanted to be left alone. I may look smart to you, but I'm one of them, the Special Ed people. I have special needs, and I expect people to see it that way.

Forget about my stupid intelligence. I was even IQ tested in college, and found to be exactly what I am telling you I am, intellectually smart and performance dumb. That's why I can't perform a job well.

I'm too dumb to figure out how to perform tasks but I'm good at the books. I have to be shown everything because I get confused over every little thing. My boss at Dollar General in 1998 through 2000 even mentioned that. If I am pushed too fast I begin having high blood pressure, rapid pulse, severe fatigue, stomach problems, sleep 15 hours a day at home, and then become so severely fatigued at work to the point that I can't remember anything I ever learned, and am almost in the state of dementia. This is why I got fired at my last job in March 2003 at the Green Forest Exxon. That state of confusion disappears, when I am left alone and allowed to do things at my own pace that makes sense to me. I'm tired of people expecting me to be something I can never be because I appear to be smart. You want to know why else I look smart. I found out I had the star voice and hung out with all these opera people that taught me their communication system which made absolutely no sense to anyone else. I thought I'd never get their mannerisms down like they wanted and when I did, I was stuck that way. I got harassed for displaying these mannerisms these people wished me to have that they trained me to have because people were considering me to be a freak because I looked like them instead of me. Have you ever seen the movie, "Princess Diaries?" These opera music instructors did the same thing to me that they did to the girl in this movie and ever since that people thought I was a freak. No one ever thought I was a freak before I was trained to look like those stiff bodied people you see at the Metropolitan Opera. That's what they made me look like. I was continually blamed for looking like that, and accused of things I never did, and was specifically told it was based on my body language. Well, let me tell you something. It was not my body language. It was their body language. They trained me to such a point that I got stuck looking like them and then got accused of being a freak for having their mannerisms, not mine, theirs. As soon as I finally broke loose of their stupid facade they got me stuck looking like, people liked me again.

I never want to look like them again. I want to be left alone, and I want everything back the way it was, before I busted my head off to get smart for no reason. I'm an individual with special needs who only acquired a book intelligence that never came naturally.

I wish to be treated with the exact same accommodations as the retarded people and the borderline normal Special Ed people who are not retarded, but are not far from it. I was one of the borderline normal people from ages 10 to 13. My IQ ratings at that age range were Intellectual 74 and performance 67, with an overall IQ of 70. I never wanted to leave their world, and I expect to be treated like one of them.

I want all my nurses everywhere to treat me as if I was one of their kids. When I left the Special Ed world in the 8th grade, after loving their world, I've resented it ever since. The people I went to Special Ed with were not actually retarded, but they were borderline normal. Some may have had a certain amount of mild retardation in an area or two, but they were basically smarter than the retarded people, but still well below the normal average intelligence level of everyday people. That's about the level of intellectual functioning I had. I had a barely normal (borderline normal) 74 intellectual intelligence and a mildly retarded, but almost normal 67, social and performance intelligence. I was right close to the borderline normal cut off of 70 on both ends, slightly below the cut off in one area and slightly above the cut off in the other. After being educated to death, by age 23 my IQ went up to Intellectual 84 and Performance 77. At age 29, my IQ went up again to Intellectual 92, but Performance remained the same at a 77 IQ putting me at an overall IQ of 85. Notice the incredible jaggedness. I am 15 points intellectually smarter than I am performance smart and social smart. That's pretty bad. People see the higher mark and expect the performance to be on the same level as the intellectual, not 15 points lower. People use this against you, and demand you perform and socialize on the level of someone with 15 points higher of a social level and performance level, just because your intellectual level is up there. It's thanks to this, that all these bullheads out there expect me to be sociably up to their par, and be as performance smart as they are as well.

They think you're either one number or the other. Dumb or smart.
It's pretty bad when your book smart and performance dumb, and
sociably dumb, and you're expected to act like someone that is a
social genius. It's not right, and it's not fair.

Some people in certain towns may say, "We need to teach him that
it is not right to hug."

Others, say, "There is nothing wrong with hugging people. The
world would be a better place if everybody hugged everybody."

Bertha and I are the town huggers in our town, and people love it.
I tend to go with the second opinion. You can't teach me to not do
something that I need; because some sophisticated bullhead thinks
you have to learn to do what they think is appropriate. A need is a
need. And for their information, the less I'm able to hug people,
and the less I am able to be my special needs self, like the Special
Ed people I wanted to be with in the first place, the more I lose my
will to live, because I cannot function without it, because it is a
need and not just a want. It's not something you teach me not to
do. It's something you deal with because it is a genuine need that
has to be met. I know a couple with an autistic daughter who has
to constantly roll play dough in her hands to calm her nerves and if
she can't do that it will make her uneasy and send her into a
depression. Just as this girl is uneasy not rolling play dough in her
hands constantly, it makes me uneasy and uncomfortable not to be
able to hug somebody I like, and sends me into a depression
because it is a genuine need that needs met. I'm autistic, and
autistic people don't do things like this because they don't know
any better, if that's what people think. People with autism do it
because they have to do it, because it will throw them out of kilter
not to be able to do what they need to do.

People need to get off of the "What's proper and what's not"
scenario and think about "What does this autistic person need?"

They never think about the possibility it might **hurt** the autistic person that craves touch not to be able to hug somebody they like, especially when they are being taken care of by nurses that are doing something that terrifies them, and they need this to comfort them. Asking me to not hug somebody is like telling someone that accidentally burned their hand on a stove that they can't pour water on their burnt hand to cool the burn, or like telling someone to not scratch something that itches them, or telling them not to turn the air conditioner on when they are burning up, or telling someone not to brush their teeth when they got stink in their mouth.

How would you like it if every time you burned your hand on a stove somebody said, "You can't cool your hand in the sink. That's not allowed. You need to let it burn."?

How would you like it if every time you itched someone said, "You can't scratch your arm. That's not allowed. You're going to have to let it itch."?

How would you like it if every time you burned up from the summer heat someone said, "You're not allowed to turn the air conditioner on. You'll have to burn up."?

How would you like it if every time you have a yucky taste in your mouth someone said, "You can't brush your teeth. That's not allowed. You'll just have to deal with the yucky taste in your mouth."?

You know what happens when someone has an acidic reaction in their stomach and they take Pepto Bismol to soothe it and tame it down. That's what a hug feels like to me when I put my ear on somebody's cheek. It's like hugging a pillow, because I have a stimulus in my right ear somehow that is only soothed by pressing it on somebody's cheek, and when I do so, I feel comforted and it feels better. Without this, the stimulus drives me up the wall, and I cannot handle it. Pressing my ear on another person's cheek is like taking the Pepto Bismol for an acidic stomach to tame it down and soothe it.

Big City Hospitals Don't Like Cowards   Brian Evans

I visited the State School once in Abilene, Texas when I was in my 20's, and a retarded girl kept running her hand up my arm. That seemed different yes, but I let her because that is what she needed to do, and it would have messed up her emotional state to not be able to do it, and it is what she needed to stay calm. I realized that myself, and let her do this to me without complaint, because I knew this is what she needed to stabilize herself.

I'd like to ask that no one ever drag someone out of Special Ed to turn them into some normal person to make some big accomplishment they can never make and can never be the person you want them to be. A lot of misunderstandings have occurred on account of throwing me in a world that was not mine, and if I would have been left alone, this whole thing would have never happened. If I would have continued to look as airheaded as I did then, people would have understood me, but because I'm quote "Intelligent", the bullheads out there think I am without excuse.

Let me tell you, I am only book smart, and nothing else. I am dumb at everything that is not in a book. And the shocking truth is I watch kid movies and Christmas movies, and 1800s classics. Regular TV depresses me. I like bath salts, and candles, and Christmas trinkets, and bright colors, and flowers, etc. I like shopping in gift shops that have pretty stuff and antique stuff in them. Notice, I didn't say I liked football or automobile mechanics. I am not a manly person at all, and I can barely carry something weighing 30 pounds without straining. I even like Antique Dolls and Christmas movies. I like hiking trails and taking pictures and making greeting cards and calendars with them and then painting pictures from the photographs I took on big canvases. My cards are photographs, not paintings. My paintings are all on canvases sizes 16X20 to 24X36. I paint with oils when I am in the mood and feel like it. I like pretty pillows, pretty blankets and bright colored walls. I crave touch, and have a need to be hugged by everybody I know. I'm also a picky eater with my foods, and my local nurses know it. I have an incredible oversensitivity to pain, a shot feels like a steak knife, an IV feels like a butcher knife, and a catheter feels like a sword being run through me.

388

Yes, I get anxious before I get stuck, but the pain is very real, and there are other autistics that have this same problem. People with autism can either be over sensitive to pain like me, or be undersensitive to pain like my sister, who you have to watch because she can't feel it when she hurts herself. I am not a manly person at all, and I can barely carry something weighing 30 pounds without straining. That's right. I like what girls like, and I like what kids like. I'm just like a kid, regardless of my age and I wish to keep it that way, so I'd like all these bullheaded people to back off, and let me be myself and treat me like a kid. My local hospital did this for me back when they understood, and had no problem with it, and if they knew other people were harassing me about it they would have be mad as a hornet. My local hospital understood me, unlike the hospital that did my Transesophageal Echocardiogram and Heart Catherization in 2014. And anytime I've ever had problems with any other facility, and told my nurses at the local hospital I go to about it, they were not happy about it, because they know me, and know I'm special. It made some of my nurses at my local hospital mad when nurses at a different hospital treat me mean or take advantage of me.

My local hospital's nurses knew I was easy to take advantage of. They know that when put in the path of an evil person that they can run right over me, and my not be able to do anything about it. When people take advantage of this knowledge and use it to torture me, or kick me around, my nurses at the local hospital I go to get angry about it because they like me the way I am, and think I am special. It makes them feel like they want to tell somebody to back off because I didn't do anything to anybody.

My nurses at my local hospital I've told about other hospitals and clinics giving me trouble think that some of these bullies at some of these other hospitals needed to leave me alone. I hope you see my point. I may ask strange requests, but they are what I need to get through invasive procedures because of my oversensitivity to pain, and my needle phobia, and because of my autism. The nurses at my local hospital knew this until recently and met my every need every time. I just wish all these other places could figure that out.

I don't really know whether the other hospital I just went to considered me intelligent and without excuse to be different or whether they thought I was retarded. I've gotten both depending on the audience I'm around. Some of the people in the town we used to live in thought I was without excuse for being different and wanting to hug people because they thought I was intelligent. The people we live around in our current location could care less, and consider me a Special needs individual who needs extra attention. Some other places think I am an absolute retard. It just depends on the place or the people. They probably thought I was retarded. I don't know what they thought, but they sure didn't understand my need for hugs and for comfort through invasive procedures. I need all these things met everywhere by everybody and I think they should accept me the way I am and meet them. There are patients out there that are in so great agony and despair when they are in the hospital that they need this kind of care, and me being autistic with an oversensitivity to pain and a need to hug my nurses and be comforted in the way you would comfort a child during IV sticks and other invasive procedures should be able to receive this level of care from nurses I am comfortable with that are both *bubbly acting* and affectionate with their patients. These nurses need to do what they can to make their patients feel better, not shun them for wanting their comfort. You're not their business executive at a firm, you're their caregiver, and you should do everything necessary to meet the physical and emotional well being of all your patients. I would do this for other patients in my situation if I were a nurse and I feel like they should meet me with the same accommodations I would be willing to meet for someone else in my position seeing I need these accommodations because of my Autism. Right now, I'm on Social Security Disability, and have been since 2003, because my medical problems became so severe that I could no longer function on a job. I feel like the big city hospital I just went to at their cath lab wanted to punish me for not getting through the first two IV sticks, but get this. I even apologized to one of my nurses at my own local hospital the last time I had trouble getting through an IV at their hospital and she said, "Don't worry about me. I'm here for you."

390

As a matter of fact, this nurse at the hospital I normally go to at my own local hospital said this after they had to stick me twice, when the IV tech in their GI department there was unable to thread the needle through a vein in my right arm at my normal hospital.

At this hospital I normally go to for my procedures, when they had to do a second stick, I pleaded with a nurse not to stick me again and she said, "I'm sorry honey, we have to do this. I'm sorry we have to stick you again, but we have to. Just try the best you can, okay."

This was the reaction I got at my local hospital when they had trouble getting an IV in on the first try.

And by the way, the nurse there "rubbed my head to calm me down" and held my hand to comfort me and never complained about anything at this hospital.

She was the one that said, "Don't worry about me. I'm here for you." when I apologized to her for having so much trouble.

That should have been the attitude of the hospital that did the Heart Catherization test and Transesophageal Echocardiogram on me. The doctor there and her head Cath Lab nurse and her office nurse all three promised all of my needs would be met.

All three of these ladies said all the nurses there got my list of accommodations, and they had no problem with any of them, and all my needs would be met before I even went in for the procedure.

Well, they weren't. They quit meeting them half way through when I threw the doctor off a patient and from that point on.

They refused to hug me or rub my head to calm me down and hold my hand and acted ugly and got rough with me and stuck me hard and everything and then took it out on my wife for having to meet them.

Big City Hospitals Don't Like Cowards   Brian Evans

If they would have reacted to me like my own hospital reacted to me when they dealt with me, they would have had a win-win situation, but instead the whole situation was nothing but chaos and they were lucky they didn't kill me in the process with my oversensitivity to pain and my fear of nurses that don't treat you right. If I hadn't fell asleep just before the heart cath tube was stuck in, there would have been one really big nightmare situation and if they would have continued being rough and mean through that as well if I would have been awake to feel the pain, the situation would have been too overwhelming for me and would have probably killed me. It was already too overwhelming for me to handle. Lucky for me, I fell asleep before they went too far with their cruel behaviors.

Chapter Thirty Six
Misunderstandings I sometimes have with Nurses
Or Fear I Will Have with Nurses

I've had some misunderstandings by nurses that were just minor that they figured out were just misunderstandings but I've also had greater misunderstandings with other nurses that were drastic misunderstandings.

Some of the minor misunderstands with some of my nurses have been things like informative things I tell them they didn't know anything about. I got the feeling they thought that I made some of these things up and when Bertha got their attention they realized I wasn't making them up after all.

Examples of this would be:

1. I told one nurse I worked with that a heart monitor sticky thing they put on my chest in the hospital setting got loose, they just kind of looked at me funny and walked off.

    They acted really nice to me before that, but then they acted like they got the wrong idea when I told them this, and just ignored me.

    I told Bertha that it was loose. She asked me, "That doesn't really matter does it?   It's still on there."

    And I said, "Well, actually, I think it's supposed to stick better to my chest in order for them to monitor me on their heart monitor machine accurately.

    When Bertha finally got this nurse's attention and said, "Hey, I think you need to adjust this heart monitor lead on his chest. It looks like it's loose." Then, the nurse realized I wasn't joking after all and readjusted the lead to make it stick better.

2. There was another nurse I tried to show a square of white at
    the bottom of my leg, just above my foot where my hair
    disappeared suddenly in one day, just months before my
    hospital visit there.

    This girl had also been nice to me.

    This girl even gave me a sponge bath before I even
    mentioned this, and thought nothing bad of me at all, and I
    was relieved she was able to trust me, and not act funny,
    like "Why do I have to give him a bath?" As a matter of
    fact, I think she volunteered to do this. However, after I
    already put a new gown on, and got redressed, she still
    acted fine with me, and said, "If you need anything else,
    just let me know."

    I told her about the square place at the bottom of my leg
    where the hair disappeared, and told her I thought my
    Thyroid was responsible for it.

    I was actually hoping she would notice it, and say, "Hey,
    you got a point there. Let, me tell the head nurse." but
    instead, when I said, "I guess there is one thing you could
    do for me. I could use another water or coffee", she said,
    "I'll be right back."

    She never came back, and a few minutes later, a guy nurse
    came in there to give me my drink.

    When I asked my head nurse where this girl was, she said,
    "She had to go to the 3rd floor to work up there a while."

    I thought the girl was upset because she took me wrong.

    We demanded another *female* nurse come in there as her
    substitute until she came back and we told my head nurse
    we want this girl back when she gets back.

I finally saw her several hours later, and she still acted really nice. I was so relieved. I started telling her how glad I was I got to see her, and that she actually came back, because I thought she was upset with me.

She said, "Oh, no. I'm not upset. I just had to go to the 3rd floor to take care of things up there for a while."

I said, "I thought when I showed you that place at the bottom of my leg above my foot that I offended you. I was really worried. I'm sorry if I upset you."

The girl said, "Oh no, I wasn't worried about that. That didn't bother me at all. I just had to go take care of some patients on the other floor because they called me to 3rd floor for two or three hours."

I said, "Am I ever glad you're back. I was scared to death. I thought surely I said something wrong and I felt really bad."

She said, "No. No. No. I'm right here. You didn't run me off. Everything's just fine. I'm right here. I'll be leaving in a couple of hours, but while I'm here, I'll still come in here if you need me, so, you should see me a couple of more times."

I was really relieved and said, "Okay."

3. I had a problem with swelling and edema around the ankles, most of the edema is behind the ankles and some of it is above the ankles on the top of my feet. The other edema was just above the heels, where the spoon ladle indentions are supposed to be behind your ankles.

Every time I've told a nurse about it, they act like they are reluctant to look at it. I think they think I'm making it up.

The first time, it was slight, and one nurse, the nurse practitioner that used to work at my current doctor's office did notice I was correct.

She said, "It's not too bad yet, but keep a watch on it, and if it got worse let her know. She thought it might be a vascular problem."

Later, the problem was mild, a little puffier than it was. I was worried about telling the nurse I had at the current time about this because I was afraid she would feel this way too.

I was afraid to show anybody, because I'm afraid they'll either think I'm being inappropriate, or wind up scolding me for inappropriate behavior by wanting to show it to them, one of the two, because I'd have to take my shoes and socks off for them to see it, and they would probably think, "I really don't want to see your feet." and think I was just trying to get them to look at me a certain way, but it really is there, and I'm really not joking.

It was even worse on the left foot, and a lot of veins busted in the very place the edema is at in that foot, a few more busted down the edge on the side.

If I did show a nurse my ankles, and they looked straight up and down at my legs and my feet while I'm standing up or sitting down, they would probably not see anything, and think, "Is this some kind of a joke?" but if I cross my feet over my legs one at a time, then, if a nurse looked at it and saw it, they would probably say, "Oh my word! How long has this been going on?" My answer would be, "Since March 5, 2013."

Then, they would probably say, "When did it get worse, since you said it was slight before it got mild?" My answer would be, "In the past month."

Then, they'd probably say, "Oh my word. We may need to do something about this. Let me see what I can do."

4.   In 1994, I got a rash in my groin from going through termite eaten files. I already had problems with people thinking bad enough things about me as it was and then I had to tell these two girl nurses I had back then when they asked me, "What's the problem?"

I said, "I have a rash in my groin area."

The one girl acted like, "Oh, boy. How did we get stuck having to deal with this problem?" I felt really bad.

It wasn't my fault I had a rash in the groin area. It just happened.

They went and showed it to the head nurse and she said, "This is really bad."

When they got the cream they needed from the head nurse, one of the two younger nurses held the tube, and squeezed it, while the other girl put it in my groin area, and they were not happy about it.

I think they may have gotten over it, a week or so later, but, they acted like they were really unhappy with me, and gave me the terrible feeling they thought I got it on purpose, so, they'd have to look at me down there.

I thought, "It's not my fault I got the rash. If I hadn't had to mess with those termite eaten files, I would have never got the rash. Now, I have two nurses down on me for having one."

Now, I'm afraid if I ever get a rash in the groin again, and tell a nurse about it, they will either think I am being inappropriate, or scold me for being inappropriate, because they think I am making it up, when I am telling the truth.

Right now, I don't have one, but I'd hate to get one again, and be treated like I was being inappropriate for wanting to show a nurse what the problem is.

5. I also have knots all over my upper legs, and some on my arms, and stomach, and back.
    One time, I told a nurse about the knots, and I had to pull down my pants to show her how huge the knots on my legs were.

    I was worried she thought I was just being inappropriate, but she actually noted those knots, plus two or three others on my lower legs, and said, "That is pretty big alright. What did they tell you it was?"
    Bertha told her, "In the past, they just said it was fatty tumors."

    This nurse, believe it or not, said, "I don't know. I'm not so sure. It doesn't look right to me. If they get any bigger let me know."

6. One time I had to show this nurse a knot to the side of my breast on the left side of my chest that was hurting me.

    She measured it, and everything, and sent me to get a mammogram right away, because it had her worried.

    After it turned out normal, I was supposed to see her in a month.

    She was supposed to be a nurse practitioner.

    I kept having other things go wrong, and tried to schedule other things with her to check on me, because of how thorough she was.

    She kept trying to get out of it, and I got the feeling she had the wrong idea about the breast thing.

However, things turned out, I wound up having to see her for a different reason a month later, and she got to recheck it anyway. I think she was okay then.

7. I kept having a bleeding problem in my urinary tract that actually started in 1994 that lasted all the way to 2012.

Five different years my current Urologist did a Retrograde Cystoscopy. The first four times he found absolutely nothing.

I kept saying, "Do I need to bring my blood spotted underwear with the big spots on it to prove it?"

Bertha said, "No, don't do that."

After those four times, I gave up and decided I wasn't going to tell my Urologist I was still having bleeding problems.

Then, he said, "Are you still bleeding?" I said, "Yes."

He set me up for the test, but I quit bleeding before the day of the test, and I said, "Maybe you ought to wait 6 months for it to happen again and test it then. I'm afraid it won't show up."

He said, "No boss, I think we need to go ahead and go in there and check it out. I really do."

By some miracle, he found it this time, a polyp that had been growing in my urinary tract was causing the bleeding and he thought it was really bizarre, but he found it.

How many times over do you think his nurse must have thought I was full of it, because he didn't find anything, and they didn't see anything themselves, because nothing ever showed up on a urine sample either?

It was there, and on the 5th try he found it.

He did this test in 2005, 2007, 2009, and 2011 and found nothing.

In 2012, he found the culprit and took it out, then the bleeding problem stopped.

8. Recently, I told a physical therapist I had in January that I occasionally get cramps above the ankles and/or behind the ankles in both feet that sometimes lock, and when they do, it immobilizes me, but it only happens about once every six months for about three or four weeks, off and on, at unpredictable times.

    I reluctantly asked her how they gave therapy for something like that; worried she'd get the wrong idea.

    She doesn't know this, but if I had started having problems with my feet locking up above or behind my ankles, and I would have had to go barefoot to let her do what she needed to do, I probably would have been really embarrassed if a lot of people standing around saw me in my bare feet, because I am shy of my feet. For some reason, it doesn't bother me if I'm going swimming at a swimming pool or lake, but anywhere else in public, if someone sees me in my bare feet I feel ashamed of myself and feel inferior and want to hide somewhere because somebody saw my feet.
    I think my Autism makes me like this. She tried to tell me what they did for it, but it was difficult to explain what they did. I'm hoping she didn't think I was being inappropriate when I told her this.

I've told nurses about it, too, and they give me the feeling they think I'm putting them on too, but I'm not.

9. One nurse recently forgot at my local hospital that I liked the bubbly, chipper, peppy acting fe*male* nurses to be my nurse when Bertha told her "Don't give him any men, only fe*male* nurses."

Bertha forgot to specify what kind, and this lady forgot, too, and a lady from Express that was far from chipper, that acted straight faced, and almost grumpy-like, that had a very serious personality, came after me, and about spooked me to death, when I had to go with her, and this other nurse came in there that was a straight faced nurse that was tall, and looked like they could pass for a man, helped with seeing what was wrong with my left waist and left leg when it swelled up and gave me pain.

I was actually relieved when a CCU nurse came in, saying she wanted to give the record to my Cardiologist and my family doctor, who had a much more spiffed up personality.

Bertha said, "Is he ever glad you're here! These other ladies make him really nervous! He's scared of them! They didn't give him a chipper one like they normally do! It's a good thing you walked in!"

9d. It's also a good thing they didn't stick me with an IV because I could tell by the way they acted, and the way they handled me, that they would have got rough, and probably would not have understood my oversensitivity to pain, and not been nice about it, plus, I would have felt no comfort from them when I needed the motherly comfort of a bubbly, chipper, peppy, happy go lucky *female* nurse.

So please make sure this is what I get in the future. Mediocre nurses scare me too. And the ones that don't are boring, and are of no comfort to me.

9.   One day, Bertha had to go to the ER for her leg, and she had three different men come after her to look at her leg.

One man came to get her, one man did her vitals, and another man came to check on her. When this happened I was really spooked. I was breathing tightly, with my air going tightly to my throat from my chest in almost a hyperventilate state, that I was trying to hide. When the girls in the ER saw this, they gave me the feeling they got the feeling I was a little freaked out.

My new favorite ER nurse must have noticed from the distance, my not even seeing her, because she came in to the room a few minutes after we got there, and I was about to croak.

Bertha told her, "It's a good thing you're here. He was about to croak. Men scare him, and he was afraid a *female* nurse wasn't going to come in here."

The girl said, "Yeah, there's a lot of guys out there, isn't there."

I said, "Am I ever glad you're here! I was scared to death! I didn't think we'd get a fe*male* nurse in here!"

She said, "Yeah. I'm here. I'll be coming back. Don't worry. You'll have plenty of girls come in."

Then her, and two other girls took turns coming in, and she came in three times. No men came in after that ever again except for the doctor. I was really relieved. So please next time, no men, unless it's the doctor himself. All the nurses have to be *female*s only.

These nurses have to be the chipper, peppy, bouncy, happy go lucky *female* nurses, too. Not the other kind.

If you are a nurse, and you read this book, when I try to tell you about something that's wrong, no matter what it is, or what you have to see, please do not hold this against me, and think I am being inappropriate, but understand that I am being informative, and what I am telling you is genuine, and that I would not point out certain things, or ask you to check certain things, or look at certain things to see what you think might be wrong, if there wasn't anything wrong. If I try to show you something, or point something out, I'm actually telling the truth, because I'm not going to make up something that isn't true. There are times when I am afraid to show nurses problems I think they need to see because I'm worried they'll not believe me, and think I'm putting them on, so I'm reluctant to show them whatever the problem is, because I'm afraid they'll not want to be my friend anymore, and shun me away, or run off, and never came back, because I told them about something that was genuinely wrong that they thought I was faking about. I usually take a chance on telling someone the first time when this happens, but if they act the least bit apprehensive about what I said, I think, "I'm not telling them that again. I almost lost a good nurse. I'm not saying something this time."

If they act funny, I usually get worried, and say something like, "I hope I didn't make you upset when I tried to show you this. I didn't mean to make you upset."

If I tell them I'm worried about it, which I am, they usually figure out I didn't mean anything, but, if they have the least notion that I meant something wrong by something, and act like their going to turn on me because of it, then, I get to where I don't say anything about anything, no matter how major it is, because I don't want to lose their friendship.

Sometimes I think, "Do I show them this problem? And then, I think, What if they don't believe me? What if they think I'm making it up or just trying to get inappropriate attention?"

I feel like, "If I want to stay on good terms with this person and be friends, maybe I ought to not say anything. Maybe, later they'll figure out something's wrong."

If they do figure out something is wrong, they'll probably say, "Why didn't you tell me? Or, "Why didn't you show me?" This is terrible. I needed to see this. I can't treat you if you don't tell me what's wrong."

Then they say, "Now, I have to do something more major than I would have had to do to fix the problem."

And that's when I wind up saying, "I didn't think you believed me, so I just gave up, and decided not to say anything, because I thought you wouldn't understand me, and think I was making it up?"

It's really sad that every time I have something I feel like I need to show a "chipper acting female nurse" I like that I'm comfortable with like a rash in the groin or busted veins in the feet or knots on the legs or lumps or knots in the breast area etc. that they act like, "I don't want to have to see him like that." And they react like this because I might have to pull my pants down to let them see a rash, or take my shoes and socks off to let them see my busted veins, or pull my shirt up to let them see and feel the lumps I sometimes get in my breasts or something of that nature. But yet, if I told a "serious trended female nurse" the same things, who I am not comfortable with at all by the way, they would be like, "What's the problem?! Where's it at?! What are we looking at?! You better show me what the problem is or I'll rip your clothes right off of you!" That's because they are controlling, and they don't care what they see. These serious types would strip me completely naked if they had their way and then come at me with needles as hard as they could and scrape the tar out of me with blades if they found out they needed to scrape at something or do biopsies as roughly as they could. Those people are mean. Yet, when I ask someone I'm not afraid of they're like "I don't want to have to look at him like that, I might have to see his feet or I might have to see his private area or something. I don't want to see him undressed." I don't feel comfortable doing this for a "male doctor or male nurse" or a "serious trended female nurse".

The "Chipper acting female nurses" are the only ones I am comfortable with.

Please, just get over it, and do what you need to do when I need you to do it. I promise I'm not going to tell you something is wrong unless it really is, or unless I think something is wrong, but am not sure, and want you to check it out. Please take my word for it, and think of me as one of your kids. If it makes you feel better, think of me as just a baby in diapers if something bothers you.

]Just treat it like it is just another thing you have to do, like when you are taking care of a kid.

More Major Misunderstandings

(Already in Stories you Read)

1. Director of Speech Language Pathology Department can't really tell I actually have a Language Learning Disorder and gets the wrong idea when I asked for a *female* therapist, not understanding I've had several bad experiences with *male* nurses in my past and I'm not understood well by *male* therapists either.

2. Favorite IV nurse gets the wrong idea when I write her a letter defending myself against what I believe he is going to make her think of me, based on his own biased opinions, when he never even met me before, and did not know me personally enough to judge me so quickly.

3. Hospital I went to recently, where I normally don't go, after promising to meet my accommodations, breaks their promise half way through and complains about it.

> 3b. A nurse thought that my screaming was an act of misbehaving myself, rather than realizing that my pain was real. It was excruciating, and my reaction was an automatic reaction, which should have emphasized the amount of pain I was in.

3c. A nurse did not understand that I had a need for hugs, and not just a want.

3d. A nurse thought they were above meeting my needs, and showing compassion.

3e. A nurse thought if she punished me by having someone jab me with an IV like a shot, that it would correct unwanted behavior that wasn't even misbehavior, because it is not my fault I have an over sensitivity to pain due to my Autism.

3f. The head nurse getting the security guard after my wife, because she was crying over my traumatic experiencing in fear of her life of what was going to happen to me, because of the cruelty of the other nurses.

4. The policeman at a different hospital who frisked me in the hospital, not understanding that Bertha just went to talk to my IV helper to clear up a terrible misunderstanding, so she would forgive me for overreacting to my situation, and understand that the letter I wrote her was written in panic in order to defend myself against the man who had the wrong idea about me, because of fears he would turn her against me, and all that.

5. Nurses in some bigger city hospitals or clinics that think I'm horrible for insisting on *female* nurses, and refusing to have *male* nurses, not realizing my traumatic past with *male* nurses.

5b. Most nurses know better than this, and know that I need a *bubbly acting, chipper, cheerful female* nurse who will be more compassionate and comfort and console me through needle sticks, and invasive procedures, where men cannot, and would scare me if they even entered my room.

6. Some nurses stereotype Autistic people, who think all autistic people don't like to be touched, when in fact, some are the opposite, like me, who crave touch and need touch.

7. Some nurses think that just because the average person doesn't feel anything, or barely anything, when they are stuck with an IV or blood test, that I shouldn't feel anything either, and get mad when I scream, because I am in agony in excruciating pain. Nurses that make me nervous that want to control me, and force me to do whatever they ask, or manhandle me, because they cannot stand my reaction to pain, and are not generous enough to find a nurse that I would feel more comfortable helping me.

8. Some nurses don't understand why I want *bubbly acting female* nurses, that automatically assume that I'm just after them, when in reality I'm just looking for a *bubbly acting female* nurse to comfort and console me through needle sticks, and invasive things, and to treat me like I'm one of their kids.

9. In some instances, nurses at the bigger city hospitals think that I am being inappropriate when I ask them to rub my head to calm me down and hold my hand but I desperately need them to do this for me, because needle sticks and invasive procedures are very traumatic for me, and I need motherly acting, compassionate, bubbly *female* nurses to help me with this.

9b. Nobody ever complained about having to do this for me at my own local hospital until recently. They did this for me several times before and never had a problem for years, but now I think they are just backing down so they don't look bad to other patients coming in. Some of the other nurses that aren't used to doing this for me are complaining they think it is too intimate for them. All the other nurses that did this in the past, did not care, and considered me to be a child and saw it as stroking the head of a child to keep them calm when they are scared even if I am an adult because I have the mind of a child. I may be intellectually smart, only because of memorized book knowledge, but in reality I am sociably and emotionally like a child, and have also been diagnosed as having the social and emotional mind of a child. To everybody's bewilderment, I also am incapable of knowing what to do in an emergency situation. Therapists have constantly had to drill me in this area and said it was my worst area of language development. So, in that way, I am also a child.

There are many who would look at me when I say, "Help, I don't know what to do!" that would say out of ignorance that I was just trying to get attention but if they saw for themselves how it really is, especially if they left me in the dark and expected me to figure out all my emergency situations alone without help they would get the shock of their life when they found out I really didn't know what to do.

They would see I was not joking, and when disaster took place, they would be like, "Why did we not listen to him? He tried to tell us. He looked smarter than that to me, but I guess not. He really didn't know what to do, and whatever he asked me to do for him blew up in his face because he didn't have a clue how to solve his emergency situation."

That's a lot of the reason I get so misunderstood.

I look so smart to people because of my book knowledge that they can't see how I could possibly need or can't figure out the things I really can't figure out. And then, when misunderstandings take place disasters happen. Either I get in trouble for them for asking for help. Or, I go off and try to do something myself because someone else doesn't want bothered with it and thinks I should figure it out all myself and then I blow it all over the place because I didn't have a clue, and they find out later, bewildered when it happens. You've got to give me a break. I'm not as with it as you think I am, and I really do have needs that would normally be needs you would only think that children would have, and when they're not met, I'm sunk, and nobody knows what to do. I may seem smart to you, but I am also an ex-Special Ed student who got thrown into the normal world trying to make it and failed miserably because I didn't have a clue.

9c. I don't know why these other hospitals can't understand that I need them to meet my needs and follow suite with what my own local hospital does for me.

By the way, for the information of this Director of Speech Pathology that thought I was after the women just because I asked for a *female* therapist to do my Speech-Language Therapy at the bigger city hospital I went to at the time of my TURP surgery, and his staff members, it just so happens I went to a *female* therapist at my own local hospital recently for a whole year, and she was totally fine with me, and we did really well together.

 I also told her how this man acted, and what happened with his staff, and the rest of his hospital's staff on account of my asking for a *female* therapist at his hospital, and she thought the whole thing was absolutely ridiculous, and couldn't believe someone could be so stupid.

And they may have not been able to tell I had a Language Learning Disorder, but she could. She was totally happy with the way the therapy went, and thought I was very well behaved. She had no problem with me at all, and thought I was just fine, in that regard.

I was happy to have this lady for my therapist, and she did exactly what I asked these people to do, by taking over where the ACU Speech and Hearing Center in Abilene, Texas left off, and continuing from there.

My improvements were only mild, because I've gotten about as far as I'm ever going to get, but, she herself admitted, that technically, because of my Autism, I really needed Speech-Language Therapy from a therapist for the rest of my life, because no matter what they accomplish, there will always be something that has me stumped I need their help with. I really enjoyed our therapy while it lasted, and she did too. We worked on Memory and Sequencing Games, Problem Solving Skills and Two Way Conversation Skills. It was really nice, and she thought so, too.

Chapter Thirty Seven
My Future Desires

I applied for the AAPD Medicaid Waiver three years ago, and the person working on my case thought it would be the end of August, or beginning of September before I had an answer as to whether I can be approved for the Physical Disability in order to get this or not. He said that if I did get it, he would send a Nurse Reviewer out here to ask me questions and then I believed I could set up Home Health Services for myself with whatever Home Health Agency I have in mind. I got a denial letter for it, and planned to appeal it but didn't get it after all.

The reason I applied for it is, I may have seemed energetic at times, yes, but the majority of the time I was laying on the couch trying to fight this horrible fatigue I have that weakens me to the point that it's even a project to shave or comb my hair, etc. What's weird is, on some days I'll be this weak throughout the day and suddenly become the energizer bunny at 9am and feel like I can take on the world for 3 hours and go on a cleaning spree and then I crash and I wind up feeling like I can barely get around to do anything. I suspected I had Grave's Disease but couldn't really prove it. Plus, I've had trouble getting out of breath within 20 minutes if I decide to go plant flowers and wind up getting overheated and feeling weak. Last Spring, I had a heat stroke in only 80 degree weather after only attempting to plant flowers for 20 minutes. Many days I stare at the boxes of flowers I buy to plant for days because I am too weak and tired to plant them and then I plant them 4 to 5 days later but have to stop after only 20 minutes because it knocks it out of me. There have been many days I have felt physically taxed just by running errands and doing groceries and it can knock me out for the next week or two just to do so and make me feel incredibly tired and puny and weak if I do it for more days or longer than I feel like. Sometimes, I may even get chest pain or stomach pain from overdoing it after not doing much at all.

I thought something has to be terribly wrong and I had to prove it because my doctors did not believe me that this was happening so I thought if a home health nurse came to my home on an almost continual basis she would suddenly notice something wasn't right and think, "We've got to try to do something about this. Something is terribly wrong. This isn't normal."

I even volunteered for Bingo 4 hours a day on Mondays this past year and am dragging, desperate to go home after 2 hours when all we're doing is sitting there playing a game. I've even delayed my paintings and barely work on them once or twice a year now, where I did them 10 or 15 times a month about 3 or 4 years ago before I got tired again.

Vacuuming and washing dishes is a project in the morning but a breeze the first part of the night. Then I crash.

There has to be something terribly wrong with this.

Sometimes I felt like I was knocked down with waves to the couch feeling too weak to get around or do much of anything. I felt like the only way to find out for sure what was wrong and take care of it was to get Home Health and let the home nurses see for themselves what was going on so they could try to fix it. I feared if they did not, I would go down until one day I would be as bad off as the people in the nursing homes you see.

Even seniors normally get around better than me now; except for the days I have a sudden energy spurt and get around like nothing ever happened.

Most days this doesn't happen, so most days I'm like this. The problem is, the doctors never see it happen for themselves because I'm always well when I see them, but after I leave and before I go, I'm like this again, so what do you do?

The only way to get down to the bottom of it and see what to do and nurses be able to help me is to get Home Health and let them see for themselves what happens.

That's why I went for this.

I am not crippled, no, but physically taxed, yes.

What's wrong? Who knows? That's what I was hoping they could figure out if they came. That's what I wanted them to do and that's why I applied for their service.
 I also tried for the DDS waiver instead since I am also mentally disabled, due to my Autism but I was denied that too because I wasn't diagnosed before age 22.

The Rehab Center I went to as a child did diagnose me with mental retardation at first, and then language delay and language developmental delay, and eventually decided I had a severe language learning disorder.

Minimal brain damage was mentioned several times in my records but no one ever said the word Autism in their diagnoses before I turned 35 years and 10 months old.

It was really ridiculous, and the lady that did diagnose me with Autism said, "Why in the world did these people not diagnose you with Autism when you were 10 years old? It's so obvious just reading you're Childhood Rehab Records that you have it. What on earth were those people thinking?"

I said, "My mother tried to tell a doctor when I was 10 years old she thought I had autism after seeing a movie about a kid with autism who's symptoms matched perfectly.

The doctor said, "Oh, your kid doesn't have autism. Autism is a little kid's disease."

Thanks to him doing that to me I can't get DDS Medicaid Waiver because they think that there's nothing before age 22 that indicates it when the symptoms of it are all over the pages of the record, just not the diagnosis.

412

We visited a Home Healthy Agency last year that had two very friendly ladies working there that reminded me more of my local hospital nurses than does anybody anywhere else. We wanted a Patient Advocate to help us talk to the people at the bigger hospitals through their service, which we can do but they said I would have to qualify for the Medicaid waiver to get it. If I did get his service I want a *bubbly acting female* Home Health Aide, and a *bubbly acting female* Nurse, and a *bubbly acting female* nurse advocate. I want lots of hugs from all of them and I want them to all meet my accommodations asked nurses to meet for me in the hospital setting.

I also want any Physical Therapists, Occupational Therapists, Rehab Therapists, Radiologists, Speech-Language Pathologists, Lab Techs, EMT's, Paramedics, Emergency Room Nurses, all nurses and techs, to be *bubbly acting female*s, no men.

I want lots of hugs from all of them, and I want all my accommodations to be met by these people I asked for the nurses to meet for me in the hospital setting.

I hope if I ever get this service, the Home Health Aide, Nurse, and Advocate all three will understand me well, and give me lots of hugs, and be open to my needs that I have on account of my disability. I hope every therapist that works with me will be this way, as well.

I don't ever plan to go to a nursing home, but if I'm ever placed in one, even if it's only for a month, for rehab, like what some of my church members have run into that had to have temporary rehabilitation after leaving the hospital, I want all my nurses to be *bubbly acting female* nurses, no mediocre acting *female* nurses, *bubbly, chipper acting, cheerful female nurses* only, and no men (no *male* nurses at all). I have to be able to get lots of hugs from all the nurses that work with me in a nursing home, if I ever go to one, and be accommodated by their nurses in the same way as the hospital including with any needle sticks or invasive procedures.

I don't plan to go to one, but if I go to one, they have to do everything for me I asked the hospital nurses to do for me.

If the issue comes up, "Yes, but what if they have to give you a bath?" I don't care. If I get disabled enough to the point a *female* nurse has to give me a bath, then so be it. I want a *bubbly, chipper acting, cheerful female* nurse to be my nurse even if they have to give me a bath, no men. Besides that, I've had to be bathed by *female* nurses at the hospital before. And the last one that gave me a bath was a chipper acting cheery nurse too. It didn't bother her. If that's what happens, oh well, I don't care. I do not want a *male* nurse, and I never want a *male* nurse, or any other man, to take care of me in the medical setting, ever. Only chipper, *bubbly acting*, happy go lucky *female* nurses are allowed to deal with me everywhere, no matter where it is, or what they have to do, I want *females* only, no men ever.

If anybody ever comes up with the complaint over this specific issue stating, "Since you're a guy, you need to have a guy give you a bath instead of a girl." I don't care. I never want a guy to take care of me ever. I always want a chipper acting cheery female nurse. I would rather a female nurse see me naked than a guy. The reason why is, after "male doctors and nurses" sternly asked me to undress for them at the military hospital and then glared at me like I was dirt to them and they looked at me like it pleasured them for me to be naked because it made me feel inferior to them and defenseless against them I feel like a naked little peon piece of trash next to them and feel as if I am at their mercy and am like a slave to them as I was back then. They used my nakedness to lower my defenses when they decided to torture me with needles. The "male mental health staff" did the same thing to humiliate me in front of a room full of boys to make me feel low, at the institution as well as one "serious trended female" mental health staff person. I feel inferior around men when they ask me to undress for them because I feel like a peon slave piece of dirt to them.

When a "chipper acting cheery female nurse" asks me to undress for them, I feel like someone they consider to be a baby in diapers who they dress and undress like a doll and clean me up when they need to when they have bathed me in the hospital setting in the past.

But, if a "serious trended female nurse" does the bathing, I feel like a peon slave piece of dirt to them too, because they did the same thing to me as the men when I was younger to make me defenseless against them while they also pursued me with needles and treated me like I was a piece of dirt to them also.

Don't ever give me a "male nurse" or a "serious trended female nurse" for anything, including giving me a bath or toileting, or anything else, whether it requires they do something that causes them to have to see me naked or not. One way or the other I want them to be it, the "Chipper acting female nurses". If they see something they would not normally see, I want them to be it. If they don't have to see anything they normally wouldn't have to see, I still want them to be it. Naked or not naked, I want them to be my nurses and them only.

I want the Home Health Advocate to get the bigger hospitals to meet all my needs, and give me all bubbly, peppy, happy go lucky *female* nurses and no men.

When I go for IV sticks, I want one *bubbly acting female* nurse to rub my head to calm me down and hold my hand while another *bubbly acting female* nurse does the stick. I want lots of hugs from all my nurses.

I'd like them to check in ever so often in inpatient care, every few minutes to see how I am, and give me a hug, and let me know they haven't left me, and I haven't been abandoned, say, once every 20 to 30 minutes. One hour at the longest. Or, I will start to worry I've been left.

I need to be able to put Lidocaine/Prilocaine (Emla) on my arm on the site they chose to do the stick one hour before they start. I need my nurses to comfort and console me through all invasive procedures, or anything scary, anything that might cause sharp pain.

I need to be put to sleep for all invasive procedures, including having a urinary catheter put in, and especially, a heart catheter, that's too much to ask to do awake, and so is the urinary catheter. The pain from a urinary catheter is so overbearing, it is worse than an IV, and there is no way I can handle it awake, and they will probably have a nightmare on their hands if they even think about doing it awake.

Although, I appear normal to most people, I am a special needs person. I'm not really retarded, but I still have special needs. As I said, I used to have a borderline normal IQ and with lots of drilling in school work and struggling with sequencing on jobs, I finally went up one deficit. So, now instead of two deficits below normal, I am one deficit below normal. However, as far as social and performance are concerned I am still about 1 ¼ to 1 ½ deficits below normal. It's hard to tell I'm this bad off by looking at me, but after you get around me a while you start to notice the same thing as my ex-boss at Dollar General told me in 1998.

He said, "You want to know something. You're book smart, but you're not street smart. I hope you don't mind my telling you that, but I just wanted you to know. I'm really afraid somebody is going to take advantage of you one of these days. I really am."

To back up my case for wishing to be comforted and consoled by all my nurses and being allowed to receive physical touch to comfort me, instead of a stander by just talking, I would like to show the nursing world what their nursing oath or creed says. Nurses are actually required to do everything I am asking them to do, and if they read one of their creeds, or oaths, they would see that I am right, and hopefully conform to doing what I need them to do for me.

416

As I said, if a nurse is not willing to put themselves in the position to be ready to have to comfort their patients in the way a mother comforts her child or cares for her baby, then they need to not be a nurse, and find another profession.

I am hoping that these nurses reading their oaths and creeds verifies that for me for them to see I am right, and I hope it causes them to treat me in this manner, like I'm one of their kids, and they begin to comfort and console me the way a mother comforts her child and baby. If you are a nurse reading this book, and I wind up having you for my nurse one of these days, please do not persecute me if I fail you by not getting through the first two IV stick attempts like this one hospital did, I mentioned. Please, treat me like I'm one of your own kids, and have mercy on me, and show me compassion, and keep trying. I am sorry I am so difficult to get through needles, but if you just bear with me, I'll do the best I can and surely you can get it in my arm eventually. I only want you to stick me with the IV, or comfort me through the IV, if you are a *bubbly acting female* nurse, because that is what I am comfortable with.

So, if you are not a *chipper acting female* nurse, please do not even attempt to do anything with me, because you will make me nervous, and you will scare me. I want Bubbly, Peppy, Chipper, Happy Go Lucky, Motherly acting *female* nurses only. Thanks.

Also, if you ever see me have an emergency, and you're tempted to call an ambulance make sure the paramedic is a *female* also, thanks. Check to see if you can find Bertha around first, and have her take me. If not, make sure the paramedic is a *female*.

I never want a *male* nurse to take care of me period, even if they are an EMT or Paramedic, *female* nurses only. Men with this particular job are usually macho and make me especially nervous, and the more macho they are the more they will make me nervous. They will anyway, so make sure it's a *female* every time no matter what. Thanks.

Big City Hospitals Don't Like Cowards   Brian Evans

I have just recently found another family doctor. She is a *chipper acting female* APN nurse with *chipper acting female* assistant under her who will understand me and meet all my emotional needs. I really like her. She is the most wonderful doctor I have ever had. I hope she continues to understand me and continues to meet my needs from now on.

From what I understand she always will. I also have a new circle of doctors who are understanding of me and are willing to meet my needs. If there are any other doctors I need she will advocate for me to them so they understand me as well.

If I ever have trouble with anyone not understanding me that I already go to, she will set me up with someone who does understand and will send me to places my needs will be met. What I need from all my doctors and hospitals I go to is to be given nurses with chipper, fun loving personalities, who don't mind giving me hugs or rubbing my head to calm me down and hold my hand through needle sticks.

I also want them to take me seriously about my medical conditions and not blow me off because they don't believe me about any of my medical knowledge of my own conditions, most of which were already previously diagnosed up to 20 years ago, conditions that other family doctors and even some specialists out there just refuse to believe exist. It is very important I get this. This is what I really need badly. Thank you for understanding.

Chapter Thirty Eight
The Nurses' Creed and Recourse List
It is Their Responsibility to Comfort and Console Their
Patients

Here is the Nurses' Creed I found.

The Nurses Creed by M.A. Haggerty, RN says, "Lord, let me begin today with your blessing to provide care for those who need me. Give me the patience to listen, intuition to see beyond the visible, knowledge to practice the art of nursing, and the attitude to deliver care with humility. Help me to see every patient clearly unbiased, and with individual respect help me to face fear and anxiety with kind words and a gentle touch. Help me to see the joy and wonder each new day brings. And let your healing light shine through my hands."

Here are some resources that verify the fact that nurses are supposed to comfort their patients in the hospital setting.

According to Glencoe Health a Certified Surgical Technologist (CST) will demonstrate the following upon completion of an approved program:

1. Knowledge of surgical aseptic (cleansing) techniques;

2. Familiarity with basic surgical procedures, with anatomy, physiology, and microbiology, and with pathological processes;

3. The ability to meet patient's need for comfort, safety, and reassurance;

4. The ability to anticipate and meet the needs of the surgical team and function in areas where qualified.

Notice this says, "Ability to meet the patient's comfort" in number 3. It also says to meet their need for "reassurance".

This book directs its nurses to the American Medical Association's Committee on Allied Health Education and Accreditation, or the Association of Surgical Technologists.

This is on page 265 of the Glenco Health textbook for Health students.

Also, according to Glenco Health, LPNs and LVNs perform many of the patient-care duties, teaching them good health practices, assisting with rehabilitation, and offering comfort and emotional reassurance during times of suffering and crisis.

Notice it says "Perform Patient duties", one of which is to "Comfort" their patients and give them "emotional reassurance". This is on page 441 of the Glenco Health textbook for Health Students.

Glenco, McGraw-Hill, 1989.

CODE OF ETHICS for the Medical Assistant:

"The Code of Ethics of this Association shall set forth principles of ethical and moral conduct as they relate to the medical profession and the particular practice of medical assisting. Members of this Association dedicated to the conscientious pursuit of their profession, and thus desiring to merit the high regard of the entire medical profession and the respect of the general public which they serve, do pledge themselves to strive always to render service to humanity with full respect for the dignity of each person; respect confidential information gained through employment unless legally authorized or required by responsible performance of duty to divulge such information; uphold the honor and high principles of the profession and accept its disciplines; seek to continually improve our knowledge and skills of medical assisting for the benefit of patients and professional colleagues; and participate in additional service activities which aim toward improving the health and well-being for the community."

The Administrative Medical Assistant, Mary E. Kein, 1988, 2nd Edition, page36.

"Much of what you do as a nurse is based on sympathy, empathy, compassion and your want to care."
>How to Books –Working as a Nurse, Esther Bartlett and Marion Field, 1999. Page 32

The Florence Nightingale Pledge goes like this, "I solemnly pledge myself before God and in the presence of this assembly, to pass my life in purity and to practice my profession faithfully. I will abstain from whatever is deleterious and mischievous, and will not take or knowingly administer any harmful drug. I will do all in my power to maintain and elevate the standard of my profession, and will hold in confidence all personal matters committed to my keeping and all family affairs coming to my knowledge in the practice of my calling. With loyalty will I endeavor to aid the physician in his work, and devote myself to the welfare of those committed to my care."
>American Nurses Association
>The Nightingale Tribute (Kansas State Nurses Association Website)

Comfort: Nurse's First and Last Consideration

"Nowadays, you can see nurses in hospitals receiving a number of patients. Unaware of their actions during initial interaction comfort has been forgotten and out of priority."
>By Grepaz Isaac, RN
>Quezon City, Philippines

"While a lot is written about the bullying that can go on within the nursing profession, Christine Szweda RN, BSN, MS, NE-BC, director of nursing education for competency and assessment at the Cleveland Clinic believes nurses can instead provide each other with a powerful support network."
>Nursezone.com
>For Work for Life

"When it comes to patient care, nurses consistently play the role or advocate as they support each patient's emotional well-being, contribute to the healing process and speak on their patient's behalf. Nurses can also put their advocacy skills to work in advocating for each other and for the profession as a whole"

Meagan M. Krishka,
Nursezone.com
For Work or For Life

"Everyone is capable of showing care and giving comfort…whether it is for someone so close to you or even for a bystander needing help or assistance…Giving comfort or showing care is not stated in books, it comes out naturally…
They say you cannot be a nurse when you don't know how to care and you don't care at all…I definitely agree to that… A nurse is always judged by her ability to make her patients comfortable.
As nurses, we are the comfort providers…we don't simply follow doctor's orders and give medications in an instant, instead, we dig deeper…we empathize…we do our own interventions within our scope of responsibility giving emphasis on provided simple comfort measures."

Dianne Kristin G. Pella., R.N.
Calcoon City, Philippines
Sunday, July 11, 2010
A Novice Nurse

Hospice Patients Alliance
Standards of Care-Nursing

Hospices must provide adequate nursing care to meet the needs of the patient. That is the law. "All nurses, including hospice nurses, are trained to provide care according to the accepted standards of practice within the nursing field. Standards of nursing practice and the "Code of Nurses" can be found by contacting your State's nursing association. The nurse's license authorizes her to perform professional assessments of her patients, create nursing plans of care, perform many skilled nursing procedures, provide all necessary aspects of nursing bedside care, and many other tasks.

The nurse's license requires her to make sure the patient's needs are met."
Hospice Patients Alliance

Comfort Behaviors Checklist

I actually found a Comfort Behaviors Checklist on the Internet for Nurses observing their patients.

Number 11 on this list is how well a patient responds to "rubbing of an area"
Number 14 on this list is how well the patient "accepts kindness".
Number 15 on this list is how well the patient "likes touch/hand holding".

This was on Dr. Katharine Kolcaba's "Comfort Care in Nursing.

"Comfort is a concept that has a strong association with nursing. Nurses traditionally provide comfort to patients and their families through interventions that can be called comfort measures. The intentional comforting actions of nurses strengthen patients and their families. When patients and families are strengthened by actions of health care personnel (nurses), they can better engage in health seeking behavior.
Dr. Katharine Kolcaba's Comfort Care in Nursing

"For Centuries nurses have helped care for the sick and injured. The word "nurse" is from the Latin word nutrire, "to nourish" or "cherish".
The New Book of Knowledge, N13, page 409, 1970

"What a nurse does depends upon the needs of patients in the hospital units in which she works."
The New Book of Knowledge, N13, page 410, 1970

"Nursing is a career of service and dedication. It is a career that demands intelligence, dependability, warmth, patience, and an awareness of the feelings of others. In return, nursing offers the deep satisfaction of helping people in need and sharing closely in the joys and sorrows of others."

The New Book of Knowledge, N13, page 412, 1970

Since nurses are supposed to treat their patients like children, I'd like to point out what this book says about empathy toward babies.

"Simply put, to develop empathy, a baby needs warm, nurturing attention from one or two reliable, central caregivers who touch, interact with, and respond attentively to his or her unique emotions and needs."

> The Art of Empathy: A Complete Guide to Life's Most Essential Skill, page 215, Karla McLaren, Sounds True Incorporated, 2013

"Babies, especially in their first year, need as much warm, emotive, and intimate human interaction as they can get" and that's how I am.

> The Art of Empathy: A complete Guide to Life's Most Essential Skill, page 215, Karla Mc Laren, Sounds True Incorporated, 2013

I'm autistic and I have childlike needs and these needs need to be met.

"Nurses offer patients "comfort" and advice".

> What Do They Do? Nurses, Jennifer Zeiger, page 8, Cherry Lane Publishing, 2010

"Sometimes patients need extra care. They might need special tests. Nurses help run the tests. They also prepare patients for operations. They also 'help people feel less scared' and help their pain go away."

> What Do They Do? Nurses, Jennifer Zeiger, page 8, Cherry Lane Publishing, 2010

On page 11 of the book, "What Do They DO? Nurses" you will see a friendly female nurse smiling and holding a girl patient's hand.

>What Do They Do? Nurses, page 11, Jennifer Zeiger, Cherry Lane Publishing, 2010

On page 15 of the book, "What Do They Do? Nurses" you will notice a nurse puts one hand behind the back of a male patient in a wheel chair and puts his other hand on his shoulder and looks at him and smiles.

>What Do They Do? Nurses, page 15, Jennifer Zeiger, Cherry Lane Publishing, 2010

The lady nurse on the cover of the book, "What Do They Do? Nurses" is also smiling cheerfully at a girl patient as she takes her temperature.

>What Do They Do? Nurses, Jennifer Zeiger, Book Cover, July 2010

"Nursing is a profession that provides care to the sick, the injured and other people in need of medical assistance."

>World Book Encyclopedia Online, 2016

"Patients often get most of their direct health care through nurses. Nurses record patient medical histories and symptoms help perform medical tests, administer treatment and medications, operate medical machinery, and help with follow up care and rehabilitation. They also provide advice and "emotional support" to patients and their families.

>World Book Encyclopedia Online, 2016

"The Well Being of Patients is of first importance to nurses. RNs are taught to "recognize and understand patients' needs." They provide 'emotional support' as well as physical care, taking time to 'reassure worried patients and boost their morale'".

>World Book Encyclopedia Online, 2016

"Each type of patient has 'special needs' requiring nurses with 'specialized knowledge and training'".

>World Book Encyclopedia Online, 2016

"Nurses must really care about people and want to help them. People who are ill may feel alone and afraid, and nurses can give them confidence."

The New Book of Knowledge, N13, page 412, 1970

"Nursing is also good preparation for raising a family. Nurses learn about health, illness, child care, and relationships among people."

The New Book of Knowledge, N13, page 412, 1970

"Lisa H. Newton in her defense of the traditional role of the nurse appeals to an argument based on the patient's needs. Because a patient may not be able to take care of himself Newton points out, 'his entire self concept of an independent human being may be threatened'…He needs 'comfort', 'reassurance', 'someone to talk to', the person he really needs, who would be taking care of all these problems is his mother, and 'the first job of the nurse is to be a mother surrogate.'"

Caring: Nurses, Women, and Ethics, Helga Kuhse, page 58, Blackwell Publishers, 1997

"Nursing care needs to provide mental and physical stimulation, particularly for a young child."

Fundamentals of Nursing, 7th Edition, page 1250, Potter and Perry, Mosby Elsevier, 2009

"Nurses can use touch and eye contact to enhance a client's self-esteem."

Fundamentals of Nursing, 7th Edition, page 417, Potter and Perry, Mosby Elsevier, 2009

"Touch is a primal need, as necessary as food, growth, or shelter. Think of touch as a nutrient transmitted through the skin and "skin hunger" as a form of malnutrition that has reached epidemic proportions in the United States, especially among older adults (Fontaine, 2005).

Fundamentals of Nursing, 7th Edition, page 784, Potter and Perry, Mosby Elsevier, 2009

"Older adults need touch as much as or more than any other age-group. However, skin hunger or poverty of touch is often acute among older adults. It is an unfortunate coincidence that older adults often have fewer family members or friends to touch them at a time when simple touch could be an enhanced form of communication when other senses are reduced (Dossey and others, 2005). Simple touch helps older adult clients feel more connected to and accepted by those around them and to their environment. Touch enhances self-esteem and sense of worth. A nurse who reacts adversely to the skin changes of older people often finds it difficult to touch an older client. The nurse's reluctance then communicates a negative message to the older adult (Dossey and others, 2005).

> Fundamentals of Nursing, 7th Edition, Box 36-5, page 784, Potter and Perry, Mosby Elsevier, 2009

A holistic nursing approach to care of older adults also includes the caregivers, who often experience poor health or have neglected their own health, encounter their own psychological issues as they relate to the care giving experience, feel the effects of multiple stressors, or feel spiritual distress. (Eliopoulos, 2004)."

> Fundamentals of Nursing, 7th Edition, Box 36-5, page 784, Potter and Perry, Mosby Elsevier, 2009

"The ability to attend to the learning process depends on physical comfort and anxiety levels and the presence of environmental distractions. The nurse ensures that clients, families, and communities receive information needed to promote, restore, and maintain optimal health. In today's fast-paced technical environments, nurses are required more than ever to bring the sense of caring and human connection to their clients (see Chapter 8). Touch is one of the nurse's most potent forms of communication. Nurses are privileged to experience more of this 'intimate' form of personal contact than almost any other professional. Touch conveys many messages, such as "affection", emotional support, encouragement, "tenderness", and "personal attention".

> Fundamentals of Nursing, 7th Edition, pages 353,354, Potter and Perry, Mosby Elsevier, 2009

"Comfort touch, such as holding a hand, is especially important for vulnerable clients who are experiencing severe illness with its accompanying physical and emotional losses. In older persons, touch increases a sense of safety, increases self-confidence, and decreases anxiety (Geleeson and Timmons, 2004). Research has found that in children having a lumbar puncture, a medical procedure, a nurse's soothing nonessential touch decreased anxiety and lowered the child's distress (Bannorshdall and others, 2004). Students may initially find giving intimate care stressful, especially when caring for clients of the opposite gender (Seed 1995). Students learn to cope with intimate contact by changing their perception of the situation. Since much of what nurses do involves touching, you need to learn to be sensitive to others' reactions to touch and use it wisely. Touch should be as gentle or as firm as needed and delivered in a comforting, nonthreatening manner."
> Fundamentals of Nursing, 7th Edition, pages 353,354,
> Potter and Perry, Mosby Elsevier, 2009

"The nurse uses touch to communicate." (Figure 24-02), page 354
> Fundamentals of Nursing, 7th Edition, page 354, Figure 24-2, Potter and Perry, Mosby Elsevier, 2009

"The nurse establishes, directs, and takes responsibility for the interaction, and the client's needs take priority over the nurses' needs. The nurse's nonjudgmental acceptance of the client is an important characteristic of the relationship. Acceptance conveys a willingness to hear a message or to acknowledge feelings. It does not mean you always agree with the other person or approve of the client's decisions or actions. A helping relationship between nurses and client does not just happen – you create it with care, skill, and trust. Therapeutic interactions increase feelings of personal control by helping the person feel secure, informed, and valued. Creating a therapeutic environment depends on your ability to communicate, to comfort, and to help clients meet their needs."
> Fundamentals of Nursing, 7th Edition, page 346, Potter and Perry, Mosby Elsevier, 2009

"Health is a "state of complete physical, mental, and social well-being, not merely the absence of disease or infirmity. Health is a state of being that people define in relation to their own values, personality, and lifestyle. Each person has a personal concept of health. Health and illness must be defined in terms of the individual."

> Fundamentals of Nursing, 7th Edition, page 748, Potter and Perry, Mosby Elsevier, 2009

"The nurse's presence helps to calm anxiety and fear related to stressful situations. Giving reassurance and thorough explanations about a procedure, "remaining at the client's side", and coaching the client through the experience all convey a presence that is invaluable to the client's well being."

> Fundamentals of Nursing, 7th Edition, page 784, Box 36-5, Potter and Perry, Mosby Elsevier, 2009

"A Hospital is an institution for the treatment and care of persons who need medical attention. Night and day, the members of the hospital staff work as a well-drilled team to provide for the comfort and health of patients."

> The World Book Encyclopedia, H, page 332, 1967

"In the hospital corridors, white-uniformed nurses move quickly and quietly from room to room, bringing comfort to their patients."

> The World Book Encyclopedia, H, page 332, 1967

"A modern hospital is designed to provide for a patient's comfort as well as his health."

> The World Book Encyclopedia, H, page 332, 1967

"Professional Services staff consists of hospital personnel directly concerned with the care of patients."

> The World Book Encyclopedia, H, page 332, 1967

"The word hospital comes from the Latin word hospitium, which means a house or institution for guests."

> The World Book Encyclopedia, H, page 335, 1967

"The hospital offers a large variety of careers for persons interested in helping the sick. Those who like to help other people will find hospital work a good life. This work is hard and demanding on a person's time and energy. However, there is compensation for all the day to day problems and hardships – the conviction that this work is essential to humanity."

The World Book Encyclopedia, H, page 335, 1967

"The emphasis on comfort and the role it plays in health care has changed in the last 10 decades. From 1900 to 1929, comfort was the central focus and moral imperative of nursing: from 1930 to 1959, comfort was considered a strategy for achieving fundamental requirements of nursing care: and from 1960 to 1980, comfort fell out of favor, to become only a minor aspect of nursing, and was significant only to people who received no medical treatment. During the last 3 decades, comfort has been relegated to end-of-life care where it is equated with the simplest aspects of care, which could be just as easily be provided by nonprofessional caregivers. Today, as always, comfort remains a substantive need throughout our oncology nurses play an important role in promoting comfort through their lives. Comfort is not a novel idea and has been cited by prestigious and cancer patients. In conclusion, comfort should not be relegated to end-of-life care. There is a powerful need for an increase in translational research to promote comfort in every stage of patient care. When comfort is emphasized in nursing care and when promoting comfort becomes an important core value of nursing, I believe that nurses will gain more respect from their patients, the families of patients, and our colleagues in the field of medicine."

Chia-Chia, Lin, PhD, RN
School of Nursing
Taiwan
Comfort: A Value Forgotten in Nursing-Lin,Chia-Chia PhD, RN
Cancer, Nursing: November/December 2010-Volume 33-Issue 6-pp409-410

"Most nurses work in hospitals, where they help comfort and care for people who are sick, injured, or recovering from surgery."
World Book Encyclopedia, Number 14, N, page 618, 2006

"Nursing offers daily satisfaction to those who have a genuine desire to help others."
World Book, Number 14, N, page 619, 2006

"A nurse must like people and want to help them and must also have self-reliance and good judgment. Patience, tact, honesty, responsibility, and ability to work easily with others are valuable traits. Good health is another must."
World Book, Number 14, N, page 619, 2006

"In all schools of nursing, classroom work or theory is interwoven with practice. Clinical experience, or practice, means the time that the student spends in learning to spend with different types of patients."
World Book, Number 14, N, page 619, 2006

"In selecting a nursing home, it is important to match both the medical and psychological needs of a person with the recourses of the care giving institution. Nursing homes also should provide for the psychological needs of their residents."
World Book, Number 14, N, page 620, 2006

"Nursing students study such subjects as anatomy, chemistry, nutrition, pharmacology, physiology, psychology, and sociology, as well as the fundamentals of nursing care. They learn to care for the sick by working in the nursing laboratory. Frequently, the students practice on one another."
World Book, Number 14, N, page 619, 2006

You would think with these nurses practicing on each other and seeing how much pain it puts them in to give each other IVs and whatever else they do to each other that is painful that they would understand what pain their patients are feeling when they do this to them.

I just found the following quote in one of my medical assisting books that proves some patients can't handle pain well.

"A patient who has excruciating pain will require a larger dose of analgesic than a patient who has intermittent pain."
     Clinical Skills and Assisting Techniques for the Medical Assistant, Sharon M. Zakus, RN, BA, MS, CMA, page 248, 1988.

This proves that there are some patients out there with oversensitivity to pain and I am one of them. I'm not a cash register. I'm not a grill. I'm not a car. I'm a person and I have feelings and I have needs that need to be met and they are not being met. It hurts to be stuck with needles and have other invasive things done to me and I need to be comforted by my nurses when they do this stuff to me because it is what I need to keep me calm and make me feel more at ease. I need the comfort to emotionally stabilize myself through the traumatic situation. I normally feel the pain tremendously when stuck with shots, blood tests, and IVs but even when I get lucky and don't feel the pain I still need your comfort because this is what helps me. I'm at total chaos without it whether I feel the pain or not, but the chaos is even worse if I am feeling the pain, especially if it is as severe as it normally is for me. If there were not any patients like this around this that felt this much pain when they were put through needle sticks and procedures this comment would not be in this nurse's book written for Medical Assistants.

The following comment was made for medical assistants assisting doctors with minor surgeries in a doctor's office.

"Remember, any surgical procedure is an invasion into body parts not normally interfered with; and although it may be a minor surgical procedure, it often does not appear minor to the patient. Many patients are somewhat anxious, nervous, or concerned about what is going to happen."
          Clinical Skills and Assisting Techniques for the Medical Assistant, Sharon M. Zakus, RN, BA, MS, CMA, page 161, 1988.

"The medical assistant can and must help the patient relax and ally any fears of apprehensions. On arrival of the patient in the office, greet and usher the patient into the treatment room. Attend to the patient's needs for comfort and communication, and give emotional support and reassurance. The best of care can be enhanced by evaluating every patient and situation individually."

Clinical Skills and Assisting Techniques for the Medical Assistant, Sharon M. Zakus, RN, BA, MS, CMA, page 161, 1988.

"Nursing is a profession the members of which provide auxiliary care to the sick and disabled under the direction of physician's or other medical specialists."

Funk and Wagnall's Encyclopedia, page 6243, The Universal Standard Encyclopedia, 1988.

"Most nursing schools require the candidates be graduated from high school and have two years of science as well as good health and a personality suited to the demands of service to the sick."

Funk and Wagnall's Encyclopedia, page 6243, The Universal Standard Encyclopedia, 1958.

"Among the rewards of nursing are the challenges it offers. A badly injured person may need immediate and expert care. Medicines and equipment must be rushed to the patient's bedside. The family must be comforted and the doctor must be given a detailed report on the patient's condition. A nurse's greatest reward often is the knowledge that his or her skill has helped to relieve suffering or to save a life."

World Book, Number 14, N, page 619, 2006.

"The well-being of patients is of first importance to nurses. They take time to reassure worried patients and boost the patient's morale. Nurses are taught to recognize and understand patients' needs and provide emotional support as well as physical care."

World Book, Number 14, N, page 617, 2006

"The well being of patients is of first importance to nurses. RNs are taught to recognized and understand patients' needs. They provide emotional support as well as physical care, taking time to reassure worried patients and boost their moral. Each type of patient has special needs, requiring nurses with specialized knowledge or training. As a result, hospital nurses typically choose an area of specialty just as most doctors develop a specialty. Nurses' specialties range from basic primary care to fields requiring highly developed technical skills. Patients often get most of their direct care through nurses."
          World Book, N-O, Volume 414, 616, 2014

"Nurse's aides give important social and emotional support to patients as the registered nurses may not have enough time to spend with the patients. Nurse's aides help by answering patient calls; feeding, washing, and walking patients; and recording vital signs and other indications of a patient's care. If a patient's aides go along they may help support patients during treatment of help move them onto or off of beds and stretchers."
          World Book, N-O, Volume 14, page 616, 2014

"Nurses aides give important social and emotional support to patients as the registered nurses may not have enough time to spend with the patients. Nurse's aides help by answering patient calls; feeding, washing, and walking patients; and recording vital signs and other indications of a patient's care. If a patient's aides go along they may help support patients during treatment or help move them onto or off of beds and stretchers."
          World Book, N-O, Volume 14, 616, 2014

"Most nurses work in hospitals where they comfort and care for people who are sick, injured, or are recovering from surgery."
          World Book, N-O, Volume 14, 616, 2014

"Nursing offers satisfaction to those who desire to help. A nurse must like people and want to help them."
          World Book, N-O, Volume 14, 616, 2014

"Good nursing consists in securing as much physical comfort as possible for the patient in rendering prompt first aid in emergencies that may arise, and in soothing and cheering the patient's mind."

> Victor Robinson, Ph.C., M.D., Modern Home Physician, Wise, 1968

"Nursing is also good preparation for raising a family. Nurses learn about health, illness, child care, and relationships among people."

> The New Book of Knowledge, N13, page 412, 1970

I noted these two things on a chart of Watson's 10 Carative Factors, one carative factor was "forming a human – altruistic value system. An example in practice for this is to "use loving kindness to extend yourself." You use self-disclosure appropriately to "promote a therapeutic alliance with your client." Another example in practice in promoting and expressing positive and negative feelings is to "support and accept your clients' feelings. In connecting with your clients you show a willingness to take risks in what you share with one another." It also says another carative factor is "providing a supportive, protective and/or corrective mental, physical, societal, and spiritual environment." An example of this would be to "create a healing environment at all levels, physical and nonphysical. This promotes wholeness, beauty, "comfort", dignity, and peace."

> Fundamentals of Nursing, 7th Edition, page 98, Table 8-1, Potter and Perry, Mosby Elsevier, 2009

On page 131, Figure 10-3 a nurse holds a patient's hand and puts her other hand just below her shoulder on her arm as she talks to her.

> Fundamentals of Nursing, 7th Edition, page 131, Figure 10-3, Potter and Perry, Mosby Elsevier, 2009

A nurse on page 129 in Figure 10-2, possibly at a nursing home is observing family interactions when they put a puzzle together actually leans over and helps them put some of the pieces of the puzzle together. She assists in understanding family functioning by doing this.

Fundamentals of Nursing, 7th Edition, page 129, Figure 10-2, Potter and Perry, Mosby Elsevier, 2009

This is an example of just how relational a nurse is supposed to be. Some nurses may just stand off to the side and think, "I'm just going to mind my own business while this family puts a puzzle together" but this nurse interacts with her patients and tries to make them feel at home and helps to entertain them.

Fundamentals of Nursing, 7th Edition, page 129, Figure 10-2, Potter and Perry, Mosby Elsevier, 2009

Try to learn to be more involved with your patients and interact with them and do everything you can to keep them happy and comfort them affectionately when they need you to. Don't just act standoffish, be a good nurse and show motherly compassion to all those in your care and put their minds at ease when they come to you.

The Fundamentals of Nursing Book says this about Emotional Comfort on page 347, Box 24-5. "Recently hospitalized clients described emotional comfort as a pleasant positive feeling and state of relaxation that resulted from therapeutic interactions. Clients described emotional discomfort as unpleasant negative feelings and tension. Personal control over the situation contributed to emotional comfort. Therapeutic interactions helped the client achieve control and were associated with emotional comfort. Clients perceived a positive link between emotional comfort and recovery" It goes on to say the following about Application to Nursing Practice: "Clients perceive a connection between the mind and body. Increased emotional comfort increases physical comfort and enhances recovery. Nurse-clients therapeutic interactions improve the client's emotional and physical comfort. Using therapeutic communication to increase the client's perceived control of the situation and the environment increases comfort." (Williams AM, Irurita VF: Emotional comfort: the patient's perspective of a therapeutic context, Int J Nurse Study 43 (4); 405; 2006.

Fundamentals of Nursing, 7th Edition, page 347, Box 24-5, Potter and Perry, Mosby Elsevier, 2009

In the Fundamentals of Nursing book on page 131 you will see in Figure 10-3 that a female nurse is holding a patient's hand and puts her other hand just below her shoulder on her arm as she talks to her.

> Fundamentals of Nursing, 7th Edition, page 131, Figure 10-3, Potter and Perry, Mosby Elsevier, 2009

In Figure 25-3 on page 377 a female nurse puts her arm on a male patient's back when they walk them down the hall.

> Fundamentals of Nursing, 7th Edition, page 377, Figure 25-3, Potter and Perry, Mosby Elsevier, 2009

In Figure 27-4 on page 417 a female nurse touches a male patient on the arm with her hand. The statement under this picture says, "Nurses can use touch and eye contact to enhance a client's self esteem."

> Fundamentals of Nursing, 7th Edition, page 417, Figure 27-4, Potter and Perry, Mosby Elsevier, 2009

On page 482 in Figure 30-7 a female nurse puts her arm around their colleague during time of loss to support them. This is a nurse comforting a nurse. The same should go for nurses toward patients in their loss as well.

> Fundamentals of Nursing, 7th Edition, page 482, Figure 30-7, Potter and Perry, Mosby Elsevier, 2009

In the Reader's Digest: "Your Body Your Health, The Heart" there is a friendly female nurse on page 128 that puts one hand under a male patient's shoulder while checking his heart with a stethoscope with the other hand.

On page 131 of "Your Body, Your Health, The Heart" there is a female nurse putting her arms around the arm of a male patient to help him walk forward. She seems to be guiding him along so he won't fall.

> Reader's Digest: "Your Body Your Health – The Heart", page 128, Reader's Digest Association, London, 2002

This nurse may have not necessarily done this to comfort this patient, but at least she was showing compassion by being willing to put her arms around his arm to hold him up instead of standing back and saying, "I'm a professional. I can't do that. I'm not touching anybody. You'll just to have to hold on to a guard rail and walk on your own."

I've never heard anyone make that particular statement in this area of care before, but, they have said similar things to me in similar circumstances. And this is what it feels like when nurses act like they think they are so professional to the point they refuse to touch you or let you touch them. The more they act like this, the more you begin to get the feeling one of them might actually do something like this if they wanted to get out of touching you. Nurses are supposed to comfort their patients and any nurse that thinks they are not supposed to comfort their patients is wrong. Any nurse that thinks this way needs to go back and reread their own books. Even the college text book I found on nursing says this several times. It even comes out and tells you how to comfort your patients in several instances and actually tells you to use "touch therapy" to comfort your patients.

In other words, this book is also telling you to comfort your patients with the hand holds and the head rubs and some of this other stuff I'm asking you to do.

And, the Nursing Career CD I found with a book for nurses seeking careers in nursing it showed nurses rubbing the heads of patients, stroking their face, and holding their hands several times. And, they weren't old people or children either, they were my age. I'm 47 years old and these people appeared to be in their 30's, 40's, and 50's.

 Seeing that, it is not just limited to seniors and children, and it shouldn't be.

Comfort from nurses should be for all stages of life, and one of the recourses I quoted said so as well.

Comfort should not be delegated to end of life care as they said and people of all ages should be comforted by their nurses.

 Believe it or not, even though some nurses have been picky about comforting me I've run into the past couple of years, there are some that I've run into over the past 10 years that are more than happy to meet my needs. Many of them even call me sweetie, or honey, or bud, or buddy. I've ran into some people in the public that will complain and say, "I just can't stand it when they do that. I'm not their honey. And, I'm not their sweetheart."

And, you know what I have to say to them, "What's wrong with you? I like it when my nurses call me honey and sweetheart, and buddy. I think it's sweet, and I feel like they think I am special to them when they do this for me. I think it's great."

They all give me lots of hugs that are like this and they will rub my head to calm me down and hold my hand through a needle stick. The problem was that only certain departments would go along with this in my old hospital and I needed nurses in all departments to be this way instead of acting all pompous and stoic and standoffish refusing to comfort me because they thought they were some kind of a professional that worked for a business somewhere like it was a firm or something, when in fact they were a nurse, not my business associate.

I didn't come to do business with them, I came to be "cared for" by them because they are supposed to "take care of me" because they are my "caretakers" and nurses are your caretakers, not your business associates.

In a doctor's office or hospital setting, and especially the hospital setting, the nurses are basically supposed to take the place of your mother and treat you as if you were one of their own kids and comfort you in the same manner as they would their own child or baby, because they are "taking care of you" as a mother would "take care" of a child, and you are their patient, and they are now supposed to take on the role of the parent, and supply all the comfort you need in the way you need them to comfort you and not the way they decide they want to comfort you.

Nursing a patient is not about the nurse, but the patient. It's not about the nurse's rights, it's the patients, and when you read your own college books as I did mine when I went to school, you will see when you read it that it tells you in your own school book, "It's not about the nurse's rights. It's about the patient's rights." It's the patient that matters and you need to be willing to resort to doing whatever they need you to do for them like a mother would a child. Nurse means to nurture, and any nurse that is not willing to comfort their patients like they would their own child or baby should not be a nurse and should find a different profession to work in.

"As nurses deal with health and illness in their practice they grow in the ability to care. Nursing behaviors related to caring include providing presence, a "caring touch", and "listening". Nurses who demonstrate caring use a caring approach in each encounter with clients."

> Fundamentals of Nursing, 7th Edition, page 100, Potter and Perry, Mosby Elsevier, 2009

"Caring facilitates healing and improves client satisfaction with nursing care. However, does the instructional process influence human caring? Do nurse educators present instructional methods that improve students' caring practices? Undergraduate nursing students received a 15 week educational module on nursing as human caring. The purpose of the module was to improve students' understanding of caring practices and to thus make them more caring practitioners.

Researchers interviewed the students before and after completing the module to understand the effect of this module on their caring practices. For example, they asked students about factors that facilitated and impeded their caring practices. The students reported an increased self-awareness in regard to (1) connecting in relationships with self and others, (2) finding purpose and meaning in life, and (3) clarifying values. Several students spoke of becoming more tolerant of others, recognizing persons' uniqueness and appreciating their perspectives. By recognizing themselves as caring persons, the students gained meaning in their lives. Many were able to relate a great deal of satisfaction in recognizing that they were caring persons and how nursing allowed them to express that. Students worked through the emotional issues and practical constraints, which allowed them to grow spiritually and connect with clients at a deeper level. Finally, students also expressed and enhanced appreciation of what they valued."

> Fundamentals of Nursing, 7th Edition, page 98, Box 8-2, Perry and Potter, Mosby Elsevier, 2009

"Application to Nursing Practice in enhancing caring is increasing knowledge and understanding of caring helps nurses begin to understand a client's world and to change their approach to nursing care. The use of caring in nursing practice encourages a more therapeutic approach to nursing care. As nurses use caring, they get to know their clients and therefore better meet their needs. The caring model involves a closeness, commitment, and involvement in the nurse-client relationship."

> Fundamentals of Nursing, 7th Edition, page 98, Box 8-2, Potter and Perry, Elsevier, 2009

"Clients face situations that are embarrassing, frightening, and painful. Whatever the feeling or symptom, clients look to nurses to "provide comfort". The "use of touch" is one "comforting approach" where the nurse "reaches out to clients to communicate concern and support."

> Fundamentals of Nursing, 7th Edition, page 101, Potter and Perry, Mosby Elsevier, 2009

"Touch is relational and leads to a connection between nurse and client. Touch involves contact and noncontact touch (Frederickson, 1999). Contact touch involves obvious skin-to-skin contact, whereas noncontact touch refers to eye contact. It is difficult to separate the two. Both in turn are described within three categories: task-oriented touch, caring touch, and protective touch (Fredrickson 1999). Nurses use task-oriented touch when performing a task or procedure. The skillful and gentle performance of a nursing procedure conveys security and a sense of competence. An expert nurse learns that any procedure is more effective when administered carefully and in consideration of any client concern. For example, if a client is anxious about having a procedure, such as the insertion of a nasogastric tube, the nurse offers "comfort" through a full explanation of the procedure and what the client will feel."

> Fundamentals of Nursing, 7th Edition, page 101, Potter and Perry, Mosby Elsevier, 2009

"The nurse then expresses that the procedure will be performed safely, skillfully, and successfully. This is done in the way that supplies are prepared, the client is positioned, and the nasogastric tube is gently manipulated and inserted. Throughout a procedure the nurse talks quietly with the client to provide assurance and support."

> Fundamentals of Nursing, 7th Edition, page 101, Potter and Perry, Mosby Elsevier, 2009

"Caring touch is a form of nonverbal communication, which successfully influences a client's comfort and security, enhances self-esteem, and improves reality orientation (Boyek and Watson, 1994). You express this in the way you "hold a client's hand", "give a back massage", "gently position a client", "or "participate in a conversation."

> Fundamentals of Nursing, 7th Edition, page 101, Potter and Perry, Mosby Elsevier, 2009

"When using a "caring touch", the nurse is making a connection with the client and showing acceptance of the individual (Tommansini, 1990)."

> Fundamentals of Nursing, 7th Edition, page 101, Potter and Perry, Mosby Elsevier, 2009

In the movie "Love Finds a Home" Belinda, a doctor takes care of her sister or other doctor friend when she has sharp pains and is pregnant and has a fever. Belinda put her hand on her forehead to see how hot she was. Then she pulled her blanket over her body to cover her. Then, she held her hand. After that she raised her hand up and put it on the lady's face and caressed the side of the lady's face with her hand from the top of her face to the bottom of her face in a stroking motion.
She looked at her with deep sadness for her and was filled with compassion. Then she stepped back and let her rest so she could sleep.

I guess some nurses don't think nurses do things like this, but they did here and I've seen several other movies where they did the same kind of thing.

In the movie, "Awakenings", a true story about patients with encephalitis, Dr. Sayre's nurse rubs the old lady patient's head (strokes her head) when she sees how upset she is that it is not still 1922.

Another nurse stroked the top of the head of the red headed lady patient against her hair on the side of her head and then flung her fingers through the strands of her hair at the bottom of her head when she tilted her head backwards to the side in her chair.

Another nurse rubbed a lady patient's upper back in circular motion when they looked at themselves in a mirror and said, "Are you okay?"

If you'll notice, Dr. Sayer him self even gently touched each of his patients as he positioned them as if to show his love for them to make them feel comforted.

On the commercial about St. Jude's Hospital on television they show various ways nurses touch their kid patients to comfort them. I've seen them get close to them several times and either put their arm around them or put their hand on their shoulder. It's hard to remember for sure what all I saw because I haven't seen the commercial in two weeks, so because of that I looked up their commercial videos on the internet and loved what I saw.

On the internet video clips of St. Jude's hospital they showed three different nurses hugging their patients. A male nurse was shown hugging their kid patient. Then, a female nurse was shown hugging their kid patient. Then, a toddler ran up to their female nurse and their female nurse hugged them. One female nurse rubbed a kid patient's back. Another female nurse rubbed a kid patient's hand. One female nurse held a kid patient in their arms. Another female nurse let a kid patient lay their head on their shoulder. It was wonderful. I thought it was the sweetest thing they did for their kids and it should be that way.

When I looked up nurses comforting patients and clicked on "Images of Nurses Comforting their Patients", I saw a slew of pictures I had to scroll down through showing nurses doing everything for their patients I ever asked you to do. There were about two pages worth of these pictures. Several nurses held their patients' hands. Several nurses put their hands on their patient's shoulders. One nurse was putting their hand on their patient's back. Another nurse was putting her arm around one of her senior patients. Another nurse put their arm around a kid. The rest of these people were young to middle aged adults. There were a few kids in between, but there must have been at least 15 or 20 pictures of young to middle aged adults in this whole slew of pictures that were getting their hand held, or their shoulder held, and even getting their head rubbed. They even showed one nurse hugging a 37 year old woman. I clicked on this and it went to this story about a New York lady patient getting to reunite with her nurse who took care of her as an infant. The patient's name was Amanda Scrarpauil, and she finally got to meet the nurse that brought her comfort for nearly 40 years.

She had a burn she was treated for as a child and she finally got to meet her nurse who took care of her as an infant and be with her again. I have a feeling from the way the rest of the story went she stuck with this nurse from there on out because she loved her so much. This was in the New York Daily Times on the computer.

When I looked up "Nurses Hugging Patients, or Nurses Giving Patients Hugs" on the Internet and clicked on Images of Nurses Hugging Patients, there were several of them, probably two pages worth of pictures of nurses hugging their patients.

When I looked up videos on nursing it was harder to find what I was looking for because they were mainly showing the technical stuff for educational purposes to show nurse students how to take a blood test or take records for example, but there was one I found from VC San Diego Medical Center where two chipper acting female nurses were taking care of a lady while another nurse sat at her bedside and held her hand. Then, when the two chipper acting nurses began working with the lady patient one of these two chipper acting female nurses put their hands on the patient's shoulder when she asked a question. Then she put her hand on her arm to tell her something. When she wanted to check her response ability, she told this lady, "Squeeze my hand when I say "A". She began Saying, "A. S. A. S. A. A." every time she said "A" the lady patient squeezed her hand. This nurse was very sweet and had the type of personality I like in a nurse. She was very chipper and sweet and caring. I thought it was great.

On one of these videos they had a box of words to the side that said, "To Care", "To Advocate", "To Inspire", "To Be a Nurse", "Nursing."

When I looked up a video on needle phobics, one nurse was stating, "You need to be more than careful when dealing with a needle phobic patient. They need a lot of attention."

She went on to say, "When they come for me to take blood, I'm going to lay them down. I'm not going to have them sit in my chair."

I've always requested the nurses lay me down to draw blood because that works better for me. Some lab techs or nurses will do this for me, but there have been some who didn't understand and wanted to use their chair anyway because they cared more about whether it suited them or the doctor more to do it in the chair than they did about whether it suited me. It works better to lay me down on a bed to do it. And, when you do, one chipper acting female nurse needs to stand on the left side of the bed to rub my head to calm me down and hold my hand while another chipper acting female nurse does the Blood test, IV, or shot in the right arm because it hurts worse to do it in the left.

Also, when it comes to shots, I don't mean to embarrass anybody, but it hurts less to have those in the hip so anytime you can do those in the hip please do.

I haven't had a shot in the arm for close to 25 years and I have a feeling I'd jump and freak out for sure if you attempted to give me a shot there again. And, I know you probably think I'm a cry baby for this, because you're thinking, "It's only a shot", but I want a chipper acting female nurse to stand to the side of me to rub my head to calm me down while the other chipper acting female nurse does the shot too. And, all you other doctor offices and hospital staff out there, I need you to do this for me too. I need you to do this for the shot, and the blood test, and the IV, and anything else sharp, even biopsies, or anything invasive, please. It's very important you do this for me.

"Caring – As you take the NCLEX-RN, 2014 exam remember that the test is about 'caring' for people, not working with high-tech equipment or analyzing lab results."
> Kaplan Nursing, Kaplan NCLEX-RN 2014-2015, Strategies, Practices, and Review with Practice Test, page 11, Kaplan, Inc., 2014

"The first subcategory for this 'client need' is "Basic Care and Comfort" which accounts for 9 percent of the questions."

> Kaplan Nursing, Kaplan NCLEX-RN, 2014-2015, Strategies, Practices, and Review with Practice Test, page 11, Kaplan Inc., 2014

"Providing basic care and comfort for your clients is one of your most important roles."

> Kaplan Nursing, Kaplan NCLEX-RN 2014-2015, Strategies, Practice, and Review with Practice Test, page 8, Kaplan Inc., 2014

"Combining medical technology and the 'human touch', health care workers administer care around the clock, responding to the 'needs' of millions of people – from new borns to the critically ill."

> Health Care, The Big Picture, Chapter 1, Page 1, Video Number 1, JIST Works, America's Career Publisher, The Editors @ JIST, JIST Publishing, 2008

"Anyone considering a career in health care should have a strong desire to help others, genuine concern for the welfare of patients, and clients, and an ability to deal with people of diverse backgrounds in stressful situations."

> Health-Care Career Vision Book and DVD, page 17, JIST Works, America's Career Publisher, The Editors @ JIST, JIST Publishing, 2008

Here's what it says about Home Health Aides.

"Home Health Aides perform a variety of duties as requested by a client, such as obtaining household supplies or running errands. Accompanying clients to physicians' offices and on other trips from home, providing transportation, assistance, and "companionship". Administer prescribed oral medications under written direction of a physician as directed by home care nurse and aide. Care for children who are disabled or who have sick or disabled parents. Massage patients and apply preparations and treatments such as liniment, alcohol rubs, and heat lamp stimulation."

> Health Care Vision Book and DVD, page 50, JIST Works,
> America's Career Publisher, The Editors @ JIST, JIST
> Publishing, 2008

Now that's personal. Talk about me asking nurses to be personal
with me. They act like I'm in the wrong for asking for hugs, head
rubs, and hand holds. Look what these nurses have to do, the
home health aides and nurses.

Along with the long list of duties EMTs and Paramedics are given
this is included in the list, "comfort and reassure patients."

> Health Care Vision Book and DVD, page 84, JIST Works,
> America's Career Publisher, The Editors@JIST, JIST
> Publishing, 2008

Here is what the Health Care Career Vision Book has to say about
Licensed Practical and Licensed Vocational Nurses:

"Care for ill, injured or, 'disabled people', in hospitals, nursing
homes, clinics, private homes, group homes, and similar
situations."

> Quick Look, page 88, Healthy Care Career Vision Book
> and DVD, America's Career Publisher, The Editors@JIST,
> JIST Publishing, 2009

"LPNs provide basic patient care and treatments such as taking
temperatures or blood pressures, dressing wounds, treating bed
sores, giving enemas, or douches, rubbing with alcohol,
'massaging' or performing Catherizations."

> Health-Care Career Vision Book and DVD, page 88, JIST
> Works, America's Career Publisher, The Editors@JIST,
> JIST Publishing, 2008

"Registered Nurses are to 'administer nursing care to ill, injured,
convalescent, or 'disabled patients.' They are to 'assess' patient
health problems 'and needs', develop and implement nursing care
plans and maintain medical records."

Health-Care Career Vision Book and DVD, page 124,
Video 39, JIST Works, America's Career Publisher, The
Editors@ JIST, JIST Publishing, 2008

Here are some notes I took on the DVD videos presented on the
Health-Care Career Vision Book and DVD videos:

One female nurse rubbed the head of a guy patient while she and
the other nurse stood on the sides of his bed. The male patient was
wearing a face mask probably for anesthesia to be put to sleep for a
procedure.

Another female nurse held a lady patient's hand.

The narrarator made this statement on the DVD.

"For all these jobs you need to be comfortable "touching" the
people in your care."

Other things I noticed were as follows:

A female nurse pats a lady patient on the back.

A female nurse holds a guy's hand.

A female nurse put lotion on a patient's foot and rubbed the top of
their foot and bottom of their leg.

The narrarator then made this statement on the DVD about Nurse
Aides and Orderlies.

"You should have a desire to work with others and have
compassion."

On the Video about Licensed Practical Nurses I noted the
following:

A female nurse held a male patient's hand.

Another female nurse put her hand on this male patient's shoulder.

Another female nurse held another patient's hand.

The narrarator made the following statement regarding massage therapists on this DVD:

"Being comfortable touching patients is an important necessity."

I believe he also said that many RNS and LPNs give massages as well or at least that they go into massaging during their career.

The narrarator made the following comment about Sonographers:

"Sonographers need to be willing to calm an anxious patient in a comforting way."

The narrarator also made this statement regarding Nuclear Medicine Technologists:

"A friendly reassuring manner is almost more important or better than expertise."

The narrarator made this statement regarding Registered Nurses on the DVD:

"Registered nurses play a crucial role in providing physical and emotional care for the sick, injured, and handicapped."

The narrarator also said, "Registered Nurses have to have a strong desire to help others. You should be compassionate and the well being of patients must be constantly understood and evaluated."

Here are other things I noted about the video on Registered Nurses on the DVD:

A female RN nurse stroked a male patient's face.

The Narrarator said, "RNs must make patients feel at ease before surgery."

He also said, "RNs work in Hospitals, Clinics, and Nursing Homes."

Another female nurse stroked a lady patient's arm before she went for her lab stuff to draw this lady's blood.

I noticed the following on the video about the Physician's Assistants on this DVD:

The narrator said, "P. A. s must be compassionate and caring when working with other people."

About surgeons the narrator said, "Surgeons must have good bedside manner."

I also noticed a surgeon held a patient's hand and put their other hand on the patient's shoulder.

All of this was on the DVD of the Health Care Career Vision Book and DVD. And, by the way, these weren't old, dying people either. They weren't children either. They were my age. I'm 47 years old. They were everyday, middle aged people ages 30s, 40s, and 50s going for procedures and what the DVD showed the nurses do to comfort them in the same manner, by the way, I'm asking them to comfort me. Go see for yourself.

> Health-Care Career Vision Book and DVD, DVD Video Content, JIST Works, America's Career Publisher, The Editors@JIST, JIST Publishing, 2008

I also found this statement in an AARP magazine.

See next page for statement.

Here's what it says:

"When you provide another with comfort, when you lend a hand, or simply be there for someone who needs help, you transform the health of our country. Big change doesn't require a hero's effort. Just one small act of kindness can make you a hero to someone else. How will you participate?"

> Give Health A Hand, Medco Foundation, AARP Magazine, March & April 2010, page 67

In Funk & Wagnall's New Illustrated Encyclopedia of Family Health, 1 A-B, page 60, "a nurse is holding a patient's hand while giving them anesthesia with a gas mask and holding their stomach with their other hand."

> Funk & Wagnall's New Illustrated Encyclopedia of Family Health, 1, A-B, page 60, The Universal Standard Encyclopedia, 1958

"Dr. Diane Meier is quietly leading a revolution to treat patients (and their families too) as living, breathing, feeling individuals. And why is that so shocking?"

When a patient of Diane Mier, MD dies, the family receives a call or a note. "She was with me when my wife died at home", says Bert Gold of New York City still missing, Sylvia his wife of 57 years. She took me in the living room and "put her arm around me" and "started to cry." She "thanked me for letting her take care of Sylvia. Imagine."

> AARP Magazine, September & October 2007, The Comfort Connection by Joan Kenon, page 52, 122, 123

"Meier, 55, of the Mount Sinai School of Medicine in New York School of Medicine in New York City, is one of the leading exponents of a new and growing discipline known as palliative care. Palliative care means soothing the symptoms of a disease, regardless of whether the patient is seeking a cure. It's a concept that's totally transforming the way doctors and hospitals treat seriously ill patients. The ideas of easing pain and improving the quality of a patient's life may seem radical, but classic medical training focuses on attacking the disease. Most doctors simply don't have time to be supersensitive Marcus Welby's checking up on patients to see how they feel. Even if they do have time, they lack the advanced training of palliative care doctors and nurses to ease symptoms such as anxiety, pain, or severe nausea. Most are better equipped to deal with microorganisms than matters of care."
      AARP Magazine, September & October 2007, The
      Comfort Connection by Joan Kenon, page 52, 122, 123

I like Marcus Welby. I think nurses and doctors should be like this again. Besides all this, these nurses may complain they don't have time to comfort their patients but even Gentle Annie and Clara Barton took out the time to comfort their patients in the middle of trying to catch them as they fell off of horses. Soldiers were falling left and right and Clara Barton even cradled a soldier in her arms when he was dying regardless of all the other soldiers around her falling, hoping she could catch them to take care of them. You think you're busy, they were really busy and this never stopped them. They took out time to comfort their patients anyway no matter how busy they were, and that was busy if I ever saw busy.

Try keeping up with that kind of pace with your patients. That's hard for me to do, and yet I would do this for them too. I just wish you would do this for me.

"When people first hear of palliative care, they often confuse it with Hospice care. Hospice focuses on terminally ill patients, but palliative care teams consist of every one from social worker to physical therapists who can follow patients for days, months, or years."

>AARP Magazine, September & October 2007, The Comfort Connection by Joan Kenon, page 52, 122, 123

"Thanks in large part to the training and outreach programs, Meir runs as the Center for the Advancement of Palliative Care, (CAPC) in New York City, the number of hospitals has nearly doubled, from 632 in 2000 to 1,240 in 2005. Palliative care has the potential to change the way doctors and nurses address pain and emotion, how they help patients and families soothe through their choices as life nears it's end."

>AARP Magazine, September & October 2007, The Comfort Connection by Joan Kenon, page 52, 122, 123

"Bert Gold is 91, takes a lot of medicines, is frail, falls sometimes, lost a big toe, 5 years ago and still deals with pain with an awkward gait. Bert visits Meir in her office today before going back to the foot surgeon and Meir spends 'more than an hour' - yes more than an hour – reviewing his symptoms, his diet, his medications, his mood."

>AARP Magazine, September & October 2007, The Comfort Connection by Joan Kenon, page 52, 122, 123

"Meier believes strongly that palliative care should not be the 'death team', and she sees patients 'early' in the course of the disease."

>AARP Magazine, September & October 2007, The Comfort Connection by Joan Kenon, page 52, 122, 123

"Meir is pushing for more programs and she says 'too many are stuck in a medical no-where land, forced to choose between 'comfort care' and 'emotional support' in a hospice or a chance to keep fighting their illness."
          AARP Magazine, September & October 2007, The
          Comfort Connection by Joan Kenon, page 52, 122, 123

"Meier says, 'It's not human nature to accept death and agree to give up on life. With palliative care we don't have to."
          AARP Magazine, September & October 2007, The
          Comfort Connection by Joan Kenon, Health Writer in
          Washington D.C., page 52, 122, 123

I have seen doctors and nurses comfort their patients on the St. Jude Children's Hospital Commercial several times.

I've even seen a place on the internet I looked up where they had pictures of nurses hugging their patients on a website they had, a whole slew of them.

My mother wanted me to be taken care of after she dies. She wants me to be taken care of and me to be happy and have my needs met. And, even though my needs seem unusual, my needs are my needs and that is what I need. I'm autistic and I am an Ex-Special Ed student and I have the same childlike needs I had back then. They never went away and they never will and these needs need to be met for the rest of my life. In order for me to be taken care of, I have to be able to get hugs from all my church friends and from all my nurses and doctors and techs when I go to the hospital or doctor's office, and get chipper acting female nurses only who will do this for me, and rub my head to calm me down and hold my hand through all needle sticks every time they're done on me. Meet my list of needs on the list, "all of them" and we are good to go. Please meet my needs.

"The Hebrew Home has put an unusual emphasis on the power of touch and touch therapy. Beverly Herzog has been widowed for 21 years but she still can't get used to this absence. She bought a baby pillow which helps a little but it's not the same. 'I like being touched, being stroked, being held', says Herzog, who lives in the Hebrew Home at Riverdale, a skilled nursing facility in New York. "Anyone who says they don't isn't telling the truth. You feel abandoned if you haven't been touched. We all need somebody." said, Herzog." (Page 38)

    The Power of Touch, pages 37-43, AARP Magazine, December 2015-January 2016

The Hebrew Home has put an unusual emphasis on that idea. The staff here is encouraged to hold resident's hands and offer gentle caresses. Beauticians are trained to massage the feet during pedicures, as well as the scalp and neck during shampoos. And, intimate relationships between residents are not discouraged – a rarity in long term care."

    The Power of Touch, pages 37–43, AARP Magazine, December 2015-January 2016

"Herzog has taken full advantage of this ground breaking policy."

    The Power of Touch, pages 37-43, AARP Magazine, December 2015-January 2016

"When you're younger, it might be easy to take touch for granted. Old people may loose their sense of touch but ironically need to be able to receive touch all the more."

    The Power of Touch, pages 37-43, AARP Magazine, December 2015-January 2016

"Depriving newborns of touch is disaster – growth is slowed, and serious cognitive and behavioral disorders emerge that can persist into adulthood. Touch is crucial for forgoing the first emotional bond with a parent and for creating the unique human experience."

    The Power of Touch, pages 37-43, AARP Magazine, December 2015-January 2016

"Seeing believes", wrote the 18th century English Physician Thomas Fuller, "but Feeling's the truth."
>   The Power of Touch, pages 37-43, AARP Magazine,
>   December 2015-January 2016

"Doctors who touch their patients are not only considered more caring – their patients have better outcomes."
>   The Power of Touch, pages 37-43, AARP Magazine,
>   December 2015-January 2016

"Therapeutic Touch lowers levels of the stress hormone Cortisol and increases the amount of Oxytocin, the so called love hormone, which is credited with mother-and-child bonding, among other things. When we put our hands on each other, we're tapping into deep associations between touch and emotion that are kind let at the dawn of life."
>   The Power of Touch, pages 37-43, AARP Magazine,
>   December 2015-January 2016

This place did more for their residents than I am asking of you. I'm just asking for hugs (putting my right ear on your cheek) from chipper acting, cheery female nurses with motherly personalities when I need to and for you to rub my head to calm me down and hold my hand through needle sticks and I feel like I am being scolded for asking.

"A surrogate- is a substitute figure, especially a person of authority, who replaces a father or mother in one's feelings."
>   Webster's New World Dictionary, 2nd Edition, David B.
>   Garualive, Editor in Chief, William Collins + World
>   Publishing, Co, Inc., 1976

I want all of you, nurses and techs and doctors, and radiologists and anesthesiologists, etc, especially all my nurses and techs to be a surrogate mother to me, especially those working with me. This is what I need.

My whole life I've see it this way, and now some of these nurses seem to want to redefine comfort as if it is something else.

Comfort to me is what it has always been, a warm hug, a tender touch, or a rub on the head or shoulder.

None of this other stuff they come up with these days is comfort. It's just a lame excuse to get out of showing comfort so they don't have to get too personal with you when in reality that's what nursing is all about, mothering your patients helping heal their wounds and comforting them in their sorrow and pain. Even if they are not in sorrow or pain, they will be if you don't comfort them because they will feel like you don't care and they're just a number to you, and they are starved for affection because you didn't give it to them and their heart is broken. Is that really what you want? Refusing to comfort your patients is wrong, and any patient that comes to you should be able to be comforted by you if they ask you to comfort them whether you feel like they need it or not. They just need to feel loved and cared for and you are supposed to treat your patients as a mother treats their own children. Not doing so just causes chaos and fear and broken heartedness and even if you stood a chance of saving your patient you may have just lost them because of what you just did. You refused them of the very thing they needed. The comfort they needed you to give them as you would give to your own child. Please comfort your patients, especially me. It especially causes chaos when a patient has a sensory issue in their right ear like me that can only be relieved by putting it on the cheek of the people that I like, including nurses. The disabled need it worse than ever. They need their needs met even worse than normal every day people do and when you keep that from them it traumatizes them and causes them to lose their will to live.

They feel like me, like why bother getting well if my nurses are going to treat me like a stranger they just want to fix up and get rid of. They're just there for the paycheck and they don't care anything about me. Why doesn't anybody care? Please remember to show compassion in your care and comfort your patients the way they need comforted. Thank you.

Just as Solomon in the Bible told God that he wanted wisdom instead of riches, I wish to have affection instead of riches including my hugs from my church friends and my doctors and nurses and techs at all my doctor's offices and every department in the hospital that I see, especially those taking care of me.

I still want to have a feasible income, but I would rather receive all the affection I need, especially the hugs I need from everyone everywhere I go, especially at church and at the doctor's offices and hospitals I go to than to have riches galore.

I only ask I get my need for hugs and affection met and can live feasibly enough financially to get by.

In the medical setting this means I get my hugs I need from all my nurses and doctors and techs, and that the chipper acting female nurses I get rub my head to calm me down and hold my hand through needle sticks.

You give me that, and we've got it made.
Male nurses, doctors, and techs tortured me as a child, and serious trended female nurses tortured me in both childhood and adulthood.

Only the chipper ones ever showed me the compassion and comfort I needed and they are the ones I need because they have the chipperness I need to cheer me up and the compassion to comfort me the way I ask them to comfort me with motherly love. There is actually a picture of a nurse hugging an elderly woman on page 25 of the Fundamentals of Nursing textbook in Figure 2-3. It says "providing nursing services in assisted living facilities promotes physical and psychosocial health" and this nurse is doing so by giving this lady a hug just as I am asking you to do for me.
Fundamentals of Nursing, 7th Edition, page 25, Figure 2-3, Potter and Perry, Mosby Elsevier, 2009

Students may initially find giving intimate care stressful, especially when caring for clients of the opposite gender (Seed 1995). Students learn to cope with intimate contact by changing their perception of the situation. Since much of what nurses do involves touching, you need to learn to be sensitive to others' reactions to touch and use it wisely. Touch should be as gentle or as firm as needed and delivered in a comforting, nonthreatening manner."

Fundamentals of Nursing, 7th Edition, pages 353,354, Potter and Perry, Mosby Elsevier, 2009

Even the college text book I found on nursing says this several times. It even comes out and tells you how to comfort your patients in several instances and actually tells you to use "touch therapy" to comfort your patients. In other words, this book is also telling you to comfort your patients with the hand holds and the head rubs and some of this other stuff I'm asking you to do. And, the Nursing Career CD I found with a book for nurses seeking careers in nursing it showed nurses rubbing the heads of patients, stroking their face, and holding their hands several times. And, they weren't old people or children either, they were my age. I'm 47 years old and these people appeared to be in their 30's, 40's, and 50's. Seeing that, it is not just limited to seniors and children, and it shouldn't be. Comfort from nurses should be for all stages of life, and one of the recourses I quoted said so as well. Comfort should not be delegated to end of life care as they said and people of all ages should be comforted by their nurses. Believe it or not, even though some nurses have been picky about comforting me I've run into the past couple of years, there are some that I've run into over the past 10 years that are more than happy to meet my needs. Many of them even call me sweetie, or honey, or bud, or buddy. I've ran into some people in the public that will complain and say, "I just can't stand it when they do that. I'm not their honey. And, I'm not their sweetheart." And, you know what I have to say to them, "What's wrong with you? I like it when my nurses call me honey and sweetheart, and buddy. I think it's sweet, and I feel like they think I am special to them when they do this for me. I think it's great." They all give me lots of hugs that are like this and they will rub my head to calm me down and hold my hand through a needle stick.

The problem was that only certain departments would go along
with this in my old hospital and I needed nurses in all departments
to be this way instead of acting all pompous and stoic and
standoffish refusing to comfort me because they thought they were
some kind of a professional that worked for a business somewhere
like it was a firm or something, when in fact they were a nurse, not
my business associate. I didn't come to do business with them, I
came to be "cared for" by them because they are supposed to "take
care of me" because they are my "caretakers" and nurses are your
caretakers, not your business associates. In a doctor's office or
hospital setting, and especially the hospital setting, the nurses are
basically supposed to take the place of your mother and treat you
as if you were one of their own kids and comfort you in the same
manner as they would their own child or baby, because they are
"taking care of you" as a mother would "take care" of a child, and
you are their patient, and they are now supposed to take on the role
of the parent, and supply all the comfort you need in the way you
need them to comfort you and not the way they decide they want to
comfort you. Nursing a patient is not about the nurse, but the
patient. It's not about the nurse's rights, it's the patients, and when
you read your own college books as I did mine when I went to
school, you will see when you read it that it tells you in your own
school book, "It's not about the nurse's rights. It's about the
patient's rights." It's the patient that matters and you need to be
willing to resort to doing whatever they need you to do for them
like a mother would a child. Nurse means to nurture, and any
nurse that is not willing to comfort their patients like they would
their own child or baby should not be a nurse and should find a
different profession to work in.

"Caring facilitates healing and improves client satisfaction with nursing care. However, does the instructional process influence human caring? Do nurse educators present instructional methods that improve students' caring practices? Undergraduate nursing students received a 15 week educational module on nursing as human caring. The purpose of the module was to improve students' understanding of caring practices and to thus make them more caring practitioners. Researchers interviewed the students before and after completing the module to understand the effect of this module on their caring practices. For example, they asked students about factors that facilitated and impeded their caring practices. The students reported an increased self-awareness in regard to (1) connecting in relationships with self and others, (2) finding purpose and meaning in life, and (3) clarifying values. Several students spoke of becoming more tolerant of others, recognizing persons' uniqueness and appreciating their perspectives. By recognizing themselves as caring persons, the students gained meaning in their lives. Many were able to relate a great deal of satisfaction in recognizing that they were caring persons and how nursing allowed them to express that. Students worked through the emotional issues and practical constraints, which allowed them to grow spiritually and connect with clients at a deeper level. Finally, students also expressed and enhanced appreciation of what they valued."

> Fundamentals of Nursing, 7th Edition, page 98, Box 8-2, Perry and Potter, Mosby Elsevier, 2009

"Application to Nursing Practice in enhancing caring is increasing knowledge and understanding of caring helps nurses begin to understand a client's world and to change their approach to nursing care. The use of caring in nursing practice encourages a more therapeutic approach to nursing care. As nurses use caring, they get to know their clients and therefore better meet their needs. The caring model involves a closeness, commitment, and involvement in the nurse-client relationship."

> Fundamentals of Nursing, 7th Edition, page 98, Box 8-2, Potter and Perry, Elsevier, 2009

To Nurse means to nurture. Nurture in the dictionary also means nourish. I like a spelling thesaurus gadget a friend gave me. I don't really have trouble spelling. I just play with it for kicks to get meanings of words. According to this thesaurus gadget a friend at bingo gave me, the word nurse means "to act as a parent to." I've been looking for this definition the whole time. That's what I thought it meant. So, you see, nurses are actually supposed to treat their patients as if they were their own children and provide the same love and affection toward their patients as they would their own child. To those who wish to be nurses, you are not just taking on a profession where you stick patients with a bunch of needles and help with surgeries and then receive a paycheck for it. You are acting as a parent to these people. You are their caregivers and you are actually supposed to treat these people that are your patients like they are your children while they are under your care. Anything you would do for your child from a comforting standpoint needs to be done for your patients. That's why I believe one of the people I copied the quote of in my book said that being a nurse is a great teaching tool for how to raise your kids. I think they meant that you were supposed to comfort them and console them in their fear and pain with great compassion. And they did say in their quote that you are supposed to comfort your patients, by the way. That means if they need you to pat them on the shoulder, or give them a hug, or rub their head to calm them down and hold their hand you need to do so. You would do this for your kids wouldn't you? Your patients need you to do the same for them no matter what their age. In case you think I am the only one emphasizing age one of the people I quoted said that comfort should not be left to end of life care but that people of all ages should be comforted by their nurses. This fact is found in one of the quotes found in this Chapter by your own medical professionals. So, please remember to reevaluate your responsibility as a nurse and remember that comforting your patients is the key to good patient care.

By the way, one of your own medical professionals also made this quote almost exactly. I'm just confirming it. You didn't know I knew all this did you?

So, you see, nurses were supposed to comfort their patients all along. It's just that some of the nurses in the bigger hospitals have let pride get in the way of their jobs as comforters, and have stopped meeting their patients' needs, abandoning the earlier practices of nursing where comfort was the main key. Instead they think of themselves as someone above having to meet the needs of their patients, like they think they are business executives, when in fact, they are caregivers that are responsible for meeting the needs of their patients, including comforting and consoling them in their fear and pain. Please make sure to remember to comfort me and all your patients when they come your way. Thank you.

To Read more about my life as a person with autism, be sure to read Autism Undiagnosed Part I – What Happened? , Autism Undiagnosed Part II- Will I Always Be An Outcast? and Autism Undiagnosed Part III- Joys and Sorrows of Living with Adult Autism, a three part series by my wife, Bertha Marie Evans.

Thank you. I hope you had a nice read and I hope this book gave you a better understanding of the needs I have that I need met by all my nurses in the medical field.

Sincerely,

Brian Gene Evans

Also available are…

"Victory: What Everybody Wants" by Bertha Marie Evans

"How to Have a Happy Marriage: Getting Past the Differences"
By Bertha Marie Evans

To schedule Bertha Marie to talk to your church group or
organization, contact her at (870) 416-1030 or (870) 416-8912.

I have also written four other books you can read:

"Mainstreaming a Disabled Person into the Normal World is a Big
Mistake" by Brian Gene Evans

"What Language Therapy Really Entails" by Brian Gene Evans

"Compassion for Disabled Peers in College is Needed" by Brian
Gene Evans

"To Nurse Means to Nurture" by Brian Gene Evans

"To Nurse Means to Nurture Part Two" by Brian Gene Evans

"To Nurse Means to Nurture Part Three" by Brian Gene Evans

"Touch: The Most Important Role of the Nurse in Caring For a
Patient" by Brian Gene Evans

www.ingramcontent.com/pod-product-compliance
Lightning Source LLC
Chambersburg PA
CBHW051437170526
45166CB00001B/15